SBAs for the Final FRCR 2A

SBAs for the Final FRCR 2A

RWK Lindsay MB BCh BAO MRCS FRCR
Clinical Fellow in Interventional Radiology, McGill University Hospital, Montreal, Canada

JSJ Gillespie MB BCh BAO (Hons) MRCP FRCR
Consultant Radiologist, Royal Victoria Hospital, Belfast, Northern Ireland

RM Kelly, MB BCh BAO (Hons) MRCP FRCR
Consultant Radiologist, Antrim Area Hospital, Antrim, Northern Ireland

R Sathyanarayana, MB BS MRCS FRCR
Clinical Fellow in Interventional Radiology, Auckland City Hospital, Auckland, New Zealand

PA Burns BSc MB BCh BAO (Hons) MRCP FRCR
Specialty Registrar, Royal Victoria Hospital, Belfast, Northern Ireland

OXFORD
UNIVERSITY PRESS

OXFORD
UNIVERSITY PRESS

Great Clarendon Street, Oxford OX2 6DP
United Kingdom

Oxford University Press is a department of the University of Oxford.
It furthers the University's objective of excellence in research, scholarship,
and education by publishing worldwide. Oxford is a registered trade mark of
Oxford University Press in the UK and in certain other countries

First Edition published in 2012
Reprinted 2013

British Library Cataloguing in Publication Data
Data available

Library of Congress Cataloging in Publication Data
Library of Control Number: 2012934790

ISBN 978-0-19-960776-1

To my wife Maura and my children Peter,
Charlotte, and Alexander

RWKL

To my wife Janice and my children
Katie, Harry, and Johnny

JSJG

To my wife Jane

RMK

To my wife Bharathi and my children
Riya and Keshav

RS

To my wife Ciara and my son Oisin

PAB

PREFACE

In view of the recent changes in the FRCR 2A examination format from multiple true/false to single best answer (SBA), we decided to write *SBAs for the Final FRCR 2A*, appreciating that success very much depends on acquisition and repeated testing of knowledge. We feel well placed to write such a book due to our own recent examination success. In addition, included in our authors are a previous FRCR 2A gold medallist and a past chairman of a Regional MCQ panel for the FRCR part 2 examination.

The questions have been written in the format of the new FRCR 2A examination and are extensively referenced from current literature and leading radiology texts. As the book is divided into system modules, each chapter can be taken as a practice examination if desired. When preparing for the exam we found that those questions which were of most benefit were those which were set at a level of difficulty slightly above that of the actual exam and also provided detailed answers and explanations. There is little to be gleaned from undertaking questions the answers to which one already knows. Therefore do not be disheartened if some of the questions seem overly difficult. We hope that this book will not only provide a challenging test of knowledge but also, through the detailed answers, give a broad overview of radiology in general. Finally, we wish you all the best in your forthcoming exam!

RWKL
JSJG
RMK
RS
PAB

CONTENTS

ABBREVIATIONS

A&E	accident and emergency
AAA	abdominal aortic aneurysm
AAST	American Association for the Surgery of Trauma
ABC	aneurysmal bone cyst
ABPA	allergic bronchopulmonary aspergillosis
ACC	agenesis of the corpus callosum
ACL	anterior cruciate ligament
ACTH	adrenocorticotropic hormone
ADC	apparent diffusion coefficient
ADEM	acute disseminated encephalomyelitis
ADI	atlanto-dens interval
AF	atrial fibrillation
AFP	alphafetoprotein
AH	autoimmune hypophysitis
ALCAPA	anomalous origin of the coronary artery from the pulmonary artery
AP	antero-posterior
APACHE II	Acute Physiology and Chronic Health Evaluation II
APW	absolute percentage washout
ARDS	acute respiratory distress syndrome
ARPKD	autosomal recessive polycystic kidney disease
ASD	atrial septal defect
ASO	arterial switch operation
ATN	acute tubular necrosis
AV	atrioventricular
AVN	avascular necrosis
AVM	arteriovenous malformation
AXR	abdominal x-ray
BAE	bronchial artery embolization
BAL	bronchoalveolar lavage
BHL	bilateral hilar lymphadenopathy
BMI	body mass index
BOOP	bronchiolitis obliterans organizing pneumonia
BPD	bronchopulmonary dysplasia
bpm	beats per minute
CAD	coronary artery disease
CAH	congenital adrenal hyperplasia
CBD	common bile duct
CBF	cerebral blood flow
CBV	cerebral blood volume
CCA	common carotid artery

CCAM	congenital cystic adenomatoid malformations
CDH	congenital diaphragmatic hernia
CEA	carcino-embryonic antigen
CF	cystic fibrosis
CHD	common hepatic duct
Cho/Cr	choline/creatine
CMC	carpometacarpal
CMV	cytomegalovirus
CNS	central nervous system
COP	cryptogenic organizing pneumonia
COPD	chronic obstructive pulmonary disease
CPA	cerebellopontine angle
CPPD	calcium pyrophosphate deposition
CRMO	chronic recurrent multifocal osteomyelitis
CRP	C-reactive protein
CSF	cerebrospinal fluid
CSP	cavum septum pellucidum
CT	computed tomography
CTA	CT angiogram
CTP	CT perfusion
CTPA	CT pulmonary angiography
CV	cavum vergae
CVI	cavum vellum interpositum
CXR	chest X-ray
DAD	diffuse alveolar damage
DAI	diffuse axonal injury
DAVF	dural arteriovenous fistula
DCIS	ductal carcinoma in situ
DIG	desmoplastic infantile ganglioglioma
DIP	desquamative interstitial pneumonia
DNET	dysembryoplastic neuroepithelial tumour
DRE	digital rectal examination
DRUJ	distal radio-ulnar joint
DSA	digital subtraction angiography
DVA	developmental venous anomaly
DWI	diffusion-weighted imaging
ECA	external carotid artery
ECG	electrocardiogram
EDH	extradural haematoma
EEA	extrinsic allergic alveolitis
EEG	electroencephalogram
eGRF	estimated glomerular filtration rate
ENT	ear, nose, and throat
ERCP	endoscopic retrograde cholangiopancreatography
ESR	erythrocyte sedimentation rate
ESWL	extracorporeal shock wave lithotripsy
ET	endotracheal
EUS	endoscopic ultrasound
FAP	familial adenomatous polyposis
FDG	fluorodeoxyglucose

FESS	functional endoscopic sinus surgery
FLAIR	fluid attenuated inversion recovery
FNA	fine needle aspiration
FFNH	focal nodular hyperplasia
FSE	fast spin echo
GBM	glioblastoma multiforme
GCS	Glasgow Coma Scale
GCT	giant cell tumour
GDA	gastroduodenal artery
GFR	glomerular filtration rate
GGO	ground-glass opacification
GI	gastrointestinal
GIST	gastrointestinal stromal tumour
GP	general practitioner
GSF	greater sciatic foramen
HAART	highly active antiretroviral therapy
Hb	haemoglobin
HCC	hepatocellular carcinoma
β-HCG	beta human chorionic gonadotrophin
HCM	hypertrophic cardiomyopathy
HHT	hereditary haemorrhagic telangiectasia
HIDA	hepatobiliary iminodiacetic acid
HIFU	high-intensity focused ultrasound
HIV	human immunodeficiency virus
HLA	human leucocyte antigen
HMPAO	hexamethylpropylene amine oxime
HPOA	hypertrophic pulmonary osteoarthropathy
HPV	human papilloma virus
HRCT	high-resolution CT
HSG	hysterosalpingogram
HSV	herpes simplex virus
HU	Hounsfield unit
IAC	internal auditory canal
IAM	internal auditory meatus
ICA	internal carotid artery
ICU	intensive care unit
IEE	idiopathic eosinophilic oesophagitis
ILC	invasive lobular carcinoma
IP	interphalangeal
IUCD	intrauterine contraceptive device
IV	intravenous
IVC	inferior vena cava
IVU	intravenous urogram
JGC	juxtaglomerular cell
JRA	juvenile rheumatoid arthritis
JVP	jugular venous pressure
KUB	kidneys, ureters, and bladder
LAD	left anterior descending
LAO	left anterior oblique
LBBB	left bundle branch block

LCH	Langerhans cell histiocytosis
LCx	left circumflex
LDH	lactate dehydrogenase
LFT	liver function test
LIP	lymphocytic interstitial pneumonia
LMP	last menstrual period
LMS	left main stem
LSF	lesser sciatic foramen
MAA	macro-aggregated albumin
MCA	middle cerebral artery
MCDK	multicystic dysplastic kidney
MCL	medial collateral ligament
MCP	metacarpophalangeal
MCUG	micturating cystourethrogram
MDCT	multidetector CT
MDCTA	multidetector CT mesenteric angiogram
MDP	methylene-diphosphonate
MIBG	meta-iodobenzyl-guanidine
MIP	maximum intensity projection
MISME	multiple intracranial schwannomas, meningiomas and ependymomas
MLA	minimal luminal area
MM	multiple myeloma
MMSE	mini mental state examination
MPS	mucopolysaccharidoses
MRA	magnetic resonance angiogram
MRCP	magnetic resonance cholangiopancreatography
MRI	magnetic resonance imaging
MRS	magnetic resonance spectroscopy
MS	multiple sclerosis
MSA	multisystem atrophy
MSK	musculo-skeletal
MTT	mean transit time
NA	neuropathic arthropathy
NAA	N-acetyl aspartate
NAI	non-accidental injury
NBCCS	nevoid basal cell carcinoma syndrome
NEC	necrotizing enterocolitis
NF-1	neurofibromatosis type 1
NF-2	neurofibromatosis type 2
NHL	non-Hodgkin lymphoma
NOF	non-ossifying fibroma
NPH	normal pressure hydrocephalus
NSAID	non-steroidal anti-inflammatory drug
NSCLC	non small cell lung cancer
NSIP	non-specific interstitial pneumonia
OA	osteoarthritis
OCG	oral cholecystogram
OGD	oesophago-gastro-duodenoscopy
PA	postero-anterior
PACS	picture archiving and communication system

PAES	popliteal artery entrapment syndrome
PaO_2	partial pressure of arterial O_2
PCI	percutaneous coronary intervention
PCL	posterior cruciate ligament
PCOS	polycystic ovarian syndrome
PCP	*P carinii* pneumonia
PDA	patent ductus arteriosus
PIE	pulmonary interstitial emphysema
PIOPED	Prospective Investigation of Pulmonary Embolism Diagnosis
PE	Pulmonary embolism
PET	positron emission tomography
PET-CT	positron emission tomography-computed tomography
PHPV	persistent hyperplastic primary vitreous
PI	pulsatility index
PML	progressive multifocal leucoencephalopathy
POEMS	polyneuropathy, organomegally, endocrinopathy, monoclonal gammopathy and skin changes
PPH	primary (idiopathic) pulmonary hypertension
PR	per rectum
PRES	posterior reversible encephalopathy syndrome
PSA	prostate specific antigen
PSP	progressive supranuclear palsy
PTC	percutaneous transhepatic cholangiography
PTH	parathyroid hormone
PVNS	pigmented villonodular synovitis
PXA	pleomorphic xanthoastrocytoma
RA	rheumatoid arthritis
RAO	right anterior oblique
RAS	renal artery stenosis
RBILD	respiratory bronchiolitis interstitial lung disease
RCA	right coronary artery
rCBV	relative cerebral blood volume
RCC	renal cell carcinoma
RCJ	radiocarpal joint
RFA	radiofrequency ablation
RI	resistive index
RIF	right iliac fossa
RPF	retroperitoneal fibrosis
RPW	relative percentage washout
RTA	road traffic accident
RUQ	right upper quadrant
SAH	subarachnoid haemorrhage
SAPHO	synovitis, acne, pustulosis, hyperostosis, and osteitis
SBA	single best answer
SCBU	Special Care Baby Unit
SDH	subdural haematoma
SE	spin echo
SI	sacroiliac
SLE	systemic lupus erythematosis
SMA	superior mesenteric artery

SPECT	single photon emission computed tomography
SPIO	super paramagnetic iron oxide
SPN	solitary pulmonary nodule
SSPE	subacute sclerosing panencephalitis
STIR	short tau inversion recovery
SUFE	slipped upper femoral epiphysis
SUV	standard uptake value
SUV_{max}	maximum standard uptake value
SVC	superior vena cava
T2WI	T2 weighted imaging
TAPVR	total anomalous pulmonary venous return
TASC	trans-Atlantic intersociety consensus
TB	tuberculosis
TCC	transitional cell carcinoma
TE	time-to-echo
TFCC	triangular fibrocartilage complex
TGA	transposition of the great arteries
THAD	transient hepatic attenuation difference
THID	transient hepatic intensity difference
TIA	transient ischaemic attack
TNM	tumour, nodes, metastases
TOL	tracheo-oesophageal line
TRUC	trans-rectal ultrasound
TS	tuberous sclerosis
TTN	transient tachypnoea of the newborn
TVUS	transvaginal ultrasound
UAC	umbilical arterial line
UES	undifferentiated embryonal sarcoma
UIP	usual interstitial pneumonia
USS	ultrasound scan
UTI	urinary tract infection
UVC	umbilical venous catheter
VCUG	voiding cystourethrogram
VHL	von Hippel–Lindau
VSD	ventricular septal defect
VZV	varicella zoster virus
WCC	white cell count
WHO	World Health Organization
XGC	xanthogranulomatous cholecystitis

chapter 1 CARDIOTHORACIC AND VASCULAR

QUESTIONS

1. **A 33-year-old driver is severely injured in a motor vehicle accident. He develops increasing dyspnoea and hypoxia, and requires intubation. A chest x-ray (CXR) was normal on admission and his pulmonary capillary wedge pressure is normal. A repeat CXR performed at over 24 hours after the trauma is not normal. He is re-imaged during his intensive care unit (ICU) stay and at one point undergoes a computed tomography pulmonary angiography (CTPA), which is negative for pulmonary embolism (PE). The clinical team suspect acute respiratory distress syndrome (ARDS). Which of the following radiographic features is inconsistent with this diagnosis?**

   A. Bronchial dilatation on computed tomography (CT).
   B. Bilateral heterogenous air-space opacities.
   C. Diffuse reticular changes.
   D. Pneumothorax.
   E. Bilateral pleural effusions.

2. **A previously well 42-year-old man is admitted with acute left-sided pleuritic chest pain. His SaO_2 is recorded as 92%. D-Dimer assay is elevated. His mother had died suddenly at the age of 58 years. He is further investigated via CTPA, which is negative for PE. Based on his presenting symptoms, the referring consultant continues to be concerned that the patient has a PE. What advice do you offer regarding this patient's management?**

   A. Refer for V/Q scanning.
   B. Refer for catheter pulmonary angiography.
   C. Commence anticoagulation for 3 months given clinical suspicion.
   D. Commence anticoagulation for 6 months given clinical suspicion.
   E. No further investigation or anticoagulation required.
   F. Repeat CTPA.

3. A 45-year-old male smoker has a 6-month history of gradually increasing shortness of breath and cough. CXR shows a mild increase in interstitial markings in the mid and upper zones. An high-resolution CT (HRCT) of chest is requested for clarification and this demonstrates ill-defined centrilobular ground-glass nodules, more pronounced in the mid and upper zones. There is no traction bronchiectasis or honeycombing. What is the most likely diagnosis?

A. Desquamative interstitial pneumonia (DIP).
B. Usual interstitial pneumonia (UIP).
C. Respiratory bronchiolitis interstitial lung disease (RBILD).
D. Non-specific interstitial pneumonia (NSIP).
E. Cryptogenic organizing pneumonia (COP).

4. A 25-year-old with a history of cystic fibrosis presents with massive haemoptysis. Bronchial artery embolization is requested. Which of the following statements regarding bronchial artery embolization is false?

A. A descending thoracic aortogram is performed prior to selective bronchial angiography.
B. Bronchial angiography is performed with manual injection of contrast medium.
C. The abnormal bronchial artery is embolized at its origin.
D. Polyvinyl alcohol particles (diameter of 350–500 μm) may be used as the embolic material.
E. Chest pain is the most common complication.

5. A 73-year-old patient is involved in a road traffic accident (RTA) and sustains a head injury. He is intubated at the scene due to a low Glasgow Coma Scale (GCS). The patient is transferred for a CT chest as he is hypoxic. On reviewing the CT scan you note widespread emphysema, consistent with the history of smoking. He has a narrowing of the trachea, immediately inferior to the distal margin of the endotracheal (ET) tube. This narrowing is caused by an endoluminal mass associated with a circumferential area of soft tissue that extends into the paratracheal space. There is no pneumomediastinum and no other lung injury is seen. What is the most likely cause?

A. Post-intubation stenosis.
B. Tracheal papilloma.
C. Non small cell lung cancer.
D. Adenoid cystic carcinoma.
E. Squamous cell carcinoma.

6. **A patient is admitted with a comminuted femoral fracture. Initially he is quite well, but goes to theatre for internal fixation of the fracture. His clinical condition deteriorates after 24 hours and he develops fever, hypoxia, and confusion. The clinical team have noted a rash and at the same time as requesting a CT chest, request a CT brain '?meningitis secondary to epidural'. The CT chest reveals widespread peripheral areas of ground-glass opacification (GGO) and air-space consolidation. There are no septal lines or pleural effusions. A follow-up radiograph 10 days later reveals complete resolution. What is the most likely diagnosis?**

   A. Multiple pulmonary contusions.
   B. Pulmonary oedema secondary to anaesthetic medication.
   C. Fat embolism.
   D. ARDS.
   E. Pneumococcal meningitis.

7. **A 50-year-old woman presents with gradually increasing shortness of breath. A CXR and HRCT of chest show subpleural reticulation, more marked in the lower zones. Which of the following further findings on HRCT is most likely to support the diagnosis of NSIP?**

   A. Centrilobular nodules.
   B. Air-trapping.
   C. GGO.
   D. Cystic changes.
   E. Pleural effusions.

8. **A 60-year-old man presents with a history of headache, vertigo, ataxia, and intermittent pain and weakness in his left arm initiated by using the left arm for daily activities. On examination, the left radial pulse is weak and the systolic blood pressure on the left side is reduced by 30 mmHg. Doppler ultrasound reveals reversal of flow in the left vertebral artery. What is the likely underlying pathology?**

   A. Critical stenosis of right middle cerebral artery (MCA).
   B. Critical stenosis of left MCA.
   C. Critical stenosis of third part of left subclavian artery.
   D. Critical stenosis of left vertebral artery.
   E. Critical stenosis of the origin of left subclavian artery.

9. You are carrying out a CT chest scan on a patient who is under the joint care of the respiratory physicians and the rheumatologists. The patient reports slowly progressing stridor. The patient has already been assessed by ear, nose and throat (ENT) due to collapse of the nasal turbinates, but this is felt to be unconnected to his stridor. His inflammatory markers are elevated. A nasal biopsy showed an inflammatory infiltrate in the cartilage causing dissolution, but no granuloma formation or vasculitis. The CT shows smooth thickening of the anterior trachea, with early calcium deposition, with relative sparing of the posterior trachea. This pattern is most marked in the subglottic region. There is narrowing of the airway. This pattern is unaffected on the expiratory scan as compared to the inspiratory scan. The transverse diameter of the trachea is 60% of the sagittal diameter. What is the likely cause?

A. Wegener's granulomatosis.
B. Amyloidosis.
C. Relapsing polychondritis.
D. Mounier–Kuhn disease.
E. Tracheobronchomalacia.

10. A 56-year-old man is admitted via the accident and emergency (A&E) department. He has a past medical history of mitral valve disease. He is complaining of shortness of breath and the clinical team believe he has pulmonary oedema, but ask for your opinion on his CXR to rule out infection. The presence of which of the follow features could not be attributed to cardiac failure and would make you doubt the diagnosis?

A. Perihilar alveolar opacities.
B. Sparing of the lung periphery.
C. A unilateral pleural effusion.
D. Unilateral regional oligaemia.
E. Right upper lobe opacification.

11. A 62-year-old man undergoes lung scintigraphy for investigation of PE. There is no prior history of PE. Which of the following scan patterns would be in keeping with a low probability for PE?

A. Triple matched defect in the lower lung zone.
B. Single moderate matched V/Q defect with a normal CXR.
C. Perfusion defect with a rim of surrounding normally perfused lung.
D. No defects present on perfusion scan.
E. Four moderate segmental defects.

12. A 65-year-old man has kept pigeons for over 20 years. He is complaining of gradually worsening shortness of breath. A CXR shows increased interstitial markings, with reduction in lung volumes. A subsequent HRCT of chest shows quite marked pulmonary fibrosis with areas of honeycomb formation. Which part of the lung is likely to be relatively spared by the fibrotic process?

A. Upper zones.
B. Mid zones.
C. Posterior costophrenic sulci.
D. Central peribronchovascular regions.
E. Subpleural lung.

13. A 70-year-old male undergoes endovascular stent graft repair of an infra-renal abdominal aortic aneurysm. A follow-up CT at 1 year demonstrates increasing aneurysm sac diameter without any evidence of endoleak. What is the diagnosis?

A. Type I endoleak.
B. Type II endoleak.
C. Type III endoleak.
D. Type IV endoleak.
E. Type V endoleak.

14. A patient is referred to radiology with a diagnosis of a mass in the lung which is adjacent to, but not overtly invading, the pleura. The clinical team need a tissue type to decide on treatment. There is a history of colorectal carcinoma. You are undecided as to whether to carry out a core biopsy with a coaxial system or a fine needle aspiration (FNA). Which of these factors should have the greatest influence on your decision?

A. Pneumothorax risk.
B. Availability of a cytopathologist.
C. Tumour seeding risk.
D. Suspected cell type of the lesion.
E. Risk of air embolism.

15. A 28-year-old man is being investigated for haemoptysis. He has a history of sinusitis. Full blood picture is normal. He is referred for a CT of chest during which intravenous (IV) contrast was withheld by the radiographer due to a reduction in estimated glomerular filtration rate (eGFR). It reveals bilateral nodules in a peribronchovascular distribution, some of which show cavitation. There are peripheral wedge-shaped areas of consolidation. There are also areas of bronchial stenosis and thickening. No mediastinal or hilar adenopathy is present. What is the most likely diagnosis?

A. Goodpasture's syndrome.
B. Sarcoidosis.
C. Churg–Strauss syndrome.
D. Wegener's granulomatosis.
E. Pulmonary tuberculosis.

16. A 50-year-old woman presents with progressive exertional dyspnoea, fatigue and atypical chest pain. Her jugular venous pressure (JVP) is elevated on examination. Her CXR reveals prominence of the right side of the heart with asymmetric enlargement of the central pulmonary arteries. Patchy oligaemic vascularity is also evident. What is the most likely diagnosis?

A. Atrial septal defect.
B. Primary pulmonary hypertension.
C. Chronic thromboembolic pulmonary hypertension.
D. Cardiopulmonary schistosomiasis.
E. Pulmonary veno-occlusive disease.

17. A 34-year-old woman presents with a 4-month history of gradually increasing dyspnoea and cough. A CXR and subsequent CT scan show multiple cavitating lung lesions. On the CT scan, some of these lesions are noted to have surrounding ground-glass attenuation. No other abnormality is seen. Which of the following diagnoses are the findings most compatible with?

A. Rheumatoid lung.
B. Lung abscesses.
C. Eosinophilic granuloma.
D. Churg–Strauss syndrome.
E. Melanoma metastases.

18. A 45-year-old woman presents with significant ongoing melaena, tachycardia and hypotension. Multidetector CT mesenteric angiography (MDCTA) is requested prior to consideration of mesenteric embolization. Which of the following statements regarding gastrointestinal (GI) bleeding and MDCTA is true?

A. Oral contrast should be administered to identify the causative lesion.
B. Scans are usually performed in the arterial phase only from diaphragm to ischial tuberosity.
C. Acute GI bleeding can be intermittent. Failure to demonstrate active bleeding does not prove cessation of bleeding.
D. Suture material, dense foreign bodies or faecolith can be easily distinguished from contrast extravasation.
E. The lowest detectable bleeding rate with MDCTA is 2 ml/min.

19. You are taking the respiratory multidisciplinary team meeting. A respiratory physician has asked you to present two patients, both with incidentally detected solitary pulmonary nodules. Patient A is a 64-year-old male patient. He is a non-smoker. The lesion is 7 mm in diameter and smooth. Patient B is also a 64-year-old male, who smokes 30 cigarettes per day. His lesion is 5 mm in diameter. What follow-up would you recommend for these patients?

A. Urgent positron emission tomography (PET) scan for both. Reassess with result.
B. CT within 6 months for Patient A. If unchanged repeat within 12 months. PET scan for Patient B and reassess with result.
C. CT scan within 12 months for Patient A. If unchanged further CT within a further 12 months. Serial 6 monthly CT scans for Patient B for 2 years.
D. CT scan within 12 months for both. If unchanged, both need a follow-up CT within a further 12 months.
E. Follow-up CT at 12 months for both. If unchanged, no further follow-up.

20. A 64-year-old smoker is referred by his GP for persisting consolidation which has failed to resolve despite multiple antibiotic therapies. Of note he has been apyrexic and inflammatory markers have not been particularly raised. The respiratory team request a CT of chest, which shows GGO and consolidation of almost the entire left lower lobe, delineated by the major fissure, which is not displaced. Air bronchograms are present, but there is no significant loss of volume or expansion of the lobe and no mediastinal or hilar adenopathy. No mass obstructing the left lower lobe bronchus (either endoluminal or extrinsic) is demonstrated and the bronchoscopy findings corroborate this (results from washings not yet available). A PET-CT is normal. What is the most likely pathology?

A. Carcinoid tumour.
B. Bronchioloalveolar carcinoma.
C. Small cell carcinoma.
D. Tuberculosis (TB).
E. Klebsiella pneumonia.

21. A 34-year-old woman with a preceding history of chronic cough, weight loss and intermittent chest tightness presents with acute shortness of breath. CTPA reveals a large filling defect within the left pulmonary artery. Which radiological feature would most suggest a diagnosis of pulmonary artery sarcoma as opposed to pulmonary embolism?

A. Mosaic lung perfusion.
B. Peripheral filling defect forming acute angle with arterial wall.
C. Peripheral filling defect forming obtuse angle with arterial wall.
D. Low attenuation filling defect occupying and expanding the entire luminal diameter.
E. Partial filling defect surrounded by areas of intravascular contrast enhancement.

22. A 45-year-old male smoker has a history of fatigue and mild shortness of breath. He also keeps pigeons. A CXR shows mildly increased interstitial markings in the upper zones. An HRCT of chest demonstrates multiple small pulmonary nodules and reticulation, more marked in the upper lungs. What location of the nodularity is more likely to suggest a diagnosis of subacute extrinsic alveolitis or respiratory bronchiolitis interstitial lung disease as opposed to sarcoidosis?

A. Bronchovascular bundle.
B. Centrilobular region.
C. Fissural.
D. Subpleural region.
E. Interlobular septa.

23. A 40-year-old male presents with a history of severe epigastric pain and raised amylase. CT demonstrates acute pancreatitis complicated by a 2.5-cm pseudoaneurysm of the gastroduodenal artery (GDA). Embolization of the GDA is requested. What is the accepted method of embolization?

A. Coil embolization proximal to the pseudoaneurysm.
B. Coil embolization distal and proximal to the pseudoaneurysm.
C. Embolization with polyvinyl alcohol (PVA) particles.
D. Amplatzer plug occlusion of common hepatic artery.
E. Embolization with gelfoam.

24. A 72-year-old former ship builder has presented with increasing shortness of breath to the respiratory physicians. A CXR reveals a pleural mass. You carry out a CT scan, which shows a 1cm diameter area of pleural thickening extending along the lateral chest wall inferiorly to the diaphragm. On coronal reconstructions the diaphragm appears smooth. There are a number of >1-cm nodes noted in the ipsilateral hilum as well as a solitary 1.2-cm node noted in the contralateral hilum. Following discussion with thoracic surgery a core biopsy is done, which confirms the diagnosis of malignant mesothelioma. A magnetic resonance imaging (MRI) scan is carried out. The lesion is increased signal on T2 weighted imaging (T2WI). The enlarged nodes are also identified. On post-gadolinium coronal fat saturation sequences a focus of high signal is noted to extend from the parietal pleura through the diaphragm to involve the peritoneum. A single focus of chest wall invasion is also noted. PET-CT shows high uptake in the lesion with a standard uptake value maximum (SUV max) of 25. All nodes with the exception of the contralateral node demonstrate uptake. Which of these factors means this tumour is inoperable?

A. The contralateral enlarged node noted on CT and MRI.
B. The tissue diagnosis of malignant mesothelioma.
C. The high SUV max.
D. The chest wall disease noted on MRI.
E. The diaphragmatic disease noted on MRI.

25. A 61-year-old man has a history of chronic myeloid leukaemia. He presents with mild dyspnoea and dry cough. A CXR shows symmetrical, perihilar reticulo-nodular opacities with relative sparing of the apices and costophrenic angles, without cardiomegaly or pleural effusion. An HRCT reveals smoothly thickened septal lines with intervening GGO and sharply marginated areas of geographic sparing. Bronchoalveolar lavage (BAL) is negative for organisms. What is the most likely diagnosis?

A. Pulmonary haemorrhage.
B. Left ventricular failure.
C. Pulmonary alveolar proteinosis.
D. Pneumocystis pneumonia.
E. Radiation fibrosis.

26. A 28-year-old Asian male immigrant presents with low-grade fever, weight loss and productive cough. There is no history of immunosuppression. Which of the following CXR findings is most in keeping with post-primary TB?

A. Unilateral hilar lymphadenopathy.
B. Cavitating parenchymal opacity.
C. Pleural effusion.
D. Multiple bilateral non-calcified nodules <3 mm diameter.
E. Right lower lobe atelectasis.

27. A 65-year-old man has a history of liver cirrhosis. He presents with increasing dyspnoea. A CXR shows some basal reticulo-nodular opacities. An HRCT of chest demonstrates distal vascular dilatation and subpleural telangiectasia. You suspect he may have hepato-pulmonary syndrome. Which of the following nuclear medicine techniques is most likely to prove the presence of right-to-left shunting?

A. ^{99m}Tc-labelled sulphur colloid scan.
B. ^{99m}Tc-labelled red blood cell scan.
C. ^{99m}Tc-labelled pertechnetate scan.
D. ^{99m}Tc-labelled HMPAO scan.
E. ^{99m}Tc-labelled macro-aggregated albumin scan.

28. A 55-year-old man with a recent diagnosis of multifocal hepatocellular carcinoma is referred for transarterial chemoembolisation. Which of the following statements regarding hepatic arterial anatomy is true?

A. The classic hepatic arterial anatomy, with the proper and hepatic artery dividing into the right and left hepatic arteries, is seen in approximately 80% of the population.
B. Accessory left hepatic artery from left gastric artery is seen in 25% of cases.
C. Replaced right hepatic artery commonly arises from the gastroduodenal artery.
D. Replaced left hepatic artery commonly arises from the left gastric artery.
E. The common hepatic artery is a branch of the superior mesenteric artery.

29. A 72-year-old female patient presents with a diagnosis lung malignancy obtained from bronchial washings. The CT shows a 4cm lesion in the right upper lobe with ipsilateral hilar and mediastinal lymphadenopathy in the 4R station. There is no chest wall invasion and the lung lesion is surrounded on all sides by lung parenchyma. There is currently no evidence of infradiaphragmatic disease. What is the TNM stage of this small cell lung cancer?

A. T2a N1 M0.
B. T2b N1 M0.
C. T1b N2 M0.
D. T2a N2 M0.
E. None of these.

30. A 43-year-old patient presents with cough, shortness of breath and fever which has lasted a month. An HRCT reveals bilateral areas of consolidation, predominantly in a peripheral distribution. There are also areas of GGO, predominantly in the middle and upper zones, with band-like subpleural attenuation. The plain film findings have remained unchanged for days. What is the most likely diagnosis?

A. Chronic eosinophilic pneumonia.
B. Allergic bronchopulmonary aspergillosis (ABPA).
C. Acute eosinophilic pneumonia.
D. Löffler's syndrome.
E. Eosinophilic granuloma.

31. A 30-year-old caucasian man, recently treated with bone marrow transplantation for acute myeloid leukaemia, presents with fever and cough. HRCT chest demonstrates multiple, small centrilobular nodules of soft tissue attenuation connected to linear branching opacities. What is the most likely cause of this finding?

A. Endobronchial tuberculosis.
B. Primary pulmonary lymphoma.
C. Invasive aspergillosis.
D. Obliterative bronchiolitis.
E. Diffuse panbronchiolitis.

32. A 56-year-old woman with a history of Sjogren's syndrome complains of gradually increasing shortness of breath. A CXR has identified a mild generalized interstitial pattern, with maintained lung volumes. A subsequent HRCT of chest demonstrates a few scattered well-defined, regular lung cysts. Within the lung parenchyma there is also noted patchy ground-glass change and mild centrilobular nodularity. Mild mediastinal and hilar lymphadenopathy is present. What is the most likely diagnosis?

A. Langerhans cell histiocytosis.
B. Desquamative interstitial pneumonia.
C. Lymphangioleiomyomatosis.
D. Lymphocytic interstitial pneumonia.
E. Birt–Hogg–Dube syndrome.

33. A 70-year-old man undergoes a trans-femoral angiogram as a day procedure. Haemostasis is achieved by manual compression to the puncture site for 15 minutes. The next day he returns to A&E with a history of pain and swelling in the groin. On examination a tender, pulsatile swelling is noted in the groin at the site of femoral puncture. Doppler ultrasound confirms a femoral artery pseudo-aneurysm. Which of the following statements regarding iatrogenic femoral artery pseudoaneurysm is false?

A. It is contained only by the haematoma and surrounding tissues.
B. Patients undergoing haemodialysis are at increased risk of developing pseudoaneurysm.
C. Low femoral puncture is associated with a higher risk of developing pseudoaneurysm.
D. Ultrasound is the diagnostic method of choice.
E. Ultrasound-guided compression is the treatment of choice.

34. A 68-year-old patient has a CXR carried out due to a recurrent chest infection. The patient is a smoker. The CXR shows a solitary pulmonary nodule. A CT is carried out which demonstrates a 2.8-cm lesion in the right lower lobe as noted on CXR. This lesion is spiculated. There is a second lesion noted in the right lower lobe that is 1.2 cm in size and was not visible on the CXR. There is a 0.8-cm ipsilateral peribronchial lymph node identified. There are no evident metastases. A PET-CT is carried out which shows an SUV max of 8 in both pulmonary lesions. There is no uptake in the lymph node. No metastases are identified. A biopsy confirms non-small cell lung cancer. Based on the available imaging, what is the stage of this lesion?

A. Stage 1A.
B. Stage 1B.
C. Stage 2A.
D. Stage 2B.
E. Stage 3A.

35. A specialty trainee from the medical ward shows you a CXR of a breathless patient. You observe splaying of the carina and a 'double right heart border'. What is the most likely underlying diagnosis?

A. Mitral stenosis.
B. Aortic stenosis.
C. Tricuspid incompetence.
D. Left ventricular aneurysm.
E. Coarctation of the aorta.

36. A 64-year-old man with a history of alcoholism presents with acute onset fever and productive cough. What feature on his admission CXR would be in keeping with *Klebsiella* pneumonia as opposed to pneumococcal pneumonia?

A. Lobar consolidation.
B. Parapneumonic effusion.
C. Reticulonodular opacity.
D. Bulging interlobar fissure.
E. Spherical opacity.

37. A 67-year-old man who was previously a manual worker presents with chest pain, which subsequently turns out to be due to myocardial ischaemia. He has a CXR performed which shows numerous small nodular densities and you suspect he has an occupational lung disease, as these densities are unchanged from previous radiographs. A subsequent HRCT of chest shows no evidence of linear interstitial change or fibrosis. Pulmonary function tests are normal. Which of the following possible causes is least likely to result in functional lung impairment?

A. Coal workers' pneumoconiosis.
B. Silicosis.
C. Berylliosis.
D. Siderosis.
E. Asbestosis.

38. A 35-year-old male smoker presents with a history of progressive dyspnoea and rapidly deteriorating lung function. CXR shows hyperinflated lungs and decreased pulmonary vascular markings. High-resolution CT of chest shows well-defined foci of reduced lung attenuation without definable wall, decreased pulmonary vascular markings and bullae with basilar predominance. What is the likely diagnosis?

A. Centrilobular emphysema.
B. Paraseptal emphysema.
C. Alpha-1 antitrypsin deficiency.
D. Congenital lobar emphysema.
E. Chronic obstructive pulmonary disease (COPD).

39. You are attending a lecture on lung cancer, but unfortunately you arrive late so you have missed the introduction. The lecturer is describing a subtype of lung cancer. The description is of a tumour that comprises 30% of all lung cancers. It typically occurs peripherally, but can be central. This tumour can cavitate, but this occurs in only 4% of cases. Hilar and/or mediastinal involvement is seen in over half of cases on plain film radiography. What subtype of lung cancer is being described?

A. Adenocarcinoma.
B. Bronchoalveolar carcinoma.
C. Squamous cell carcinoma.
D. Small cell carcinoma.
E. Giant cell carcinoma.

40. A 63-year-old male has a complex past medical history including testicular carcinoma, cardiac disease, rheumatoid arthritis (RA) and diabetes mellitus. He presents with shortness of breath and is referred for a CT chest. This reveals multiple areas of ground-glass attenuation, crazy-paving and consolidation in both lungs. You also notice that the spleen and liver are of increased attenuation. What is the most likely explanation for these findings?

A. RA-related lung disease.
B. Cardiac failure.
C. Amiodarone.
D. Bleomycin.
E. Methotrexate.

41. A 28-year-old HIV-positive IV drug user presents with progressive exertional dyspnoea, fever and non-productive cough. CXR demonstrates bilateral parahilar fine reticular opacities. There is no appreciable lymphadenopathy. What is the most likely diagnosis?

A. Mycobacterium avium-intracellulare.
B. *Pneumocystis jirovecii* (formerly *P. carinii*).
C. Toxoplasmosis.
D. Coccidioidomycosis.
E. Candidiasis.

42. A 50-year-old man has developed graft v host disease following a bone marrow transplant. He develops some breathlessness and has pulmonary function tests showing irreversible obstruction. Constrictive (obliterative) bronchiolitis is suspected. Which of the following findings on HRCT is likely to be most helpful in making this diagnosis?

A. 'Tree in bud' opacities.
B. Bronchiolectasis.
C. Air-trapping.
D. Centrilobular nodules.
E. Cystic change.

43. A 50-year-old female is found to have a solitary pulmonary nodule on imaging. Which of the following features suggests that it is benign?

A. Irregular, spiculated margin.
B. Central 'popcorn' calcification.
C. Doubling time of 180 days.
D. Contrast enhancement of 25 Hounsfield units(HU).
E. SUV of 8 on PET-CT.

44. A 47-year-old male patient is referred to the respiratory physicians with a 1-year history of wheeze. He is a non-smoker. A CXR reveals subtle narrowing of the bronchus intermedius. A CT scan reveals a lesion with an endobronchial component, which narrows the airway significantly. The lesion also has an extraluminal component, which is 2 cm in diameter and has smooth margins. The lesion displays stippled calcification and no cavitation. Following contrast enhancement, the lesion enhances avidly in the arterial phase. You formulate a differential diagnosis based on these imaging features. The patient is not keen for intervention. Based on your suspicions, what would be the least invasive means of follow-up imaging to help achieve a diagnosis?

A. PET-CT.
B. Bronchoscopy and biopsy.
C. Indium-111 octreotide single photon emission computed tomography (SPECT) CT.
D. MRI using T2WI and short tau inversion recovery (STIR) coronal imaging.
E. Bronchial angiography.

45. A 45-year-old male presents with a 3-month history of a non-productive cough and dyspnoea, which was preceded by a flu-like illness. Pulmonary function tests reveal a restrictive pattern and a CXR shows multifocal bilateral consolidation. HRCT of chest reveals bilateral peripheral subpleural well-defined areas of consolidation, some of which are surrounded by ground-glass opacity and some of which show an air bronchogram. There is also a focal area of GGO, which is surrounded by a smooth-walled ring of consolidation. Which of the following is the most likely diagnosis?

A. Sarcoidosis.
B. TB.
C. Cryptococcosis.
D. Obliterative bronchiolitis.
E. Cryptogenic organizing pneumonia.

46. A 24-year-old serviceman presents with insidious onset of fever, headache and worsening non-productive cough. His white cell count and erythrocyte sedimentation rate (ESR) are elevated and serum cold agglutination is positive. He had failed to improve with initial antibiotic therapy. HRCT of chest demonstrates areas of ground-glass opacity, air-space consolidation, centrilobular nodules and thickening of bronchovascular bundles. What is the most likely diagnosis?

A. Chlamydia pneumonia.
B. Mycoplasma pneumonia.
C. Pneumococcal pneumonia.
D. Legionella pneumonia.
E. Staphylococcal pneumonia.

47. A 51-year-old woman has a past history of a prolonged ICU admission following a subarachnoid haemorrhage 2 years previously. Despite the stormy course in ICU, she made a good neurological recovery, but has had persistent breathlessness on exertion since discharge. Her imaging shows interstitial fibrosis. Which part of the lung is likely to be relatively spared by the interstitial process?

A. Posterior aspect of the lungs.
B. Anterior aspect of the lungs.
C. Periphery of the lungs.
D. Lower zones of the lungs.
E. Mid-zones of the lungs.

48. A 30-year-old male smoker presents with a history of acute dyspnoea. CXR shows bilateral reticulo-nodular interstitial changes, predominantly in the upper and mid zones, with preservation of lung volume. There is a right-sided apical pneumothorax and a small right pleural effusion. HRCT of chest shows complex thin- and thick-walled cysts and irregular centrilobular nodules in a similar distribution with sparing of the bases. The intervening lung appears normal. What is the diagnosis?

A. Lymphangioleiomyomatosis.
B. Bronchiectasis.
C. Metastases.
D. Pulmonary Langerhans cell histiocytosis.
E. Idiopathic pulmonary fibrosis.

49. A 55-year-old male patient with a history of dilated cardiomyopathy has undergone a cardiac transplantation. Now 3 months post-op, the patient presents to his cardiologists with acute lethargy, dyspnoea and productive cough. A CXR is carried out, which shows a diffuse right-sided airspace infiltrate, with an ill-defined density noted in the right upper lobe. A CT scan is carried out, which shows patchy areas of air-space consolidation with surrounding ground-glass change in the right hemi thorax. There is an area of cavitation in the right upper lobe that has a surrounding halo of ground-glass change. The interstitial markings are not thickened. There is low attenuation noted around the heart, which has an attenuation value of –10 HU. There is a calibre change between the donor and recipient aorta. Based on the most likely pathology, as indicated by these features, what is the most appropriate first-line treatment?

A. Systemic amphotericin.
B. Frusemide infusion.
C. Systemic ganciclovir.
D. High-dose steroid and OKT3.
E. CT guided biopsy of lesion.

50. A 42-year-old male presents with chest pain, dyspnoea and palpitations. He undergoes cardiac MRI, which reveals extensive scattered delayed enhancement in the anterior, lateral and inferior wall and apex of the left ventricle. This enhancement occurs in the midwall with relative sparing of the subendocardial region. T2WI is unremarkable. What is the most likely diagnosis?

A. Acute myocardial infarction.
B. Sarcoidosis.
C. Myocarditis.
D. Hypertrophic cardiomyopathy.
E. Amyloidosis.

51. A 28-year-old woman presents with fever, myalgia and cough. Due to a current community outbreak, the clinical team suspect that she has H1N1 influenza (swine flu). Which finding on her admission CXR is most strongly predictive of an adverse outcome?

A. Upper lobe consolidation.
B. Bilateral central opacity.
C. Multizonal peripheral opacity.
D. Air bronchogram.
E. Pleural effusion.

52. A 56-year-old man presents with shortness of breath. He subsequently has an HRCT of chest performed. This shows a mosaic attenuation pattern throughout the lung parenchyma, but you are having some difficulty determining if the more lucent areas are normal or abnormal. Which of the following findings is most likely to be helpful in confirming that the lucent areas are the abnormal areas and you are not dealing with multifocal GGO?

A. Increased calibre of vessels in denser areas.
B. Decreased calibre of vessels in denser areas.
C. Increased calibre of vessels in lucent areas.
D. Decreased caliber of vessels in lucent areas.
E. Calibre of vessels is unhelpful and expiratory scans must be used.

53. A 60-year-old male awaiting cardiac bypass surgery undergoes Doppler assessment of leg veins to check suitability for a vein graft. On ultrasound, incidental note is made of 1.8-cm popliteal artery aneurysm with mural thrombus. Which of the following statements regarding popliteal artery aneurysm is false?

A. It is bilateral in 50–70% of cases.
B. It is associated with abdominal aortic aneurysm in 30–50% of cases.
C. Symptomatic patients present with effects of distal embolization.
D. It may be missed on conventional angiography.
E. It should be treated only when symptomatic.

54. A 55-year-old female patient presents to the neurology service with features of myasthenia gravis. As part of the routine work-up a CXR is requested which demonstrates an anterior mediastinal mass. A CT scan is requested. This reveals a 5cm mass located centrally within the anterior mediastinum. This mass has poorly defined margins, resulting in obliteration of the mediastinal fat plane. There are areas of low attenuation within this lesion which have an attenuation value of 3 HU. There are stippled areas of calcification noted. There is also a right-sided pleural effusion. There is no evidence of disease elsewhere in the mediastinum, or invasion of the great vessels. You plan to carry out a CT guided biopsy, but at this stage what is the most likely diagnosis?

A. Benign thymoma.
B. Atypical thymoma.
C. Thymic carcinoma.
D. Thymic lymphoma.
E. Malignant thymic germ cell tumour.

55. A 34-year-old man presents with chest pain and palpitations. An electrocardiogram (ECG) reveals a ventricular tachycardia with left bundle branch block (LBBB). A T1WI sequence shows transmural high signal and thinning of the myocardium of the right ventricle, with dilatation of the right ventricle and right ventricular outflow tract. What is the most likely diagnosis?

A. Tricuspid stenosis.
B. Uhl's anomaly.
C. Pericardial effusion.
D. Arrhythmogenic right ventricular dysplasia.
E. Melanoma metastasis.

56. An 18-year-old woman with Poland syndrome is being assessed by plastic surgery for reconstruction. As part of her pre-operative work-up a CT chest is requested. What is the classic finding in this disorder?

A. Absence of the sternal head of pectoralis major.
B. Hypoplastic clavicles.
C. Anterior protrusion of the ribs.
D. Bilateral breast aplasia.
E. Anterior protrusion of the sternum.

57. A 65-year-old man presents to the A&E department with acute shortness of breath. He has a CXR performed and this demonstrates a 'bat-wing' pattern of pulmonary oedema. Which of the following is the most likely cause?

A. Fat embolism.
B. Diffuse alveolar damage.
C. Adult respiratory distress syndrome.
D. Acute mitral valve insufficiency.
E. Left ventricular failure.

58. A 25-year-old baseball player presents with a history of worsening pain, diffuse oedema and discolouration of the right upper limb following a game. Doppler ultrasound demonstrates occlusion of the axillary and subclavian veins. He undergoes catheter-directed thrombolysis successfully. Check venogram demonstrates external compression from scalenus muscle. What is the diagnosis?

A. May–Thurner syndrome.
B. Nutcracker syndrome.
C. Paget–Schroetter syndrome.
D. Trousseau syndrome.
E. Virchow syndrome.

59. A 45-year-old male patient is referred by his GP for a CXR due to a history of dyspnoea and cough. The CXR shows a convex appearance to the hila with a right paratracheal stripe that measures 1.5 cm. You are arranging follow-up and the respiratory team ask you for your top differential. What do you say?

A. TB.
B. Lymphoma.
C. Sarcoid.
D. Castleman's disease.
E. Silicosis.

60. A 58-year-old smoker with a history of hypertension and diabetes presents with chest pain typical of angina and is referred for CT coronary angiography. This reveals soft plaque in the proximal left anterior descending (LAD) artery, which is causing a 40% stenosis by area and calcified plaque in the right coronary artery (RCA), which is causing a 50% stenosis by area. Which of the following is the most appropriate next step?

A. Percutaneous coronary intervention (PCI) to the LAD.
B. PCI to the RCA.
C. PCI to both vessels.
D. Exercise stress testing.
E. Lifestyle and risk factor modification.

61. A junior doctor requests your opinion on a postero-anterior (PA) CXR of a 21-year-old man admitted with chest pain. She suspects that the patient has right middle lobe consolidation. What feature on the patient's radiograph allows you to reassure her that the imaging appearances are secondary to pectus excavatum?

A. Rightward displacement of the heart.
B. 'Sevens' appearance to ribs.
C. Indistinct right heart border.
D. Bilateral hilar enlargement.
E. Steeply angulated posterior ribs.

62. A 30-year-old male mechanic presents with digital ischaemia. Catheter angiogram demonstrates occlusion of the distal ulnar artery and abrupt occlusion of some of the digital arteries. The radial artery is patent and there is filling of the superficial palmar arch via deep palmar arch collaterals. What is the diagnosis?

A. Hypothenar hammer syndrome.
B. Peripheral embolic disease.
C. Raynaud's disease.
D. Thoracic outlet syndrome.
E. Takayasu arteritis.

63. A 57-year-old patient has a CXR carried out. This shows a mass in the left apex, adjacent to the spine. Numerous soft tissue densities are noted projected across the lungs. A lateral radiograph is carried out which projects the mass over the vertebral bodies and indicates that the smaller densities are cutaneous. You request additional information from the referring clinician. This patient has a complex history. He has type 1 neurofibromatosis, but has also recently been diagnosed with myelofibrosis. You perform a CT scan, which shows widening of the neural foramen on the left side, which is in continuity with the left apex mass. This mass measures 2 cm in diameter and has an attenuation value of 4 HU. What is the most likely diagnosis?

A. Neuroblastoma.
B. Neurofibroma.
C. Extramedullary haematopoesis.
D. Lateral meningocele.
E. Neuro-enteric cyst.

64. A 45-year-old woman presents with chest pain, typical of angina. Her ECG and troponin are normal. She is a non-smoker and does not have hypertension or diabetes. Her resting heart rate is 56 beats per minute (bpm). To best assess her further, what do you decide to perform next?

A. CT calcium score.
B. Exercise stress testing.
C. Contrast enhanced cardiac MRI.
D. Retrospectively ECG-gated CT coronary angiography.
E. Prospectively ECG-gated CT coronary angiography.

65. A 64-year-old woman presents with a 3-week history of dry cough. A CXR is performed and shows multifocal bilateral peripheral areas of consolidation. An HRCT of chest is recommended and this demonstrates bilateral peripheral areas of consolidation and GGO. There is no fibrosis. There is peripheral eosinophilia detected on routine blood tests. A careful drug history is obtained. Which of the following medications is the patient most likely to be on?

A. Nitrofurantoin.
B. Amiodarone.
C. Methotrexate.
D. Bleomycin.
E. Cyclophosphamide.

66. A 50-year-old chronic alcoholic and smoker presents with chronic cough. CXR shows bilateral upper lobe consolidation with nodular opacities and cavitation. These changes are slowly progressive over serial x-rays. A bronchoscopy is arranged and washouts from the upper lobes are negative for mycobacterial infection. Aspergillus titres are positive. How is the disease process best described?

A. Allergic bronchopulmonary aspergillosis.
B. Bilateral aspergillomas with background COPD.
C. Semi-invasive aspergillosis.
D. Invasive aspergillosis.
E. Chronic aspiration pneumonia (aspergillus titres irrelevant).

67. A 70-year-old man presents with a 6-month history of cramping pain in the left calf brought on by walking and settling with rest. For the past 3 weeks he has been experiencing pain at rest, which is relieved by dependency of the foot. On examination, the popliteal and tibial pulses are absent. There is no ulceration or gangrene. What is the diagnosis?

A. Intermittent claudication.
B. Critical limb ischaemia.
C. Acute limb ischaemia.
D. Nerve root compression.
E. Diabetic neuropathy.

68. A 4-year-old with a history of asthma is admitted with an acute exacerbation. A post-admission CXR shows evidence of pneumomediastinum. Which one of the following is a recognized sign of pneumomediastinum?

A. Spinnaker/thymic sail sign.
B. Air-crescent sign.
C. Deep sulcus sign.
D. Inverted V sign.
E. Outline of the medial diaphragm inferior to the cardiac silhouette.

69. A 25-year-old man presents with chest pain on exertion. He is referred for CT coronary angiography. Which of the following findings is most significant?

A. The RCA arises from the left coronary sinus and passes between the aorta and pulmonary artery.
B. Separate ostia of the LAD and left circumflex (LCx) coronary arteries arise from the left coronary sinus.
C. The left main stem (LMS) arises from the right coronary cusp and passes anterior to the pulmonary artery.
D. The RCA arises from the right coronary cusp and passes into the right atrioventricular (AV) groove.
E. The LMS arises from the left coronary cusp and trifurcates into an LAD, LCx and ramus intermedius branch.

70. A patient is being investigated by his GP due to a history of dysphagia and occasional stridor. A CXR has been requested, which is reported as showing possible tracheal abnormality. A lateral CXR is requested and this shows an abnormality in the retro-tracheal space (Raider triangle). Using your knowledge of the anatomy of this space and the diseases that may affect it, which of the following statements correctly describes an abnormality in this area and the effect it will have radiologically on the retro-tracheal space?

A. A thickened tracheo-oesophageal stripe of 11mm will displace the trachea posteriorly.
B. An enlarged aorta bulges into the inferior aspect of the retro-tracheal space.
C. A subclavian artery aneurysm will be noted posterior to the tracheo-oesophageal stripe and will displace this anteriorly.
D. Mediastinal extension of a retropharyngeal abscess will widen the tracheo-oesophageal stripe superiorly.
E. A thyroid goitre extending retrosternally will displace the trachea posteriorly.

71. A 50-year-old male smoker presents with a history of right-sided calf claudication. The symptoms are not settling with best medical therapy. The magnetic resonance angiogram (MRA) shows occlusion of the right common and external iliac arteries. He is otherwise well and has normal calf veins. What is the recommended treatment for this type of lesion?

A. Symptomatic relief.
B. Continue modification of risk factors and exercise therapy.
C. Percutaneous angioplasty.
D. Percutaneous stenting.
E. Surgical bypass.

72. You notice a mass within the heart on a CT thorax of a 45-year-old patient. There is contrast enhancement of the mass. Without further assessment, what is this mass most likely to be?

A. Myxoma.
B. Angiosarcoma.
C. Metastasis.
D. Rhabdomyosarcoma.
E. Primary cardiac lymphoma.

73. A 28-year-old patient is admitted from the dermatology clinic where she is being treated for basal cell carcinoma. She suffered an episode of ventricular tachycardia and imaging is requested secondary to the results of echocardiography. CXR reveals bifid ribs. Cardiac MRI reveals a well-circumscribed abnormality, which is low signal on both T1WI and T2WI and shows delayed enhancement, within the myocardium of the left ventricular free wall. CT reveals a soft-tissue attenuation mass with calcification. What is the most likely diagnosis?

A. Myxoma.
B. Paraganglioma.
C. Fibroma.
D. Fibroelastoma.
E. Lipoma.

74. A patient is referred for cardiac MRI. Which of the following is a definite contraindication?

A. Cardiac pacemaker.
B. Loop recorder.
C. Coronary artery bypass grafting 2 months ago.
D. Cardiac stenting 2 months ago.
E. None of the above.

75. A 24-year-old woman who is 28 weeks pregnant is admitted with suspected pulmonary embolism. As the on-call radiologist, her obstetrician contacts you seeking advice regarding further management. An admission CXR is normal. What investigation do you advise initially?

A. Venous ultrasound.
B. Low-dose CTPA.
C. Reduced dose lung scintigraphy.
D. MRA.
E. Catheter pulmonary angiography.

chapter 1 CARDIOTHORACIC AND VASCULAR

ANSWERS

1. E. Bilateral pleural effusions.

The underlying diagnosis is ARDS. The causes may be direct lung injury (e.g. pneumonia, toxic gas inhalation, aspiration) or indirect lung injury (e.g. trauma, sepsis, pancreatitis). Diagnostic guidelines require a partial pressure of arterial O_2/fraction of inspired O_2 (PaO_2/FiO_2) < 200 mmHg and no evidence of left heart failure, and thus the presence of a pleural effusion casts doubt on the diagnosis; the appearance of ARDS can otherwise mimic pulmonary oedema.

Bronchial dilatation is frequently seen on CT. The alveolar changes are heterogenous, showing a density gradient in both the cranio-caudal and antero-posterior directions (the dorsal/dependent and lower lobes are denser than the ventral/non-dependent and upper lobes). Radiographic changes tend to be absent for the first 24 hours (with the exception of direct lung injury), then increase to remain static for days or weeks, and then begin to resolve. Pneumothorax can occur secondary to ventilation. Reticular changes, with a predilection for non-dependent lung, may be secondary to the underlying process or to barotrauma (seen in 85% of survivors in one study; the mortality of ARDS is approximately 50%).

Desai SR. Acute respiratory distress syndrome: imaging of the injured lung. *Clinical Radiology* 2002; 57: 8–17.

2. E. No further investigation or anticoagulation required.

In the setting of a low probability clinical assessment and positive D-dimer assay, a negative CTPA has a negative predictive value of 96% and further investigation and treatment are therefore not warranted. A repeat CTPA may be indicated if the images are of poor quality. The Prospective Investigation of Pulmonary Embolism Diagnosis (PIOPED) II investigators recommend that in the setting of a high pre-test probability, a negative CTPA should be followed with either venous ultrasound or MR venography.

Stein PD, Woodard PK, Weg JG, Wakefield TW, Tapson VF, Sostman HD et al. Diagnostic pathways in acute pulmonary embolism: recommendations of the PIOPED II investigators. *Radiology* 2007; 242: 15–21.

3. C. Respiratory bronchiolitis interstitial lung disease (RBILD).

RBILD is a disease of smokers and the centrilobular nodules reflect chronic inflammation in the respiratory bronchioles. GGO may occur and is typically multifocal and upper lobe predominant. Reticulation is uncommon and fibrosis is not a typical feature.

The typical features of UIP are reticulation, honeycombing, and traction bronchiectasis, with a basal and subpleural predominance. NSIP has overlapping features with UIP, but GGO is more common and honeycombing less common. There is a similar basal and subpleural predominance on HRCT.

DIP is a rare disease and, like RBILD, associated with smoking. The cardinal feature is GGO, with a basal and peripheral predominance. Sometimes small cystic areas can be seen within the areas of GGO. Progression to fibrosis/honeycombing is rare.

COP was formerly known as bronchiolitis obliterans organizing pneumonia (BOOP). The main finding on HRCT is consolidation, which is usually multifocal and bilateral. It typically has a lower zone and peripheral predominance, but can affect any lobe. Dilated airways are often seen on HRCT with air bronchograms mimicking acute pneumonia. There may also be GGO and reticulation, but lung volumes are usually maintained.

Dixon S and Benamore R. The idiopathic interstitial pneumonias: understanding key radiological features. *Clinical Radiology* 2010; 65: 823–831.

4. C. The abnormal bronchial artery is embolized at its origin.

Bronchial artery embolization (BAE) is an established procedure in the management of massive haemoptysis. Knowledge of the bronchial artery anatomy and its variations is essential in carrying out the procedure safely. A preliminary descending thoracic aortogram is performed to identify the number and site of origin of the bronchial arteries. Abnormal bronchial arteries are visualized on the preliminary thoracic aortogram in the majority of affected patients. Selective bronchial angiography is performed with manual injection of contrast. Selective bronchial artery catheterization and safe positioning distal to the origin of spinal cord branches is essential to avoid spinal cord ischaemia/infarction. Polyvinyl alcohol particles (350–500 μm diameter) are the most frequently used embolic agent. Smaller particles can freely flow via the intrapulmonary shunts, causing pulmonary or systemic infarcts. Chest pain is the most common complication (24–91%). Other complications include dysphagia (due to embolization of oesophageal branches), dissection of the bronchial artery or aorta (usually self-limited), and spinal cord ischaemia.

Yoon W, Kim JK, Kim YH, Chung TW, and Kang HK. Bronchial and nonbronchial systemic artery embolisation for life-threatening hemoptysis: a comprehensive review. *RadioGraphics* 2002; 22: 1395–1409.

5. E. Squamous cell carcinoma.

Tracheal malignancies make up 1–2% of all adult intrathoracic tumours and as such are uncommon. Malignant lesions make up 90% of all tracheal malignancies. Of these, squamous cell carcinomas are the most common, presenting in elderly patients with a history of smoking. Adenoid cystic carcinoma is the next most common, presenting in a younger age group and associated with a better prognosis. Benign lesions account for less than 10%. Non small cell lung cancer (NSCLC) would be the leading differential diagnosis if this lesion was found endobronchially, but not in the trachea. NSCLC can cause tracheal narrowing, but as an extrinsic lesion. The history is too brief for post-intubation stenosis to be considered and this is not associated with a soft tissue mass.

Marom E, Goodman P, and McAdams H. Focal abnormalities of the trachea and main bronchi. *American Journal of Roentgenology* 2001; 176(3): 707–711.
Adam A and Dixon A. *Grainger and Allison's Diagnostic Radiology. A textbook of medical imaging, Vol 1*, 5th edn, Churchill Livingstone, 2008. Ch 16.

6. C. Fat embolism.

This is an infrequent complication of long bone fracture, occurring in 1–3% of patients with simple tibial or femoral fractures, but in up to 20% of those with more severe trauma. Less commonly it can be caused by major burns, pancreatitis, haemoglobinopathy, tumours and liposuction. A complication of pulmonary, cerebral, and cutaneous symptoms (petechiae secondary to coagulopathy), it typically occurs within 12–24 hours after the traumatic event. The time lapse between the traumatic event and the radiographic abnormalities is usually 1–2 days, which allows differentiation from traumatic contusion. The radiographic findings resemble ARDS, although a peripheral distribution of consolidation is described. V/Q scanning will reveal multiple peripheral perfusion defects. In practice it is the clinical features such as the rash, confusion, and coagulopathy, as well as the presence of a fracture, which raise the suspicion of fat embolism.

Han D, Lee KS, Franquet T, Müller NL, Kim TS, Kim H et al. Thrombotic and nonthrombotic pulmonary arterial embolism: spectrum of imaging findings. *RadioGraphics* 2003; 23: 1521–1539.

7. C. GGO.

This is a salient feature of NSIP and is seen in almost all cases. Diffuse nodules are very infrequent in NSIP. If centrilobular nodules are present, one should think of other forms of diffuse lung disease such as respiratory bronchiolitis interstitial lung disease (RBILD) or hypersensitivity pneumonitis.

If multiple cysts are present, again other diffuse lung disease should be considered, such as lymphocytic interstitial pneumonia (LIP), DIP, lymphangioleiomyomatosis, and pulmonary Langerhans cell histiocytosis.

Areas of air-trapping would be a more typical finding in hypersensitivity pneumonitis, rather than NSIP. Pleural effusions are not a typical finding in NSIP.

Kligerman SJ, Groshong S, Brown K, and Lynch DA. Non-specific interstitial pneumonia: radiological, clinical and pathologic considerations. *RadioGraphics* 2009; 29: 73–87.

8. E. Critical stenosis of the origin of the left subclavian artery.

The vertebral artery arises from the first part of the subclavian artery. Stenosis/obstruction of the subclavian artery at its origin (i.e. proximal to the origin of the vertebral artery) leads to reversal of flow in the vertebral artery to maintain circulation to the ipsilateral upper limb. This effectively 'steals' blood from the posterior cerebral circulation, resulting in symptoms of vertebro-basilar insufficiency. Exercising the ipsilateral extremity triggers the symptoms of vertebro-basilar and/or brachial insufficiency. Atherosclerosis is the most common (94%) acquired cause of subclavian steal syndrome. It is more common in males and on the left side, with a ratio of 3:1. Additional lesions of extracranial arteries are often seen (up to 81%) when symptoms of vertebro-basilar insufficiency are present. However, the underlying pathology for this syndrome is stenosis/occlusion of the origin of the subclavian artery.

Reversal of vertebral artery flow can be demonstrated by colour Doppler imaging, augmented by arm exercise/blood pressure cuff inflation above systolic pressure for 5 minutes. Aortic arch angiography/MR angiography may be performed to demonstrate the subclavian stenosis/occlusion. Percutaneous angioplasty and surgical bypass are the treatment options.

Huang BY and Castillo M. Radiological reasoning: extracranial causes of unilateral decreased brain perfusion. *American Journal of Roentgenology* 2007; 189: S49–S54.

9. C. Relapsing polychondritis.

Wegener's granulomatosis and amyloidosis can both give a similar appearance to that described. Amyloid can occur as an isolated condition or as a part of systemic amyloidosis. It gives smooth narrowing, but can also give multifocal stenoses or plaques, and is frequently associated with calcification. Wegener's commonly affects the subglottic region, giving an identical appearance, although it can cause a more irregular pattern of thickening and ulcer formation. Similarly Wegener's commonly affects the cartilage in the nose. However, histologically, Wegener's causes vasculitis and granuloma formation. Mounier–Kuhn disease is also known as tracheobronchomegaly. It can be associated with tracheobronchomalacia, which may give a similar CT appearance to that described. The key difference is that this condition is characterized by a reduction in calibre of >50% of the airway lumen during expiration, as compared to inspiration. Relapsing polychondritis is a systemic condition also affecting the cartilage of the nose, ears, and joints.

Adam A and Dixon A. *Grainger and Allison's Diagnostic Radiology. A textbook of medical imaging, Vol 1*, 5th edn, Churchill and Livingstone, 2008. Ch 16.

10. D. Unilateral regional oligaemia.

This represents Westermark's sign and is associated with PE, not pulmonary oedema. The other features are consistent with cardiac failure. In particular, focal right upper lobe oedema is associated with mitral regurgitation, where the regurgitant jet produces locally increased pressures in the right upper lobe pulmonary veins with a focal increase in oedema in that region. This can mimic consolidation on plain film, but will be seen to resolve after diuresis. Pleural effusions may be unilateral in cardiac failure.

Miller WT. *Diagnostic Thoracic Imaging*. McGraw Hill, 2006. pp. 3–6.

11. C. Perfusion defect with a rim of surrounding normally perfused lung.

Multiple bilateral perfusion defects with a normal ventilation scan are the classic diagnostic findings in PE. Occluding pulmonary emboli produce segmental perfusion defects that extend to the pleural surface. As other conditions may also produce perfusion defects, the ventilation scan improves specificity. Non-embolic lung disease will typically have both perfusion and ventilation abnormalities, resulting in matched defects. V/Q scans are categorized as normal, low, intermediate, or high probability. A perfusion defect that matches ventilation and CXR abnormalities in size and location is a triple matched defect. A triple matched defect in the middle or upper lung zones is in keeping with low probability, but rises to intermediate probability when in the lower zones. A single moderate matched V/Q defect, but with a normal CXR, is also of intermediate probability. No perfusion defect is in keeping with a normal scan and four moderate segmental defects is a high probability scan. A perfusion defect with a rim of surrounding normally perfused lung is known as the stripe sign and corresponds to low probability for PE, as PE perfusion defects should extend to the pleural surface and have no overlying stripe of perfused lung.

Brant WE and Helms CA. *Fundamentals of Diagnostic Radiology*, 3rd edn, Lippincott Williams & Wilkins, 2007. pp. 1376–1383.

12. C. Posterior costophrenic sulci.

The question is leading to chronic hypersensitivity pneumonitis as the most likely underlying diagnosis. The fibrotic process, in advanced stages, affects both the subpleural lung and the peribronchovascular interstitium. There may be honeycomb formation at the lung bases, but unlike usual interstitial pneumonia/idiopathic pulmonary fibrosis, the honeycombing typically spares the most extreme posterior costophrenic sulci. Classically, the fibrotic process is more pronounced in the mid and upper lung zones.

Hirschmann JV, Pipavath SNJ, and Godwin JD. Hypersensitivity pneumonitis: a historical, clinical and radiologic review. *RadioGraphics* 2009; 29: 1921–1938.

13. E. Type V endoleak.

The main aim of endovascular or surgical treatment of abdominal aortic aneurysm (AAA) is exclusion of the aneurysm sac from the systemic high-pressure circulation. Ongoing leakage of blood into the excluded aneurysm sac after endovascular repair is termed 'endoleak'. Identification of the type of endoleak and its effect on the aneurysm sac is important for further management.

Type I endoleak: Contrast/blood leak at the proximal or distal landing zones of the stent graft is described as type I endoleak. This is due to poor proximal or distal graft apposition, exposing the sac to systemic pressures with significant risk of aneurysm rupture. This type is further subdivided into type IA (proximal aortic attachment) and type IB (distal iliac attachment). These are most commonly seen at the time of the procedure or may develop subsequently due to graft migration. They require urgent treatment.

Type II endoleak: This is due to retrograde flow into the aneurysm sac via the inferior mesenteric artery (type IIA) or lumbar arteries (type IIB). Many of these close spontaneously and are managed expectantly. Further treatment is indicated if the sac enlarges or the patient develops symptoms of sac pressurization.

Type III endoleak: Leakage of blood through the body of the stent graft due to either poor apposition of graft components or a tear in the graft material is type III endoleak. This requires urgent management due to sac pressurization.

Type IV endoleak: Aneurysm sac opacification without an identifiable source intraprocedurally is described as type IV endoleak. These are transient and usually resolve after withdrawal of anticoagulation.

Type V endoleak: Continued growth of the sac without radiological evidence of a leak is termed type V endoleak or endotension. Continued growth of the aneurysm sac will require surgical repair due to risk of rupture.

Bashir MR, Ferral H, Jacobs C, McCarthy W, and Goldin M. Endoleaks after endovascular abdominal aortic aneurysm repair: management strategies according to CT findings. *American Journal of Roentgenology* 2009; 192: W178–W186.

14. B. Availability of a cytopathologist.

Contrary to expectations, core biopsy is not associated with a higher rate of pneumothorax as compared to FNA, especially when used to sample peripheral lesions. Overall complication rates for the two procedures are similar. The chance of tumour seeding is low and is postulated to be lower when coaxial systems are used. Air embolism is also rare, although it is more common in core biopsies and when a central lesion is being sampled. The main drawback of FNA is inadequate sampling, which frequently occurs, requiring a repeat procedure. Thus the availability of a cytopathologist to review the sample at the time, to ensure an adequate number of cells have been obtained, is essential to this being a cost-effective procedure.

Tomiyama N and Yasuhara Y, Nakajima Y, Adachi S, Arai Y, Kusumoto M et al. CT-guided needle biopsy of lung lesions: a survey of severe complications based on 9783 biopsies in Japan. *European Journal of Radiology* 2006; 59(1): 60–64.

Anderson J, Murchison J, and Patel D. CT guided lung biopsy: factors influencing diagnostic yield and complication rate. *Clinical Radiology* 2003; 58: 791–797.

15. D. Wegener's granulomatosis.

The history of sinusitis, pulmonary haemorrhage, and renal involvement (reduced eGFR) point towards Wegener's granulomatosis. This is a systemic autoimmune disease characterized by granulomatous vasculitis of the upper and lower respiratory tracts, glomerulonephritis, and small vessel vasculitis. It predominantly affects male patients. There is pulmonary involvement in most patients. The most common radiographic appearance is lung nodules or irregularly marginated masses with no zonal predilection. The nodules are solitary in up to 25% and cavitating in 50% of cases. The cavities usually have a thick, irregular wall. With treatment they may resolve or result in a scar. Peripheral areas of wedge-shaped consolidation representing infarction may occur. Pleural effusions occur in less than 10% and mediastinal/hilar adenopathy is uncommon. Tracheal and bronchial thickening can be smooth or nodular. Haemorrhage can result in focal areas of dense consolidation, patchy bilateral areas of consolidation, or diffuse consolidation (these may be difficult to distinguish from infection).

The main differential diagnosis would be Churg–Strauss syndrome, which involves asthma, eosinophilia (which would be noticed in the full blood picture), and less severe renal and sinus disease. Patchy transient consolidation, which may be peripheral, is the norm and nodules may occur, although cavitation is rare. Wegener's granulomatosis is associated with c-ANCA and Churg–Strauss with p-ANCA. Goodpasture's syndrome is associated with glomerulonephritis and pulmonary haemorrhage, but the findings are initially extensive perihilar and basal consolidation with sparing of the apices, which is subsequently replaced by an interstitial pattern. Cavitating nodules are not a feature. Haemoptysis is uncommon in sarcoidosis and cavitating nodules rare; one would typically expect perilymphatic nodules and in classic cases adenopathy. TB can produce cavitating nodules and haemoptysis, but the other features are more consistent with Wegener's granulomatosis.

Mayberry JP, Primack SL, and Müller NL. Thoracic manifestations of systemic autoimmune diseases: radiographic and high resolution CT findings. *RadioGraphics* 2000; 20: 1623–1635.

16. C. Chronic thromboembolic pulmonary hypertension.

Pulmonary hypertension is the haemodynamic consequence of vascular changes within the precapillary (arterial) or postcapillary (venous) pulmonary circulation. The diagnosis of primary (idiopathic) pulmonary hypertension (PPH) can only be made after exclusion of known secondary causes. The classical findings in advanced disease include prominent central pulmonary arteries with sharply tapering peripheral vessels and right ventricular enlargement. It typically affects younger women of childbearing age. The radiographic features of pulmonary hypertension caused by chronic shunting are similar to PPH, although a normal sized cardiac silhouette may reflect diminished shunting due to a markedly elevated pulmonary vascular resistance. Most congenital cardiac lesions that may eventually cause pulmonary hypertension are now repaired at an early age. Chronic thromboembolic pulmonary hypertension may mimic PPH clinically, making diagnosis difficult. Radiographic findings are more likely to be asymmetrical. A triangular opacity representing pulmonary infarction may also been seen. Schistosomiasis will demonstrate the radiographic features of pulmonary hypertension and may also exhibit tiny nodular granulomas. It is endemic in the Middle East, Africa, and the Atlantic coast of South America. Pulmonary veno-occlusive disease is the post-capillary counterpart of PPH. It is suggested radiographically when the features of pulmonary arterial hypertension are accompanied by evidence of diffuse pulmonary oedema and a normal sized left atrium.

Frazier AA, Galvin JR, Franks TJ, and Christenson ML. Pulmonary vasculature: hypertension and infarction. *RadioGraphics* 2000; 20: 491–524.

17. E. Melanoma metastases.

The GGO surrounding a nodule is known as the 'halo' sign and represents perilesional haemorrhage. The differential diagnosis given rests on the presence of this feature and cavitation. Melanoma metastases can both cavitate and produce perilesional haemorrhage. The halo sign may also be seen in other conditions with perilesional haemorrhage or cellular infiltration and is usually best seen on HRCT. These diagnoses include bronchoalveolar carcinoma, haemorrhagic metastases, Wegener's granulomatosis, and angio-invasive infections, such as invasive aspergillosis. Alternative correct answers would be Wegener's granulomatosis, lymphoma, bronchoalveolar carcinoma, and squamous cell carcinoma as these can produce both cavitating nodules and the halo sign. Rheumatoid lung, eosinophilic granuloma, and lung abscesses are associated with cavitating nodules but not the halo sign. Churg–Strauss syndrome is not associated with the halo sign and cavitation is rare.

LeeYR, Choi YW, Lee KJ, Jeon SC, Park CK, and Heo J-N. CT halo sign: the spectrum of pulmonary diseases. *British Journal of Radiology* 2005; 78: 862–865.

18. C. Acute GI bleeding can be intermittent and failure to demonstrate active bleeding does not prove cessation of bleeding.

Acute GI bleeding is a medical emergency associated with high mortality and morbidity, especially in those presenting with haemodynamic instability. The majority (75%) of GI bleeds cease spontaneously, but it can recur in 25% of cases. Accurate early diagnosis of the bleeding source is crucial. Endoscopy is commonly used to identify and treat the source of bleeding. However, it is of limited value in massive haemorrhage (due to difficulty in visualizing the bleeding point) and in assessing the distal duodenum and most of the small bowel.

MDCTA is a rapid and accurate diagnostic method used to identify the site and in some cases the cause of active GI bleeding. However, acute GI bleeds (even when massive) are intermittent and failure to demonstrate active bleeding does not imply cessation of bleeding. The reported lowest detectable rate of bleeding with MDCTA, in animal and *in vitro* studies, is 0.35ml/min.

Suture material, clips, foreign bodies, and faecoliths may lead to false–positive results. An unenhanced scan is therefore essential. A portal venous phase scan is useful in identifying venous bleeds, therefore the protocol should include unenhanced and post-intravenous contrast arterial and portal venous phase scans.

Geffroy Y, Rodallec MH, Boulay-Coletta I, Julles MC, Ridereau-Zins C, and Zins M. Multidetector CT angiography in acute gastrointestinal bleeding: why, when and how. *RadioGraphics* 2011; 31: E1–E12.

19. D. CT scan within 12 months for both. If unchanged, both need a follow-up CT within a further 12 months.

Due to the rapid rise in the detection of solitary pulmonary nodules (SPNs) on CT, the Fleischner Society released guidelines on the follow-up of SPNs. For SPNs below 1 cm in diameter, PET is less reliable due to the small volume of tissue being examined. These guidelines simply use the size of the lesion and knowledge of the patient's relative risk (smoker versus non-smoker) to guide follow-up. Whilst Patient B's lesion is smaller, it requires the same follow-up as the larger lesion found in Patient A because of his increased risk. Lesions less than 4mm in low-risk patients do not require any follow-up; these lesions require a single CT within 12 months in high-risk patients.

MacMahon H, Austin J, Gamsu G, Herold C, Jett J, Naidich D, Edward F, Patz E, and Swensen S. Guidelines for Management of Small Pulmonary Nodules Detected on CT Scans: a statement from the Fleischner Society. *Radiology* 2005; 237: 395–400.

20. B. Bronchioloalveolar carcinoma.

In this disease, the tumour spreads along the alveolar septa without invading alveolar walls. The air in the alveoli is replaced by tumour cells, producing consolidation and GGO. Mediastinal lymphadenopathy is rare; pleural effusion is common. Diagnosis is made by sputum/bronchial washing cytology or lung biopsy. It mimics other causes of air-space opacification such as pneumonia, haemorrhage, oedema etc. Disseminated adenocarcinoma, choriocarcinoma, or lymphoma might produce identical CT findings.

PET-CT is often negative in the case of both bronchioloalveolar carcinoma and carcinoid tumours of the lung. Carcinoid is in the form of a focal mass, not diffuse consolidation. Klebsiella pneumonia classically produces enlargement of the involved lobe, bulging of the fissures with the propensity for cavitation, and abscess formation. One would expect pyrexia and raised inflammatory markers, and consolidation usually produces some abnormality on PET-CT. Small cell carcinoma is usually positive on PET-CT. TB is usually PET positive and has a predilection for the upper lobes, or apical segments of the lower lobes if the latter are involved.

Verschakelen JA and De Wever W. *Computed Tomography of the Lung: A Pattern Approach*, Springer, 2007. pp. 112–116.
Davies S (ed.). *Aids to Radiological Differential Diagnosis*, 5th edn, Saunders, 2009. p. 73.

21. D. Low attenuation filling defect occupying and expanding the whole luminal diameter.

Pulmonary artery sarcoma is a rare malignancy arising from the intima of the pulmonary artery. It is frequently misdiagnosed as PE, although there are features that help differentiation. Findings that favour pulmonary artery sarcoma include a low attenuation filling defect occupying the entire luminal diameter of the proximal or main pulmonary artery, expansion of the involved arteries and extraluminal tumour extension. A filling defect forming an acute angle with the arterial wall is seen in acute PE, whereas a filling defect forming an obtuse angle indicates organizing thrombus in chronic PE. A partial filling defect surrounded by areas of contrast enhancement is a feature of embolus floating freely within the lumen.

Yi CA, Lee KS, Choe YH, Han D, Kwon OJ, and Kim S. Computed tomography in pulmonary artery sarcoma: distinguishing features from pulmonary embolic disease. *Journal of Computer Assisted Tomography* 2004; 28: 34–39.

22. B. Centrilobular region.

In sarcoid, the granulomatous nodules are typically distributed along the lymphatics and are therefore seen along the bronchovascular bundles, interlobular septa, major fissures, and subpleural regions. The centrilobular region of the secondary pulmonary lobule contains the bronchiole and therefore conditions that cause peribronchiolar inflammation, such as subacute extrinsic allergic alveolitis (EAA) and respiratory bronchiolitis interstitial lung disease (RBILD), more often cause centrilobular nodules. These are often ground glass in attenuation and ill-defined, unlike the more solid appearing granulomatous nodules of sarcoid. Rarely sarcoid can cause centrilobular nodules because of the presence of peribronchiolar granulomas, but the other mentioned locations are much more typical.

Hawtin KE, Roddie ME, Mauri FA, and Copley SJ. Pulmonary sarcoidosis: the 'Great Pretender'. *Clinical Radiology* 2010; 65: 642–650.

23. B. Coil embolization distal and proximal to the pseudoaneurysm.

Coil occlusion is the commonly used method for embolization of GDA. GDA territory is a classic example for the concept of occluding 'front door' and 'back door'. If only proximal occlusion is carried out then retrograde flow via the pancreatico-duodenal arcade will re-perfuse the pseudoaneurysm. It is therefore essential to embolize GDA proximal (inflow) and distal (outflow) to the pseudoaneurysm.

Gelfoam is a temporary embolic agent and is not used in GDA embolization. Particles are not used in this territory. For aneurysms of smaller arteries, branch vessel occlusion may be carried out with particles, followed by coil embolization of the proximal parent artery.

Nosher JL, Chung J, Brevetti LS, Graham AM, and Siegel RL. Visceral and renal artery aneurysms: a pictorial essay on endovascular therapy. *RadioGraphics* 2006; 26: 1687–1704.
Kessel DO and Ray CE. *Transcatheter embolisation and therapy*, Springer-Verlag, London, 2010. pp. 5–6.

24. E. The diaphragmatic disease noted on MRI.

The finding of peritoneal disease upstages this tumour to Stage 4, which is inoperable. CT is the main imaging modality in malignant mesothelioma, which is sufficient in a lot of cases that are obviously inoperable on this modality alone. MRI has been shown to be superior to CT in the detection of local invasion, hence the normal CT appearance in this case, where peritoneal disease was noted on MRI. PET or PET-CT are better at detecting nodal disease than either CT or MRI. As such, in some cases all three modalities are necessary to stage disease. As MM does not respond well to radiotherapy or chemotherapy, the key therapeutic decision is whether or not the lesion is suitable for surgery. Even then, surgery alone has poor results and combination surgery, radiotherapy, and chemotherapy are required. T3 tumours and lower are all surgically resectable. Nodal disease extending to the contralateral mediastinum or internal mammary regions, or any supraclavicular nodal disease, denotes N3 disease. N3 disease is also unresectable, as are distant metastases.

Wang Z, Reddy G, Gotway M, Higgins C, Jablons D, Ramaswamy M, Hawkins R, and Webb W. Malignant pleural mesothelioma: evaluation with CT, PET and MRI. *RadioGraphics* 2004; 24: 105–119.

25. C. Pulmonary alveolar proteinosis.

This is rare, but most commonly develops in a primary idiopathic form (90%), chiefly in middle-aged smokers, with a male predominance. It can also occur secondary to industrial dust exposure, immunodeficiency disorders (HIV and iatrogenic causes), and, as in the question, secondary to underlying haematological malignancies. There is also a congenital form.

The typical plain film appearance is that described in the question, but less commonly there can be multifocal asymmetric opacities or extensive diffuse consolidation. The radiological findings are often out of proportion with the disease severity. The HRCT findings described are those of 'crazy-paving'. There is a wide differential diagnosis for this, including pulmonary oedema, pneumocystis pneumonia, haemorrhage, bronchoalveolar carcinoma, ARDS, lymphangitis carcinomatosis, radiation or drug-induced pneumonitis, hypersensitivity pneumonitis, and pulmonary veno-occlusive disease. The distinguishing factor in our case is the history of leukaemia; this would also predispose to infection, but the BAL has ruled pneumocystis out. In alveolar proteinosis, BAL or lung biopsy reveals intra-alveolar deposits of proteinaceous material, dissolved cholesterol, or eosinophilic globules. Symptomatic treatment includes whole lung lavage and multiple procedures may be required.

Frazier AA, Franks TJ, Cooke EO, Mohammed TH, Pugatch RD, and Galvin JR. From the archives of the AFIP: pulmonary alveolar proteinosis. *RadioGraphics* 2008; 28: 883–899.

26. B. Cavitating parenchymal opacity.

In persons with normal immune function, radiologic manifestations can be categorized into the two distinct forms of primary and post-primary disease that develop in individuals without and with prior exposure and acquired specific immunity. Lymphadenopathy is the radiologic hallmark of primary TB, although the prevalence decreases with increasing age. Parenchymal involvement in primary TB commonly appears as an area of homogenous consolidation. Obstructive atelectasis may occur from compression by adjacent enlarged lymph nodes. Pleural effusion occurs in approximately 30% of adults with primary TB. The characteristic manifestation of post-primary disease is an apical parenchymal opacity associated with cavitation. Other manifestations of post-primary TB are ill-defined opacities and tuberculomas. Lymphadenopathy is uncommon and pleural effusion is seen more frequently with primary disease. Multiple non-calcified nodules <3mm in diameter are characteristic of military TB.

Leung AN. Pulmonary tuberculosis: the essentials. *Radiology* 1999; 210: 307–322.

27. E. ^{99m}Tc-labelled macro-aggregated albumin scan.

Whole-body imaging obtained after intravenous injection of ^{99m}Tc-labelled macro-aggregated albumin (MAA) shows activity in organs other than the lungs, for example the brain, liver, and spleen, findings that are consistent with an intrapulmonary right-to-left shunt. Normally only about 3% of activity is seen outside the lungs, as the MAA particles are usually efficiently trapped by the pulmonary capillaries, unless there is an intrapulmonary right-to-left shunt.

Other imaging findings suggesting hepato-pulmonary syndrome may be seen on conventional and CT angiography. These findings include multiple slightly dilated subpleural vessels that do not taper normally and thus extend to the pleural surface (subpleural telangiectasia). Alternatively, there may be the presence of individual arteriovenous malformations on angiograms and nodular dilatation of peripheral pulmonary vessels on CT scans.

^{99m}Tc-labelled sulphur colloid is usually used in splenic imaging. ^{99m}Tc-labelled red blood cells are typically used to try and identify the location of GI bleeding. ^{99m}Tc-labelled pertechnetate is used in thyroid imaging and in the identification of a Meckel's diverticulum (due to the presence within the diverticulum of ectopic gastric mucosa). ^{99m}Tc-labelled hexamethylpropylene amine oxime (HMPAO) is used in brain imaging in an attempt to differentiate different causal pathologies in dementia.

Kim YK, Kim Y, and Shim SS. Thoracic complications of liver cirrhosis: radiological findings. *RadioGraphics* 2009; 29: 825–837.

28. D. Replaced left hepatic artery commonly arises from the left gastric artery.

The classic hepatic arterial anatomy, with the proper and hepatic artery dividing into the right and left hepatic arteries, is seen in approximately 55% of the population. Variations in hepatic arterial anatomy are common. A replaced right hepatic artery from the superior mesenteric artery is seen in 11%. A replaced left hepatic artery arising from the left gastric artery is seen in 10%. The entire hepatic trunk may be replaced, which may arise from the superior mesenteric artery (4.5%) or left gastric artery (0.5%). The common hepatic artery is a branch of the coeliac axis.

Catalan OA, Singh AH, Uppot RN, Hahn PF, Ferrone CR, and Sahani DV. Vascular and biliary variants in the liver: implications for liver surgery. *RadioGraphics* 2008; 28: 359–378.

29. E. None of these.

The TNM staging of lung cancer is not commonly used for staging small cell lung cancer. This cell type is particularly aggressive and often has occult metastases at the time of malignancy. The mainstay of treatment is with chemoradiotherapy, with imaging only used to stage disease as intrathoracic (limited or extensive) or extrathoracic.

Adam A and Dixon A. *Grainger and Allison's Diagnostic Radiology. A textbook of medical imaging, Vol 1*, 5th edn, Churchill Livingstone, 2008. Ch 18.

30. A. Chronic eosinophilic pneumonia.

This has been described as the radiological 'photographic negative' of pulmonary oedema. It is a disease of middle age and affects females more commonly than males. The history is that described, with a common history of atopy. The predominant histologic finding is filling of the alveolar airspaces with an inflammatory infiltrate containing a high proportion of eosinophils. There is usually also a cellular infiltration of the interstitium and peripheral blood eosinophilia. There is a dramatic response to steroid therapy within days.

ABPA and acute eosinophilic pneumonia do produce blood eosinophilia, but the former is characterized by bronchiectasis and mucus plugging with the possibility of mosaic perfusion in addition to peripheral consolidation, while the latter is characterized by diffuse GGO, defined nodules, smooth interlobular septal thickening, and often the presence of pleural effusion. Löffler's syndrome (simple pulmonary eosinophilia) refers to predominantly peripheral *transient* parenchymal consolidation accompanied by eosinophilia. There are minimal or no pulmonary symptoms, the plain film appearances change within one to several days and spontaneous resolution occurs within one month. Eosinophilic granuloma is nodular/cystic, a pulmonary form of Langerhan's cell histiocytosis, and should not be confused with the eosinophilic pneumonias.

Johkoh T, Müller NL, Akira M, Ichikado K, Suga M, Ando M et al. Eosinophilic lung diseases: diagnostic accuracy of thin-section CT in 111 patients. *Radiology* 2000; 216: 773–780.

31. A. Endobronchial tuberculosis.

The CT findings describe the 'tree-in-bud' pattern, which results from centrilobular bronchiolar dilatation and filling by mucus, pus, or fluid that resembles a budding tree. It is usually most pronounced in the lung periphery. All of the options provided are differentials for 'tree-in-bud', although infective causes are most common, classically endobronchial spread of active TB. The patient in this case is also at risk of invasive aspergillosis, although typically the 'tree-in-bud' pattern occurs in combination with consolidation accompanied by a halo of GGO. Obliterative bronchiolitis occurs in bone marrow transplantation in the setting of chronic graft-versus-host disease. The most sensitive CT finding in this condition is air-trapping on expiratory CT. Diffuse panbronchiolitis is of unknown cause, but occurs almost exclusively in Eastern Asia. Primary pulmonary lymphoma is also a rare cause of 'tree-in-bud'. Other potential differentials of this pattern include cytomegalovirus infection, cystic fibrosis, aspiration, connective tissue disease, and tumour emboli.

Gosset N, Bankier AA, and Eisenberg RL. Tree-in-bud pattern. *American Journal of Roentgenology* 2009; 193: W472–W477.

32. D. Lymphocytic interstitial pneumonia.

The key to this question, in addition to the described imaging features, is the history of Sjogren's syndrome, which has an association with LIP.

LIP is a benign lymphoproliferative disorder that is also associated with AIDS, autoimmune thyroid disease, and Castleman's syndrome. Lymphomas may arise in some cases. On HRCT, thin-walled cysts are seen in two-thirds and are randomly distributed, occupying less than 10% of the lung parenchyma. Other features include GGO, centrilobular/subpleural nodules, and septal thickening. Eventually larger nodules (>2 cm), consolidation, and architectural distortion may develop. The presence of mediastinal and hilar lymphadenopathy (two-thirds) and septal thickening help distinguish from Langerhans cell histiocytosis. The presence of centrilobular nodules assist in the differentiation from lymphangioleiomyomatosis.

Birt–Hogg–Dube syndrome is a rare autosomal dominant condition characterized by facial fibrofolliculomas, malignant renal tumours, and the development of thin-walled pulmonary cysts and spontaneous pneumothorax.

Grant LA, Babar J, and Griffin N. Pictorial review. Cysts, cavities and honeycombing in multisystem disorder: differential diagnosis and findings on thin section CT. *Clinical Radiology* 2009; 64: 439–448.

33. E. Ultrasound-guided compression is the treatment of choice.

Femoral artery pseudoaneurysm has been reported to occur in 0.2% of diagnostic and 8% of interventional procedures. Femoral pseudoaneursym is contained only by the haematoma and the pressure of the surrounding tissues. It is therefore at a high risk of rupture.

A number of risk factors for pseudoaneurysm formation have been identified. Patient factors include obesity, anticoagulation, haemodialysis, and calcified arteries. Procedural factors include low femoral punctures, superficial femoral or profunda punctures, and inadequate compression post procedure. Doppler ultrasound is the diagnostic method of choice. A fluid collection adjacent to femoral artery puncture site with 'yin yang' internal flow is diagnostic. Ultrasound guided thrombin injection is the treatment method of choice.

Ahmad, F, Turner SA, Torrie P, and Gibson M. Iatrogenic femoral artery pseudoaneurysms—A review of current methods of diagnosis and treatment. *Clinical Radiology* 2008; 63: 1310–1316.

34. D. Stage 2B.

The TNM definitions, on which the staging system is based, were recently updated in 2010. In this update, the nodal classifications were not changed, but the T staging was updated, as was M staging. Sub-classifications were added to T1, with lesions <2 cm being T1a and lesions between 2 and 3 cm being T1b. Lesions between 3 and 5 cm are T2a and between 5 and 7 cm are T2b. Lesions over 7 cm are T3, as are synchronous lesions within the primary lobe, as in this case. Multiple lesions within the primary lobe were formerly T4. In this question, the lymph node is not enlarged by size criteria and is not FDG avid on PET. While this may yet still be involved, on imaging findings alone, this lesion should be classed as N0. The absence of metastases is obviously M0. Thus this patient is T3 N0 M0, which corresponds to stage 2b. T2b N1 tumours are also in this stage. Stage 2a lesions are T2a N1 or T2b N0. Stage 3a lesions are T3 or less with N2 disease or T3 N1 lesions.

Goldstraw P, Crowley J, Chansky K, Giroux DJ, Groome PA, Rami-Porta R et al. The IASLC lung cancer staging project: proposals for the revision of the TNM stage groupings in the forthcoming (seventh) edition of the TNM classification of malignant tumours. *Journal of Thoracic Oncology* 2007; 2(8): 706–714.

35. A. Mitral stenosis.

The findings describe left atrial enlargement, which is caused by mitral valve disease (stenosis or incompetence), venticular septal defect (VSD), patent ductus arteriosus (PDA), atrial septal defect (ASD) with shunt reversal, and left atrial myxoma. Aortic stenosis produces left ventricular hypertrophy and eventually dilatation, the latter producing a prominent left heart border with inferior displacement of the cardiac apex. A left ventricular aneurysm produces a prominent bulge of the left heart border. Tricuspid incompetence produces an enlarged right atrium and thus a prominent right heart border on plain film. Coarctation produces left ventricular enlargement and inferior rib notching of the fourth to eighth ribs bilaterally if conventional and a 'reverse figure 3' sign: a prominent ascending aorta/arch and a small descending aorta, with an intervening notch.

Chapman S and Nakielny R. *Aids to Radiological Differential Diagnosis*. 4th edn, Elsevier, 2003. pp. 53, 197–200.

36. D. Bulging interlobar fissure.

Klebsiella (Gram-negative) pneumonia occurs predominantly in older alcoholic men and debilitated hospitalized patients. On the CXR it appears as a lobar opacification with air bronchograms. A bulging interlobar fissure is secondary to inflammatory exudate, increasing the volume of the involved lobe. This sign, however, is not specific and is also seen with *Haemophilus influenzae* and *Staphylococcus aureus*. Pneumococcal (*Streptococcus*) pneumonia typically presents as lobar consolidation. Parapneumonic effusions are seen in up to 50%. Reticulonodular opacity is a recognized atypical presentation. In children it typically presents as a spherical opacity (round pneumonia).

Brant WE and Helms CA. *Fundamentals of Diagnostic Radiology*, 3rd edn, Lippincott Williams & Wilkins, 2007. pp. 461–463.

37. D. Siderosis.

Siderosis is due to the inhalation of iron oxide particles and usually occurs in welders. It causes mutiple small centrilobular nodules, but is not usually associated with any symptoms or fibrosis. If combined with silica dust it can cause silicosiderosis, which can be associated with fibrosis.

Silicosis and coal workers pneumoconiosis, secondary to inhalation of silica dust and washed coal dust, respectively, show similar features on CT. This is usually the presence of 2–5 mm nodules, mainly involving the upper and posterior lung zones. Large opacities (>1 cm) indicate progressive massive fibrosis. Calcification in lymph nodes can occur and egg shell calcification is more typical in silicosis.

Berylliosis is a chronic granulomatous lung disease caused by exposure to beryllium dust or fumes. CT findings are similar to other granulomatous lung diseases, such as sarcoid. Fibrosis may therefore occur.

Asbestosis is pulmonary fibrosis secondary to inhalation of asbestos fibres.

Chong S, Lee KS, Chung MJ, Han J, Kwon OJ, and Kim TS. Pneumoconiosis: comparison of imaging and pathologic findings. *RadioGraphics* 2006; 26: 59–77.

38. C. Alpha-1 antitrypsin deficiency.

This is a rare autosomal recessive disorder. Alpha-1 antitrypsin is a glycoprotein synthesized in the hepatocytes, which acts as a proteolytic inhibitor. In the absence of alpha-1 antitrypsin, the enzyme elastase released by neutrophils and alveolar macrophages acts unopposed and digests the basement membrane. There is rapid progressive deterioration of lung function due to severe pan-acinar emphysema, which shows basilar predominance (due to gravitational distribution of pulmonary blood flow). The alveolar destruction is accelerated in smokers. Cirrhosis of the liver is a complication.

Meyer CA, White CS, and Sherman, KE. Disease of the hepato-pulmonary axis. *RadioGraphics* 2000; 20: 687–698.

39. A. Adenocarcinoma.

These are all classical features of adenocarcinoma. Bronchoalveolar carcinoma is a subtype of adenocarcinoma. This comprises 2–10% of lung cancers. There are three subtypes: a solitary nodule (41%), multifocal nodules (36%), and peripheral consolidation (23%). Squamous cell carcinoma is only slightly less prevalent than adenocarcinoma. It cavitates in 86% of cases and typically occurs centrally. Small cell carcinoma comprises 18% of lung cancers. It usually presents on plain film radiography as hilar and/or mediastinal adenopathy. CT often detects lung opacities. Giant cell carcinoma is a poorly differentiated subtype of NSCLC that is capable of rapid growth and early metastasis.

Hollings N and Shaw P. Diagnostic imaging of lung cancer. *European Respiratory Journal* 2002; 19: 722–742.

40. C. Amiodarone.

The pulmonary findings could equally be caused by NSIP and cardiac failure, among other causes. However, the high attenuation of the liver and spleen is due to deposition of amiodarone, which contains iodine.

Amiodarone, methotrexate, and bleomycin all may cause pulmonary toxicity. Pulmonary toxicity occurs in 5–10% of patients on amiodarone, usually within months of starting therapy. The prognosis is good, with most patients improving after discontinuation of therapy. NSIP is the most common manifestation of amiodarone-induced lung disease. Pleural inflammation is an accompanying feature and can manifest as pleural effusion. COP is less common and typically occurs in association with NSIP. A distinctive feature of amiodarone toxicity is the occurrence of focal, homogenous pulmonary opacities. They are typically peripheral in location and of high attenuation at CT, due to the incorporation of amiodarone into the type II pneumocytes. The combination of high attenuation within the lung, liver, and spleen is characteristic of amiodarone toxicity.

RA can produce many pulmonary sequelae: pulmonary nodules, pleural effusion, fibrosis, obliterative bronciolitis, and COP. Methotrexate can be used to treat RA and psoriasis, and as chemotherapy for various cancers. NSIP is most common and COP is seen less frequently.

Bleomycin is a chemotherapy agent used in the treatment of testicular carcinoma, among others. Diffuse alveolar damage (DAD) is its most common manifestation, with NSIP and COP being less common. The prognosis is poor, with most patients dying of respiratory failure within 3 months of the onset of symptoms.

Rossi SE, Erasmus JJ, McAdams HP, Sporn T, and Goodman P. Pulmonary drug toxicity: radiologic and pathologic manifestations. *RadioGraphics* 2000; 20: 1249–1259.

41. B. *Pneumocystis jiroveci* (formerly *P. carinii*).

This is most common in AIDS patients, usually when CD4 <200 cells/mm^3. Despite highly active antiretroviral therapy (HAART) and prophylaxis, it remains the most common AIDS-defining opportunistic infection. The CXR may be normal initially, but eventually a fine parahilar reticular or ground-glass pattern develops. Pleural effusions and lymphadenopathy are uncommon. Mycobacterium avium-intracellulare primarily affects the GI tract, but chest involvement in disseminated disease typically manifests as lymphadenopathy. Diffuse reticular opacities and hilar lymphadenopathy are a feature of toxoplasmosis. Diffuse miliary nodules are seen in coccidioidomycosis. Candida pneumonia demonstrates diffuse, bilateral nonsegmental airspace opacities.

Brant WE and Helms CA. *Fundamentals of Diagnostic Radiology*, 3rd edn, Lippincott Williams & Wilkins, 2007. pp. 472–477.

42. C. Air-trapping.

All of the answers, apart from cystic change, are recognized HRCT features of small airways disease. Air-trapping is an indirect finding of small airway narrowing/obliteration and is the most common and identifying imaging feature of constrictive bronchiolitis. Air-trapping is accentuated on expiratory scans.

Constrictive or obliterative bronchiolitis is a category of disorders recognized by a pattern of peribronchiolar fibrosis resulting in complete cicatrization of the bronchiolar lumen. Although most commonly idiopathic, other known causes include infections, toxic fume inhalation (oxides of nitrogen, chlorine), autoimmune disorders, including RA, graft-versus-host disease, lung transplantation, inflammatory bowel disease, and drug reactions, e.g. D-penicillamine.

Pipavath SNJ and Stern EJ. Imaging of small airway disease. *Radiological Clinics of North America* 2009; 47: 307–316.

43. B. Central 'popcorn' calcification.

Irregular or spiculated margin, eccentric or stippled calcification, doubling time of 20–400 days, contrast enhancement of more than 15 HU, and high uptake (SUV > 2.5) on PET-CT are all features associated with a malignant lesion.

Diffuse, central nodular, and popcorn-like calcification, doubling time of more than 400 days, contrast enhancement of less than 15 HU, and low uptake (SUV < 2.5) on PET-CT are associated with benign lesions.

Girvin F and Ko JP. Pulmonary nodules: detection, assessment, and CAD. *American Journal of Roentgenology* 2008; 191: 1057–1069.

44. C. Indium-111 octreotide SPECT–CT.

The imaging features allude to the diagnosis of bronchial carcinoid. This tends to occur in younger patients than bronchogenic carcinoma does, and is not associated with smoking. Whilst carcinoid tumours can present as a peripheral nodule, they are more typically central, hilar, perihilar, or endobronchial, as in this case. Classical features are of a smooth nodule, narrowing or compressing the bronchus, or of an endobronchial lesion. Both commonly have stippled calcification and demonstrate avid enhancement. Carcinoid tumours in this location are classed as either typical or atypical based on pathology. All the imaging options are valid. The degree of enhancement can simulate a pulmonary vascular malformation, which can be assessed with angiography, although MR angiography would be less invasive in this case. The definitive tissue diagnosis is commonly reached with bronchoscopy, but this can be associated with massive haemorrhage because of the vascular nature of this tumour. As such radiolabelled imaging, which is sensitive in 86% of patients, is a less invasive option. FDG PET is often negative in cases of carcinoid because of the low metabolic activity of this tumour. MRI characteristics of bronchial carcinoid have been well described, but will be unlikely to significantly progress the diagnostic pathway in this case.

Jeung M, Gasser B, Gangi A, Charneau D, Ducroq X, Kessler R, Quoix E, and Roy C. Bronchial carcinoid tumors of the thorax: spectrum of radiologic findings. *RadioGraphics* 2002; 22: 351–365.

45. E. Cryptogenic organizing pneumonia.

An area of GGO surrounded by a ring of consolidation describes the 'ring halo' sign. This is not specific to COP, but has been described in tuberculosis, active sarcoidosis, cryptococcosis, and blastomycosis. However it has been found that granulomatous infectious diseases and sarcoidosis, which cause the 'ring halo' sign, result in a nodular ring, whereas COP results in a smooth-walled ring. COP is rapidly responsive to steroids, but the latter can have deleterious effects in infectious diseases. Thus it has been suggest that a nodular ring can be used as a discriminator.

COP (also known as idiopathic BOOP) is a patchy organizing pneumonia caused by bronchiolar obstruction by plugs of loose organizing connective tissue that may wax and wane. The main finding of COP is consolidation, seen in 90% and usually multifocal and bilateral. In 50% the consolidation is subpleural or peribronchovascular. It has a lower zone predominance, but can affect any lobe. Dilated airways are often seen on CT and air bronchograms give the appearance of acute pneumonia. GGO is a prominent pattern in 60%. Linear opacities occur in isolation or in association with multifocal areas of consolidation. Nodules are seen in 30–50% and lung volumes are preserved in 75%. COP is a clinical–pathological entity and is diagnosed when the correct clinical picture and radiological findings are present. If these features are uncertain, lung biopsy is required.

Organizing pneumonia can be idiopathic (COP) or secondary to viral infection, toxic fume inhalation, RA, systemic lupus erythematosis (SLE), organ transplantation, drug reaction, or chronic aspiration.

The hallmark of obliterative bronchiolitis is air-trapping and hyperinflation. It has many causes, including RA and other connective tissue diseases.

Marchiori E, Zanetti G, Hochhegger B, and Irion KL. Re: Reversed halo sign: nodular wall as criterion for differentiation between cryptogenic organising pneumonia and active granulomatous diseases. *Clinical Radiology* 2010; 65: 770–771.
Dixon S and Benamore R. The idiopathic interstitial pneumonias: understanding key radiological features. *Clinical Radiology* 2010; 65: 823–831.

46. B. Mycoplasma pneumonia.

The given clinical history is classical of mycoplasma pneumonia, which usually affects younger adults in closed populations such as prisons or the military. It is one of the most common causes of community acquired pneumonia in otherwise healthy individuals. Serum cold agglutination is positive in up to 70%. On HRCT areas of ground-glass attenuation tend to be around areas of consolidation. Centrilobular nodules and peribronchovascular thickening are common associated findings.

Reittner P, Muller NL, Heyneman L, Johkoh T, Park JS, Lee KS et al. Mycoplasma pneumoniae pneumonia. *American Journal of Roentgenology* 2000; 174: 37–41.

47. A. Posterior aspect of the lungs.

The stem of the question is pointing towards ARDS during the ICU admission, resulting in pulmonary fibrosis. Classically HRCT shows relative sparing of the posterior aspect of the lungs. This pattern of sparing is unusual in other causes of peripheral fibrosis and is an important clue to the aetiology. During the acute and subacute phases of ARDS in the supine patient, the dependent portions of the lungs usually demonstrate extensive consolidation and atelectasis. It is postulated that these areas may be protected from the long-term effects of barotrauma and high oxygen exposure as they are essentially non-aerated during the acute and subacute phases.

Murray K, Anderson M, Berger G, and Bachman E. Distribution of lung disease. *Seminars in ultrasound, CT and MRI* 2002; 23(4): 352–377.

48. D. Pulmonary Langerhans cell histiocytosis.

This is a rare isolated form of Langerhans cell histiocytosis that primarily affects young adult smokers. Most patients are symptomatic and the most frequent symptoms are non-productive cough (50–70% of cases) and dyspnoea (35–87%). Less common symptoms include fatigue, weight loss, pleuritic chest pain, and fever. The most common finding on CXR is small irregular nodules, usually bilaterally symmetric, with upper lobe predominance and sparing of the costo-phrenic angles. Coarse reticular and reticulo-nodular pattern is seen in later stages. Pneumothorax occurs in up to 25% (may be recurrent). Pleural effusion is uncommon, but may occur with pneumothorax. Lung volumes are normal or increased in most patients. HRCT of chest demonstrates the cysts and nodules in a characteristic distribution with normal intervening lung. Interstitial fibrosis and honeycombing are seen in advanced stages. Treatment consists of smoking cessation; steroids may be useful in selected patients. Chemotherapeutic agents and lung transplantation may be offered in advanced disease. The prognosis is variable. Stable disease is seen in up to 50%. Spontaneous regression is reported in up to 25%. A variably progressive, deteriorating course is seen in up to 25%.

Abbott GF, Rosado-de-Christenson ML, Franks TJ, Frazier AA, and Galvin JR. Pulmonary Langerhans cell histiocytosis. *RadioGraphics* 2004; 24: 821–841.

49. A. Systemic amphotericin.

There are two parts to this question. Firstly, identifying the pathology based on imaging features. Secondly, knowledge of the treatment required. There are numerous complications that can occur post transplantation. These can be broken down into complications of the surgery, complications of monitoring, and post-operative non-surgical complications. This question obviously involves the latter group—non-surgical complications. These are largely related to immunosuppression post transplantation and include infections, rejection, accelerated atherosclerosis of the graft, and post-transplant malignancy. In the latter group, the most commonly noted malignancies are skin carcinoma, adenocarcinoma of the lung or GI tract, Kaposi sarcoma, leukaemia, and lymphoma. Post-transplant lymphoproliferative disorder occurs in 6%. The most common cause of death, however, is infection, particularly respiratory infection. One of the most common infections, and the infection with the highest mortality, is aspergillus infection. Invasive aspergillosis is demonstrated in this case with the hallmark features of cavitary necrosis and a surrounding halo of ground-glass change representing haemorrhage. This requires urgent antifungal therapy, but still has a mortality rate of over 50%. Cytomegalovirus (CMV) pneumonitis is also common, but usually displays diffuse pulmonary air-space change. This responds better to therapy, with a mortality rate of 14%. Bacterial pneumonias tend to occur earlier in the post-operative course. Acute allograft rejection gives a radiographic appearance not dissimilar to pulmonary oedema. It is usually diagnosed on endomyocardial biopsy.

Knisely B, Mastey L, Collins J, and Kuhlman J. Imaging of cardiac transplantation complications. *RadioGraphics* 1999; 19: 321–341.

50. C. Myocarditis.

This is defined as inflammation of the heart muscle. A large variety of infections, systemic diseases, drugs, and toxins have been associated with this condition. The diagnosis is based on a combination of clinical and imaging features. The presence of focal delayed enhancement on cardiac MRI in a non-coronary artery distribution, together with wall motion abnormalities, correlates strongly with myocarditis in the correct clinical setting. Many patients present with a non-specific illness characterized by fatigue, dyspnoea, and myalgia. An antecedent viral syndrome is present in more than 50% of patients. Myocarditis lesions occur typically in the lateral free wall and originate from the epicardial quartile of the ventricular wall. The subendocardial area is spared, a pattern that is otherwise typical for myocardial infarction (in the latter case the lesion would also correspond to a coronary artery territory). In myocarditis the enhancement pattern has been described as becoming less intense and more diffuse over weeks and months.

In acute myocardial sarcoidosis, increased focal signal intensity can be observed on T2WI (secondary to oedema due to inflammation) and both early and delayed post-contrast T1 weighted imaging (T1WI). Focal myocardial thickening is often seen due to the oedema and can mimic hypertrophic cardiomyopathy (HCM).

HCM will reveal marked hypertrophy of the interventricular septum and left ventricular wall, with associated transmural delayed enhancement in the hypertrophied areas. The latter finding corresponds to the scattered fibrosis present and the amount of enhancement will inversely correlate with regional contractivity.

Cardiac amyloidosis leads to a restrictive cardimyopathy. MR imaging shows functional impairment, biventricular hypertrophy, and non-specific inhomogenous gadolinium enhancement.

Vogel-Claussen J, Rochitte CE, Wu KC, Kamel IR, Foo TK, Lima JA et al. Delayed enhancement MR imaging: utility in myocardial assessment. *RadioGraphics* 2006; 26: 795–810.

51. C. Multizonal peripheral opacity.

The majority of H1N1 influenza cases have been mild, but the 2009 strain can cause severe illness, including in young previously healthy persons. Radiological findings in four or more lung zones distributed bilaterally and peripherally, are significantly more often seen on the CXR obtained at admission in patients with poor outcome (requiring mechanical ventilation) compared to those with good clinical outcome. Central GGO is the most common radiographic abnormality, but is not significantly associated with poor outcome. Pleural effusions are uncommon, although bilateral effusions are an independent predictor of short-term mortality in community acquired pneumonia. It should be noted that an initial normal CXR does predict against a poor outcome.

Aviram G, Bar-Shai A, Sosna J, Rogowski O, Rosen G, Weinstein I et al. H1N1 Influenza: initial chest radiographic findings in helping predict patient outcome. *Radiology* 2010; 255: 252–259.

52. D. Decreased calibre of vessels in lucent areas.

When mosaic lung attenuation is observed, it often is in an extensive, but patchy, distribution and it is important to determine if it is the lucent or denser areas of lung that are abnormal. If the blood vessels in the lucent areas are smaller, then the lucent areas are probably abnormal. The paucity of vessels in these regions may be secondary to focal air-trapping or poor ventilation and subsequent reflex vasoconstriction. If areas of lucency are exaggerated on expiratory scans (air-trapping), then this is the hallmark of small airways disease.

Alternatively, if the areas of lucency do not become more prominent on the expiratory scans, small airways disease is not the likely cause. In this situation, the inhomogeneous lung attenuation is probably secondary to changes in vessel calibre, and secondary to pulmonary hypertension, including chronic PE, emphysema, or inflammatory vasculopathies.

If the blood vessels in the regions of relative lucency are equal in size to vessels in surrounding areas, the regions of relative opacity are most likely abnormal, e.g. areas of GGO.

Murray K, Anderson M, Berger G, and Bachman E. Distribution of lung disease. *Seminars in ultrasound, CT and MRI* 2002; 23(4): 352–377.

53. E. It should be treated only when symptomatic.

Popliteal artery aneurysm (>0.7 cm in diameter) is the most common peripheral artery aneurysm. It is commonly associated with aneurysms in other locations—abdominal aortic aneurysm in 30–50% and contralateral popliteal aneurysm in 50–70% of cases.

They are more common in men (10:1 to 30:1) in their sixth and seventh decades. It is important to diagnose popliteal artery aneurysms due to significant associated risk of limb-threatening thrombo-embolic complications. Due to the high risk of complications, it is recommended that popliteal aneurysms should be repaired regardless of the symptoms or size, unless the patient is high risk for surgery due to associated co-morbidity.

Wright LB, Matchett WJ, Cruz CP, James CA, Culp WC, Eidt JF et al. Popliteal artery disease: diagnosis and treatment. *RadioGraphics* 2004; 24: 467–479.

54. B. Atypical thymoma.

Whilst the ultimate differentiation between these lesions is pathological, there are a number of clinical and imaging features that can help limit the differential if present. Whilst benign thymoma, atypical thymoma, and thymic carcinoma can all present as focal mass lesions in the thymus, benign thymoma would not demonstrate the locally aggressive features found on this patient's scan. Atypical thymoma is a locally aggressive lesion with benign features on pathology; it has a better prognosis than thymic carcinoma. Atypical thymoma, thymic carcinoma, thymic lymphoma, and malignant thymic germ cell tumours can all be locally aggressive. The presence of mediastinal lymphadenopathy, invasion of the great vessels, or distant metastases are uncommon for atypical thymoma, but are features of the other three tumours; none of these were present in this case. The final key differentiating feature in this case to indicate atypical thymoma over the other differentials is the presence of myasthenia gravis. As thymic lymphoma and malignant germ cell tumours are not of thymic origin, they would not cause this. It is rarely a feature of thymic carcinoma.

Jung K, Lee K, Han J, Kim J, Kim T, and Kim E. Malignant thymic epithelial tumours: CT-pathologic correlation. *American Journal of Roentgenology* 2001; 176(2): 433–439.

55. D. Arrhythmogenic right ventricular dysplasia.

This is part of the group of cardiomyopathies and is characterized by fibro-fatty replacement of the right ventricular myocardium and clinically by right ventricular arrhythmias of the LBBB pattern. It has a variety of clinical presentations, including mechanical dysfunctions and ventricular arrhythmia, and is a cause of sudden cardiac death in young adults. Pathogenesis is not yet understood. Diagnosis is based on structural, histologic, electrocardiographic, and genetic factors. There are major and minor criteria for diagnosis. Angiography and echocardiography lack sensitivity and specificity. MRI provides the most important morphological, anatomic, and functional criteria for the diagnosis of ARVD with one investigation.

Findings can include fatty or fibro-fatty replacement of the right ventricular free wall myocardium (hence the high T1WI signal), dilatation of the right ventricle or right ventricular outflow tract, right ventricular aneurysms, and segmental hypokinesia. Positive MRI findings should be used as important additional criteria in the diagnosis of ARVD, but the absence of MRI findings does not exclude the diagnosis.

Uhl's anomaly is very rare (less than 100 reported cases in the 20th century) and consists of a paper-thin right ventricle, with complete absence of any musculature. It can be distinguished from ARVD as it has no gender predisposition or familial occurrence (ARVD is more common in males).

Tricuspid stenosis produces dilatation of the right atrium. A pericardial effusion will result in high T2WI and low T1WI signal (unless the effusion is proteinaceous) within the pericardium. Melanoma metastases may well be high signal on T1WI, but they are rare to the heart and would not be expected to cause myocardial thinning.

Kayser HW, van der Wall EE, Sivananthan MU, Plein S, Bloomer TN, and de Roos A. Diagnosis of arrhythmogenic right ventricular dysplasia: a review. *RadioGraphics* 2002; 22: 639–648.

56. A. Absence of the sternal head of pectoralis major.

Poland syndrome is an uncommon congenital unilateral chest wall deformity characterized by partial or total absence of the greater pectoral muscle and ipsilateral syndactyly. Associated anomalies include ipsilateral breast aplasia and atrophy of the second to fifth ribs. Hypoplastic clavicles are a feature of cleidocranial dysostosis. Anterior protrusion of the ribs gives rise to pectus excavatum, whereas anterior protrusion of the sternum is seen in pectus carinatum.

Jeung MY, Gangi A, Gasser B, Vasilescu C, Massard G, and Wihlm JM. Imaging of chest wall disorders. *RadioGraphics* 1999; 19: 617–637.

57. D. Acute mitral valve insufficiency.

'Bat-wing' oedema refers to a central, non-gravitational alveolar oedema, which is seen in less than 10% of cases of pulmonary oedema. It generally occurs with rapidly developing severe cardiac failure, such as that seen with acute mitral valve insufficiency or renal failure. It develops so rapidly that it is initially observed as an alveolar infiltrate and the preceding interstitial phase of pulmonary oedema goes undetected radiologically.

ARDS and diffuse alveolar damage may overlap pathophysiologically, and along with fat embolism show radiographic changes of a non-cardiogenic pulmonary oedema. These are similar to the standard radiographic features of cardiogenic pulmonary oedema affecting the lung parenchyma, except that GGO tends to be more confluent and consolidative, the changes tend to be less dependent, and subfissural thickening/septal lines are uncommon.

Nowers K, Rasband JD, Berges G, and Gosselin M. Approach to ground glass opacification of the lung. *Seminars in Ultrasound, CT and MRI* 2002; 23(4): 302–323.

Gluecker T, Capasso P, Schnyder P, Gudinchet F, Schaller MD, Revelly JP, Chiotero R, Vock P, and Wicky S. Clinical and radiologic features of pulmonary oedema. *RadioGraphics* 1999; 19: 1507–1531.

58. C. Paget–Schroetter syndrome.

This is also known as 'effort' syndrome and is the name given to thrombosis of the axillary and subclavian veins usually due to anatomic compression in the costoclavicular space of the thoracic outlet. It is commonly seen in young healthy adults who are involved in activities with repetitive shoulder–arm movements.

Doppler ultrasound and MR venogram are useful in diagnosis. Pharmaco-mechanical or catheter-directed thrombolysis, followed by surgical decompression of the thoracic outlet is recommended for optimal treatment.

Stepansky F, Hecht EM, Rivera R, Hirsch LE, Taouli B, Kaur M et al. Dynamic MR angiography of upper extremity vascular disease: pictorial review. *RadioGraphics* 2008; 28: e28.

59. C. Sarcoid.

There are numerous causes of bilateral hilar lymphadenopathy (BHL) and in the absence of further clinical information, sarcoid would always feature high in the list of differentials. However, the finding of BHL in association with paratracheal adenopathy is classical for this disease.

Adam A and Dixon A. *Grainger and Allison's Diagnostic Radiology. A textbook of medical imaging, Vol 1*, 5th edn, Churchill Livingstone, 2008. Ch 17.
Millar W. *Diagnostic Thoracic Imaging*, McGraw-Hill, 2006. Ch 12.

60. E. Lifestyle and risk factor modification.

A stenosis is suitable for PCI when it is greater than 75% and may be suitable when it lies between 50 and 75%, depending on the minimal luminal area (MLA) and functional significance. Those stenoses less than 50% are not generally suitable for intervention and require medical management only (however, the minimal luminal area of the LMS and proximal main vessels are also taken into account by some authors). Unfortunately the blooming artefact caused by calcium will cause overestimation of the size of a calcified plaque on CT coronary angiography and this remains a great limitation of the technique. In some cases this will make a vessel appear completely occluded by calcium when it is not and an alternative investigation, e.g. catheter angiography, is required.

In this question, the calcified plaque will appear to cause a 50% stenosis, when in fact the stenosis is much smaller, certainly less than 50%. The LAD stenosis is too small to require treatment (assuming the vessel is of adequate size). Exercise stress testing is not of any particular use, as we have shown no need for revascularization and it would not alter management, which should be aggressive treatment of hypertension, hyperlipidaemia, diabetes, and lifestyle modification.

Nakanishi T, Kayashima Y, Inoue R, Sumii K, and Gomyo Y. Pitfalls in 16-detector row CT of the coronary arteries. *RadioGraphics* 2005; 25: 425–440.
Budoff MJ and Shinbane JS (eds). *Handbook of Cardiovascular CT: Essentials for Clinical Practice*, Springer, 2008. pp. 39–44.

61. B. 'Sevens' appearance to ribs.

Pectus excavatum is a relatively common thoracic skeletal anomaly. The majority of cases are isolated, although it is associated with Marfan's syndrome and congenital heart disease. The majority of patients are asymptomatic. On the PA CXR, the heart is shifted to the left. The right heart border is indistinct (suggesting right middle lobe consolidation). The posterior ribs appear horizontal and the anterior ribs are angulated steeply, giving rise to the 'sevens' appearance.

Planner A, Uthappa M, and Misra R. *A–Z of Chest Radiology*, Cambridge University Press, 2007. pp. 152–153.

62. A. Hypothenar hammer syndrome.

This is a post-traumatic vascular insufficiency of the hand. Any form of repetitive blunt trauma to the hypothenar eminence may result in intimal injury to the terminal ulnar artery or proximal superficial palmar arch, leading to thrombotic occlusion, aneurysms, and distal thrombo-embolism.

The symptoms may be similar to Raynaud phenomenon or other causes of embolic occlusion, but the location of the abnormality on imaging is specific for hypothenar hammer syndrome. Angiography may demonstrate a 'corkscrew' appearance in the symptomatic and in the asymptomatic contralateral hand. Distal occlusion due to embolic phenomenon is seen in 50% of cases. Takayasu arteritis affects the proximal aortic branch vessels.

Stepansky F, Hecht EM, Rivera R Hirsch LE, Taouli B, Kaur M et al. Dynamic MR angiography of upper extremity vascular disease: pictorial review. *RadioGraphics* 2008; 28: e28.

63. D. Lateral meningocele.

Neuroblastoma is a tumour of childhood and would be extremely rare in a 57-year-old. Whilst the history of neurofibromatosis type 1 (NF-1) would raise the possibility of this lesion being a neurofibroma, the CT findings of a cyst discount this. Extramedullary haematopoesis is a rare feature of myelofibrosis and commonly gives bilateral soft tissue masses. Lateral meningoceles are herniations of CSF through a dilated neural foramen, most commonly in patients with a history of NF-1. As they contain cerebrospinal fluid (CSF), the attenuation value would be comparable to water. A neuro-enteric cyst can have a similar appearance. These are often symptomatic and detected in childhood, unlike lateral meningoceles, which are asymptomatic. They are associated with congenital spinal abnormalities rather than widening of the neural exit foramen as described in this case.

Millar W. *Diagnostic Thoracic Imaging*, McGraw-Hill, 2006. Ch 13.

64. A. CT calcium score.

The NICE guidelines on chest pain of recent onset were published in March 2010. Given the history typical of angina, but lack of risk factors and her age, this lady will fall into the 10–29% estimated likelihood of coronary artery disease (CAD) category (i.e. 10–29% pretest probability of CAD). NICE recommends that these patients should first undergo CT calcium scoring. If the calcium score is 0, other causes of chest pain should be investigated. If the score lies between 1 and 400, they should proceed to CT coronary angiography, in which case, because of her low resting heart rate, a prospective study is possible and would provide a significantly smaller radiation dose than a retrospective one. If the score is greater than 400, she should be treated as for 61–90% CAD risk: catheter angiography if revascularization is appropriate. It remains to be seen in practice whether clinicians will proceed to catheter angiography on the basis of the calcium score if CT coronary angiography is available to select those who will actually require intervention.

For those with uncertain results from invasive or CT coronary angiography, or a pretest probability of CAD of 30–59%, functional imaging (e.g. myocardial perfusion imaging with SPECT, stress echo, MR perfusion, or MRI to assess for stress-induced wall motion abnormalities) is advised. If the pre-test probability is >90% with typical features of angina, treatment as angina is recommended (with regard to the NICE guidelines on stable angina, to be published in 2011). If the pre-test probability is <10%, alternative causes of pain should initially be explored. The guidelines only mention standard exercise stress testing with respect to patients with known CAD, where it is uncertain if the pain is caused by myocardial ischaemia.

NICE. *Chest pain of recent onset: assessment and diagnosis of recent onset chest pain or discomfort of suspected cardiac origin. NICE guideline 95*, National Institute of Clinical Excellence, 2010. Available online at: http://guidance.nice.org.uk/CG95.

65. A. Nitrofurantoin.

The findings described on the CXR and HRCT scan are those of pulmonary eosinophilia. Drugs known to cause pulmonary eosinophilia include nitrofurantoin, penicillamine, sulphasalazine, non-steroidal anti-inflammatory drugs, and para-aminosalicylic acid.

Bleomycin and cyclophosphamide are more commonly associated with DAD. Other drugs that can cause this type of lung injury include busulphan, carmustine, gold salts, and mitomycin. In early DAD, HRCT typically shows scattered or diffuse areas of GGO. Fibrosis typically develops within 1 week and if progressive can cause marked architectural distortion and honeycombing.

Amiodarone and methotrexate are associated with an NSIP pattern on HRCT. Carmustine and chlorambucil can also cause this appearance. With early disease, HRCT scans may show only scattered or diffuse areas of GGO. Later, findings of fibrosis (traction bronchiectasis, honeycombing) predominate in a basal distribution.

Other recognized patterns of drug-induced lung injury include a COP pattern and diffuse pulmonary haemorrhage.

Rossi SE, Erasmus JJ, McAdams HP, Sporn TA, and Goodman PC. Pulmonary drug toxicity: radiologic and pathologic manifestations. *RadioGraphics* 2000; 20: 1245–1259.

66. C. Semi-invasive aspergillosis.

This is also known as chronic necrotising aspergillosis and typically runs a more indolent, but slowly progressive, course than angio-invasive aspergillosis and occurs in patients with mildly impaired immunity (e.g. chronic alcoholism). The radiographic findings consist of upper lobe consolidation, multiple nodules, and cavitatory disease. The gold standard for diagnosis of semi-invasive aspergillosis is the histological demonstration of tissue invasion by the fungus and growth of aspergillus on culture. However, in practice this is difficult to achieve and therefore the combination of the characteristic clinical and radiological features and either positive serological results for aspergillus or the isolation of aspergillus from respiratory samples is highly indicative of semi-invasive aspergillosis.

Angio-invasive aspergillosis occurs in more severely immuno-compromised patients (e.g. AIDS patients). Rapidly progressive nodular opacities occur to form single or multiple homogeneous consolidations. The lesions show a characteristic halo sign on CT, reflecting an area of alveolar haemorrhage around a central nodule.

ABPA is a hypersensitivity reaction to aspergillus fumigatus that occurs in patients with asthma or cystic fibrosis. It is characterized by inspissated mucus plugs containing aspergillus organisms and eosinophils, resulting in chronic inflammation in the airway and bronchial ectasia. The most common CT finding is central bronchiectasis with upper lobe predominance and mucus impaction.

Aspergilloma is a mycetoma (fungus ball), which typically occurs in ectatic airways or parenchymal cavities (e.g. old TB, chronic sarcoid). CT characteristically shows an intracavitatory mass with a surrounding air crescent, more commonly in the upper lobes.

Al-Alawi A, Ryan CF, Flint JD, and Muller N. Aspergillus-related lung disease. *Canadian Respiratory Journal* 2005; 12(7): 377–387.

67. B. Critical limb ischaemia.

Muscle pain or discomfort in the lower limb brought on by exercise and relieved by rest within 10 minutes is termed intermittent claudication. This is secondary to reduced perfusion, which may be enough during periods of rest, but on exercise is insufficient to meet the metabolic demand of the muscles.

With progression of disease, these symptoms may be noticed at rest. Typical ischaemic rest pain is relieved by dependency of the foot secondary to gravity-aided blood flow.

Critical limb ischaemia is the presence of rest pain or tissue loss with ulcers or gangrene. This should be distinguished from acute limb ischaemia. The term 'critical limb ischaemia' implies chronicity with symptoms being present for at least 2 weeks.

Diabetic neuropathy is associated with burning or shooting pain in the feet, which may sometimes be difficult to differentiate from atypical ischaemic rest pain. Distinguishing features include bilateral symmetric distribution, cutaneous hypersensitivity, and failure to relieve by dependency of the foot. Reduced vibration sensation and reflexes are also seen in diabetic neuropathy.

Nerve root compression may sometimes result in continuous pain but it has a dermatomal distribution and is associated with backache.

Nogren L, Hiatt WR, Dormandy JA, Nehler MR, Harris KA, and Fowkes FG. Inter-society consensus for the management of peripheral arterial disease. *Journal of Vascular Surgery* 2007; 45 (1): S5–S67.

68. A. Spinnaker/thymic sail sign.

This is due to mediastinal air outlining the thymus in children. Other features of pneumomediastinum are streaky lucencies in the thoracic inlet, air outlining the major arteries (tubular artery sign), and the continuous diaphragm sign, where air in the posterior mediastinum outlines the diaphragm. This is different to air outlining the medial diaphragm under the cardiac silhouette, which is the earliest sign of a pneumothorax in a supine patient. The deep sulcus sign is also a sign of a pneumothorax in a supine patient. The air-crescent sign is a feature to note in cavitating lung lesions and mycetomas. The inverted V sign is an indicator of pneumoperitoneum.

Dahnert W. *Radiology Review Manual*, 5th edn, Lippincott Williams & Wilkins, 2003. p. 429.

69. A. The RCA arises from the left coronary sinus and passes between the aorta and pulmonary artery.

Coronary artery anomalies are rare, but can be a cause of chest pain and sudden cardiac death. Diagnosis can be difficult via conventional catheter angiography due to both difficulty in locating the abnormal ostia and correct interpretation of the vessel course. Cardiac CT is superior in this regard.

The anomalies can be malignant or non-malignant depending on the site of origin and course. Option D gives the normal path of the RCA and option E is a common normal variant of the LMS; a bifurcation into LAD and LCx being more usual. In option A the RCA has an anomalous origin from the left coronary cusp and takes a malignant, 'interarterial' course, passing between the aorta and pulmonary artery. It is thought that when dilatation of the aorta occurs during exercise, the abnormal slit-like ostium of the RCA becomes narrower, reducing RCA perfusion and causing myocardial infarction. This variant can be associated with sudden cardiac death in 30% of patients.

In option C the LMS has an anomalous origin and path, but it is benign as it passes anterior to the pulmonary artery. The multiple ostia in option B are benign and may be beneficial, as disease in one vessel proximally would not compromise the other, as would normally occur in LMS disease.

A further malignant coronary anomaly is anomalous origin of the coronary artery from the pulmonary artery (ALCAPA), which is usually symptomatic in childhood. Myocardial bridging, in which a length of coronary artery (usually mid LAD) takes an intramyocardial course and may cause ischaemia, infarction, arrhythmia, and even death, commonly causes no symptoms.

Kim SY, Seo JB, Do KH, Heo JN, Lee JS, Song JW et al. Coronary artery anomalies: classification and ECG-gated multi-detector row CT findings with angiographic correlation. *RadioGraphics* 2006; 26: 317–334.

70. B. An enlarged aorta bulges into the inferior aspect of the retro-tracheal space.

Whilst lateral CXRs are seldom requested, when they are requested it is often the retro-tracheal space that requires assessment and thus knowledge of its borders and pathological conditions is relevant. The retro-tracheal space is bounded anteriorly by the posterior border of the trachea and posteriorly by the vertebrae. The inferior margin is the aortic arch. The space is of low density, being created by the lung posterior to the trachea. The posterior tracheal line is usually 2.5 mm thick, but can be 5.5 mm thick if the anterior wall of the oesophagus lies adjacent to the posterior wall of the trachea (the tracheo-oesophageal line (TOL)). Thus an enlarged aorta would be noted inferiorly. Extension of retro-pharyngeal abscesses usually occurs along the prevertebral space, posteriorly in the retro-tracheal space, thus not affecting the TOL. A normal retro-sternal goitre extending anterior to the trachea is not located in the retro-tracheal space. A normal subclavian artery is not present in the retro-tracheal space, but an aberrant left or right subclavian artery may be identified in the position described.

Franquet T, Erasmus J, Gimenez A, Rossi S, and Prats R. The retro-tracheal space: normal anatomic and pathologic appearances. *RadioGraphics* 2002; 22(Special): S231–S246.

71. E. Surgical bypass.

According to the trans-Atlantic intersociety consensus (TASC) for management of peripheral arterial disease, aorto-iliac lesions are classified into four groups: A, B, C, and D. For full details of TASC classification please refer to the article below.

The MR angiography findings in this case fall into group D. For TASC A lesions (generally short stenosis) endovascular therapy is the treatment of choice and for TASC D lesions (complex/long occlusions) surgical bypass is the treatment of choice. For TASC B and C lesions, the patient's co-morbidities, patient preference, and local operator's long-term success rates should be considered. TASC recommends endovascular treatment for type B lesions and surgery for good-risk patients with type C lesions.

Nogren L, Hiatt WR, Dormandy JA, Nehler MR, , Harris KA, and Fowkes FG. Inter-society consensus for the management of peripheral arterial disease. *Journal of Vascular Surgery* 2007; 45(1): S5–S67.

72. C. Metastasis.

With the exception of thrombus, metastasis is the most common cardiac mass, being 100–1000 times more common than primary tumour. Melanoma has the highest propensity for cardiac involvement. Other tumours which commonly metastasize to the heart are sarcomas, lymphoma, and bronchogenic and breast carcinoma. Primary cardiac tumours are rare and 75% are benign. The most common benign primary cardiac tumour is myxoma. The most common malignant primary cardiac tumour is angiosarcoma, followed by rhabdomyosarcoma/primary lymphoma. Primary cardiac lymphoma is much less frequent than secondary involvement and most commonly occurs in immunocompromised patients.

Thrombus is by far the most common cardiac mass and most frequent mimic of a cardiac tumour, but it does not enhance. Most thrombi occur in predictable locations, e.g. within the left atrial appendage in the setting of atrial fibrillation (AF), within the left ventricle underlying a dyskinetic segment, or in the right atrium adjacent to central venous lines.

Hoey ETD, Mankad K, Puppala S, Gopalan D, and Sivanathan MU. MRI and CT appearances of cardiac tumours in adults. *Clinical Radiology* 2009; 64: 1214–1230.

73. C. Fibroma.

This patient has Gorlin's syndrome (nevoid basal cell carcinoma syndrome, NBCCS). This may result in abnormalities of the skin (basal cell carcinoma), skeletal (jaw odontogenic keratocysts, bifid, fused, or markedly splayed ribs), and genitourinary (ovarian fibromas) systems, as well as cardiac fibroma (relatively rare) and calcification of the falx. Medulloblastoma is a relatively less common manifestation.

The imaging characteristics of cardiac fibromas reflect their fibrous nature: low signal on T1WI and T2WI with delayed enhancement on MRI. Most are well circumscribed with a surrounding rim of compressed myocardium. On CT they manifest as mildly enhancing soft tissue attenuation masses. Foci of calcification are present in up to 50% of cases. Although benign they may cause ventricular arrhythmias and even sudden death secondary to interference with conduction pathways.

Atrial myxomas are of mixed signal on T1WI and T2WI sequences. They are most commonly found within the left atrium (80%), with 15% in the right atrium. On CT a low attenuation intracavitary mass with a smooth or slightly villous surface is seen.

Cardiac paragangliomas are well encapsulated, hypervascular (intensely enhancing), and 3–8cm in size. They are isointense to myocardium on T1WI and markedly hyperintense on T2WI. Presentation is with symptoms of catecholamine excess. They are found in the posterior wall of the left atrium, atrioventricular groove, and root of the great vessels.

Fibroelastomas arise from endocardial surfaces, most commonly the aortic and mitral valves. They are a recognized cause of sudden death and immediate resection is warranted. Trans-oesophageal echocardiography is the optimal means of visualization due to their small size and highly mobile nature. Cardiac lipomas have characteristic imaging features consistent with fat on MRI and CT.

Hoey ETD, Mankad K, Puppala S, Gopalan D, and Sivanathan MU. MRI and CT appearances of cardiac tumours in adults. *Clinical Radiology* 2009; 64: 1214–1230.

74. E. None of the above.

The presence of cardiac pacemakers used to be an absolute contraindication to MRI scanning. However, with the introduction of MR-conditional pacemakers, scanning is safe under certain conditions. Among these conditions is that only a 1.5 T (Tesla) magnet can be used, and that the appropriate pacing leads for the MRI-conditional pacemaker must be *in situ*. The pacemaker and leads even have a distinctive 'wiggly' line which is projected on chest radiographs and can be used for their recognition.

Modern loop recorders are MRI compatible, although they should be interrogated in advance of the scan or information may potentially be lost. Modern metallic grafts, stents etc. are non-ferromagnetic and are generally regarded as having undergone adequate fibrosis/neo-intimal hyperplasia to become fixed within the body 6 weeks after the date of insertion. MRI is generally contraindicated in cases of cochlear implants (although there may be exceptions where the internal magnet has been surgically removed or is easily removed, or at field strengths of 0.2 T). The compatibility of any device can be verified by consulting www.mrisafety.com, but it is another matter whether the presence of a compatible device will still result in such artefact as to render the images non-diagnostic.

Wilkoff BL, Bello D, Taborsky M, Vymazal J, Kanal E, Heuer H et al. Magnetic resonance imaging in patients with a pacemaker system designed for the MR environment. *Heart Rhythm* 2011; 8(1): 65–73.

75. A. Venous ultrasound.

For pregnant patients, venous ultrasound is recommended before imaging tests with ionizing radiation are performed. Up to 29% of pregnant patients with PE will have a positive venous ultrasound, obviating the need for further imaging. The majority of the PIOPED II investigators currently recommend V/Q scanning over CTPA in the evaluation of PE in pregnant patients. The foetal dose with V/Q is similar to that with CTPA, although the effective dose per breast is much greater with CTPA. MRI requires further evaluation and gadolinium-based contrast agents have not been proven to be safe in pregnancy. The role of catheter angiography is probably limited to those patients requiring mechanical thrombectomy. It should be noted that even a combination of CXR, lung scintigraphy, CTPA, and pulmonary angiography exposes the foetus to approximately 1.5mGy of radiation, which is well below the accepted limit of 50 mGy for the induction of deterministic effects in the foetus.

Stein PD, Woodard PK, Weg JG, Wakefield TW, Tapson VF, Sostman HD et al. Diagnostic pathways in acute pulmonary embolism: recommendations of the PIOPED II investigators. *Radiology* 2007; 242: 15–21.

Pahade JK, Litmanovich D, Pedrosa I, Romero J, Bankier AA, and Boiselle PM. Imaging pregnant patients with suspected pulmonary embolism: what the radiologist needs to know. *RadioGraphics* 2009; 29: 639–654.

chapter 2

MUSCULOSKELETAL AND TRAUMA

QUESTIONS

1. **A 50-year-old man who has been previously well presents with low back pain. Plain film reveals an osteolytic midline lesion in the lower sacrum containing secondary bone sclerosis in the periphery, as well as amorphous peripheral calcifications. A lateral film shows anterior displacement of the bladder and rectum. He subsequently develops faecal incontinence. No additional lesions were discovered after imaging of the whole spine. What is the most likely diagnosis?**

   A. Osteomyelitis.
   B. Ewing's sarcoma.
   C. Chordoma.
   D. Myeloma.
   E. Sacrococcygeal teratoma.

2. **A 28-year-old male presents with soft tissue swelling, pain, and reduction of motion in the small joints of his hands. Plain films of the hands show erosions at the metacarpophalangeal (MCP) joints and distal interphalangeal joints with periosteal reaction and enthesophytes. What is the most likely diagnosis?**

   A. Psoriatic arthropathy.
   B. RA.
   C. SLE.
   D. Haemochromatosis.
   E. Calcium pyrophosphate dihydrate crystal deposition disease.

3. **A 25-year-old male presents with a history of dislocation and spontaneous relocation of the patella while playing football. An MRI of the knee is requested. Which of the following findings is consistent with the clinical history of patellar dislocation?**

   A. Bone oedema involving medial facet of patella and medial femoral condyle.
   B. Bone oedema involving posterior patella and anterior aspect of the tibial plateau.
   C. Bone oedema involving the lateral facet of patella and lateral femoral condyle.
   D. Bone oedema involving the lateral facet of patella and medial femoral condyle.
   E. Bone oedema involving the medial facet of patella and lateral femoral condyle.

4. A 63-year-old female is being worked up for a left total hip replacement. She has a history of RA. As part of the routine pre-operative assessment in your hospital a cervical spine radiograph is requested. This demonstrates that there is widening of the pre-dental space, with the anterior arch of C1 located anterior to the lower part of the body of C2. The dens is not clearly visible. This appearance is constant on the flexion view. The patient is asymptomatic. What do you think these findings represent?

A. Degenerative change.
B. Pannus erosion of dens.
C. Atlanto-axial subluxation.
D. Erosion of the occipital condyles.
E. Atlanto-axial impaction.

5. A 25-year-old man presents with a 4-month history of increasing dull lower back ache. He is otherwise systemically well. He has no neurological signs. An x-ray of the lumbar spine demonstrates a slight scoliosis, with an enlarged sclerotic left pedicle of L3. A subsequent CT scan shows a 3-cm lucent focus within the left pedicle of L3, which has expanded the bone. There is surrounding sclerosis. What is the most likely underlying diagnosis?

A. Osteoid osteoma.
B. Enostosis.
C. Osteoblastoma.
D. Osteomyelitis.
E. Intracortical haemangioma.

6. A 35-year-male presents with pain in the thigh. A plain radiograph reveals an eccentric expansile lucent lesion without a sclerotic margin but with a narrow zone of transition in the distal femoral metaphysis and epiphysis, which extends to the joint surface. What is the most likely diagnosis?

A. Osteosarcoma.
B. Giant cell tumour (GCT).
C. Metastasis.
D. Aneurysmal bone cyst.
E. Fibrous dysplasia.

7. A 34-year-old female presents to the A&E department after falling on an outstretched hand. Examination reveals tenderness at the anatomic snuff box. A scaphoid radiograph series confirms scaphoid fracture. Which of the following features is most associated with a poor prognosis?

A. Fracture of the distal third.
B. Fracture of the middle third.
C. Fracture of the proximal third.
D. Horizontal oblique fracture orientation.
E. Displacement of the scaphoid fat stripe.

8. A 44-year-old female patient presents to the rheumatologists with a history of multiple painful joints for 2 years. She has synovitis clinically, confirmed on ultrasound, which involves the MCP joints bilaterally. PA and Norgaard views of the hands are requested and show small erosions in the distal radio-ulnar joint and the piso-triquetral joint, but no erosions at the MCP joints. There is widening of the scapholunate interval on the right side. There is anklyosis of the capitate to the hamate on the left. There is periarticular osteoporosis. Which of these features is atypical of RA?

A. Symmetrical disease.
B. Synovitis on ultrasound but no erosions radiographically.
C. Erosions noted in the radio-ulnar joint and radio-carpal joint preceding MCP erosions.
D. Bony ankylosis of the carpal bones.
E. Periarticular osteoporosis.

9. A 26-year-old woman presents with a 2-year history of an enlarging soft tissue mass in her left thumb adjacent to the interphalangeal joint. An x-ray of the left thumb shows a soft tissue swelling with a large well-defined erosion seen affecting the distal metaphysis of the proximal phalanx. There is no soft tissue calcification or evidence of arthropathy at the interphalangeal joint. A subsequent MRI scan shows a 3.5-cm well-defined soft-tissue mass, which is low signal on T1WI and enhances post administration of gadolinium. The lesion is low signal on T2WI and gradient echo (GE) imaging. What is the most likely diagnosis?

A. Ganglion cyst.
B. Peripheral nerve sheath tumour.
C. Lipoma.
D. GCT of the tendon sheath.
E. Soft tissue haemangioma.

10. A 24-year-old male presents to the A&E department with pain and swelling of his right thumb after landing against his ski pole while practising at the local dry ski-slope. An avulsion fracture at the base of the proximal phalanx is noted on a radiograph of the thumb. What underlying soft tissue structure has been injured to result in this fracture?

A. Ulnar collateral ligament.
B. Radial collateral ligament.
C. Joint capsule.
D. Flexor pollicis longus tendon.
E. Extensor pollicis longus tendon.

11. A 75-year-old male with a history of backache undergoes plain radiographs of the lumbar spine, which demonstrate diffuse bone sclerosis. An MRI demonstrates diffuse low signal intensity of bone marrow on all sequences with no architectural distortion. The MRI planning sequence demonstrates splenomegaly. What is the diagnosis?

A. Sickle-cell anemia.
B. Lymphoma.
C. Osteoblastic metastasis.
D. Myelofibrosis.
E. Myeloma.

12. You are carrying out an MRI on a patient with a known history of RA. The patient has minimal erosions on plain film, but severe arthralgia. She is being considered for biologic therapy. The clinicians have requested an MRI of her hands. This reveals symmetrical disease in both hands with areas of high signal on T2WI and low signal on T1WI around the triangular fibrocartilage complex (TFCC), the radio-carpal joint (RCJ), and the distal radio-ulnar joint (DRUJ). The abnormal areas at the TFCC and RCJ enhance following administration of gadolinium, the DRUJ does not. A delayed T1WI sequence displays uniform enhancement in all joints. What do these findings indicate?

A. Hypervascular pannus at the TFCC and RUJ, with fibrous pannus at DRUJ.
B. Fibrous pannus at the TFCC and RUJ, with joint effusion at DRUJ.
C. Hypervascular pannus at the TFCC and RUJ, with joint effusion at DRUJ.
D. Fibrous pannus at the TFCC and RUJ showing differential enhancement.
E. Fibrous pannus at the TFCC and RUJ with hypervascular pannus at DRUJ.

13. A 56-year-old man has a 6-week history of dull discomfort just above his right ankle. A plain ankle radiograph is performed and this demonstrates a relatively ill-defined area of lucency in the distal tibial metaphysis. An underlying aggressive lesion is suspected and the patient is referred for an MRI of the distal right leg. This shows a rather serpiginous-shaped lesion in the distal right tibia. A parallel rim of hypo- and hyperintensity is seen on one of the imaging sequences, which is very helpful in confirming that the lesion is secondary to metadiaphyseal osteonecrosis rather than a neoplasm. On which imaging sequence is this parallel rim most likely to be seen?

A. GE T2*WI.
B. Fast spin echo (SE) T1WI.
C. Fast SE T2WI.
D. Fast SE STIR.
E. Fast SE T1WI post gadolinium.

14. A 60-year-old man presents to the A&E department with acute onset lower back pain following a relatively minor fall. A plain film reveals a collapse of the L4 vertebral body against a background of osteopenia. He has a history of renal cell carcinoma and the clinical team request an MRI to 'rule out metastatic disease'. Which of the following features would most suggest a malignant rather than a benign cause for a vertebral compression fracture?

A. Isointense signal to adjacent vertebral bodies on T2WI.
B. A band-like area of low signal adjacent to the fractured end-plate on T1WI.
C. High signal intensity adjacent to the vertebral endplate on STIR imaging.
D. Retropulsion of a posterior fragment into the spinal canal.
E. A convex bulge involving the whole of the posterior cortex of the vertebral body.

15. A 39-year-old male presents with tenderness and decreased range of movement of the right elbow after falling on an outstretched arm while playing indoor football. A radial head fracture is noted on his radiographs, but the A&E doctor asks for your opinion, suspecting an additional injury. What is the most common associated fracture with this injury?

A. Olecranon fracture.
B. Coronoid process fracture.
C. Scaphoid fracture.
D. Proximal ulna fracture.
E. Capitellum fracture.

16. A 35-year-old female with a history of flushing, pruritis, and diarrhoea is referred for a small bowel series. A barium study demonstrates irregular diffuse thickening of small bowel folds. There is also diffuse osteosclerosis. Laboratory tests reveal elevated serum tryptase level. What is the diagnosis?

A. Mastocytosis.
B. Intestinal lymphangectasia.
C. Amyloidosis.
D. Waldenstrom's macroglobulinaemia.
E. Whipple's disease.

17. You are looking at an MRI of the knees of a 16-year-old male. There is widening of the distal femoral metaphyses, with a widened intercondylar notch bilaterally. There is mild loss of joint space height in the medial tibio-femoral compartment, with subchondral cyst formation on the left, with preserved joint space but subchondral erosions on the right. The ligaments are intact. GE sequences reveal blooming artefact. Synovial enhancement causing joint erosion is noted on the enhanced T1WI sequence. What is the likely diagnosis?

A. Juvenile arthritis.
B. Pigmented villonodular synovitis (PVNS).
C. Amyloid.
D. Haemophilia.
E. Tuberculous arthritis.

18. A 75-year-old man has a cemented right total hip replacement. On routine follow-up imaging he is noted to have a progressive well-delineated, rounded, focal area of lucency at the cement bone interface adjacent to the tip of the femoral stem. Which of the following given reasons is the most appropriate for this progressive lucency?

A. Aggressive granulomatous disease.
B. Primary loosening.
C. Cement fracture.
D. Normal finding.
E. Metal bead shedding.

19. A patient attends A&E following an RTA in which she was the driver of car involved in a head-on collision. She complains of pain in both knees. Plain radiographs of the knees are unremarkable. Which of the following findings on MRI is most likely?

A. Bruising in the posterior aspect of the lateral tibial plateau and middle portion of the lateral femoral condyle.
B. Bruising at the anterior aspect of the tibia.
C. Kissing contusions in the anterior aspect of the distal femur and proximal tibia.
D. Bruising in the lateral femoral condyle with a second smaller area in the medial femoral condyle.
E. Bruising in the inferior medial patella and the anterior aspect of the lateral femoral condyle.

20. An 18-year-old motorcyclist is involved in an RTA in which he was dragged by the colliding car. He is noted to have pain in his right shoulder and neck with associated paraesthesia. An MRI is requested, suspecting brachial plexus injury. What finding is most suggestive of nerve root avulsion?

A. Pseudomeningocoele.
B. Intradural nerve root enhancement.
C. Spinal cord T2WI hyperintensity.
D. T2WI hyperintensity within the paraspinal muscles.
E. Thickening of the brachial plexus.

21. A 54-year-old man presents with a swelling in his right popliteal fossa. A Baker's cyst is suspected clinically and an ultrasound scan is arranged. This confirms a complex cystic structure with debris. To help confirm this is a Baker's cyst, you look for a communication of this cyst with fluid at the posterior aspect of the knee joint between which two tendons?

A. Semitendinosis and lateral head of gastrocnemius.
B. Semitendinosis and medial head of gastrocnemius.
C. Semitendinosis and semimembranosis.
D. Medial and lateral heads of gastrocnemius.
E. Lateral head of gastrocnemius and semimembranosis.
F. Medial head of gastrocnemius and semimembranosis.

22. An 18-year-old male patient presents to the rheumatologists with a history of proximal right tibial pain and sternal pain. The patient has a history of psoriasis and is also being seen by the dermatologists with palmoplantar pustulosis. Plain films of the sternum indicate sclerosis of the manubrium and erosive disease in the sternoclavicular joint. Plain films of the tibia show a lucent lesion in the proximal tibial metaphysis with associated periosteal reaction. An MRI shows high signal on STIR in the proximal tibial metaphysis, with a cortical defect. This area enhances on the T1 post gadolinium images, as does the periosteal region. A bone biopsy of the region is negative except for inflammatory cells. What is the most likely diagnosis?

A. Psoriatic arthropathy.
B. Synovitis, acne, pustulosis, hyperostosis, and osteitis (SAPHO) syndrome.
C. Chronic recurrent multifocal osteomyelitis (CRMO).
D. Chronic osteomyelitis.
E. Aseptic necrosis.

23. A 16-year-old boy fell playing football and hurt his left knee. He has some difficulty weight-bearing and presents to the A&E department. An x-ray of his left knee is performed. This demonstrates a small joint effusion, but no fracture is seen. An approximately 3-cm diameter, well-defined lucent bony lesion, with a thin sclerotic margin, is identified within the proximal epiphysis of the tibia. No internal calcification is evident on plain x-ray. What is the most likely diagnosis for this abnormality?

A. Chondromyxoid fibroma.
B. Enchondroma.
C. GCT.
D. Chondroblastoma.
E. Chondrosarcoma.

24. A 75-year-old man presents with bone pain. Investigations reveal anaemia, renal impairment, hypercalcaemia, proteinuria, and a monoclonal gammopathy. He undergoes radiological investigation. Which of the following is most correct in relation to the radiological features of the disease process?

A. 25% bone destruction must occur on plain film before a lesion will be apparent on plain film.
B. 75% of patients will have positive radiographic findings on plain film.
C. MRI typically reveals general hypointensity of bone marrow on T2WI sequences.
D. MRI typically reveals general hyperintensity of bone marrow on T1WI sequences.
E. The use of PET is inappropriate for imaging recurrent disease.

25. A 17-year-old female is admitted with multiple penetrating injuries to her arms after shielding her face from a nearby bomb blast while walking in the city centre. For which type of penetrating foreign body is ultrasound most superior for detection?

A. Gravel.
B. Wood.
C. Plastic.
D. Windshield glass.
E. Bottle glass.

26. A 30-year-old female runner presents with a history of pain in the legs on running. Plain radiographs are unremarkable. An isotope bone scan reveals subtle, longitudinal, linear uptake on the delayed bone scan images, with normal angiogram and blood pool images. What is the diagnosis?

A. Stress fracture.
B. Shin splints.
C. Osteoid osteoma.
D. Osteomyelitis.
E. Hypertrophic osteoarthropathy.

27. You are reporting an MRI knee on a patient with moderately severe osteoarthritis (OA), as diagnosed on plain film radiography. The patient describes significant knee pain. Which of the following statements best describes the relationship between symptoms, plain film findings, and MRI findings?

A. The MRI findings correlate well with the severity of findings on plain film radiography.
B. MRI findings correlate well with the patient's symptoms.
C. Plain film findings correlate well with the patient's symptoms, unlike MRI.
D. Plain film and MRI both correlate well with the severity of the patient's symptoms.
E. Symptoms, plain film findings, and MRI findings do not have a significant association with each other.

28. A 35-year-old man sprains his right ankle and attends the A&E department. An x-ray of the right ankle is performed. This does not show any evidence of a fracture, but the lateral view does demonstrate a well-defined radiolucent lesion with a faint sclerotic margin in the mid calcaneus. There is some central calcification within the lesion. What is the most likely diagnosis?

A. Simple bone cyst.
B. Normal variant.
C. Enchondroma.
D. Intraosseus lipoma.
E. Bone infarct.

29. A 25-year-old man presents with a painful knee. A plain film reveals a lucent area with a wide zone of transition in the distal femoral metaphysis. MRI reveals fluid–fluid levels. What is the most likely diagnosis?

A. Aneurysmal bone cyst.
B. GCT.
C. Osteosarcoma.
D. Chondroblastoma.
E. Osteoblastoma.

30. A 21-year-old rugby player presents to the A&E department with right shoulder pain and decreased range of movement following a tackle. There is obvious contour deformity on examination. Plain radiographs confirm anterior dislocation. Which additional radiographic finding is in keeping with a Hill–Sachs deformity?

A. Intra-articular loose body.
B. Greater tuberosity fracture.
C. Anterior glenoid rim fracture.
D. Anterior humeral head indentation.
E. Posterior humeral head indentation.

31. A 35-year-old male presents with a history of backache. Plain radiograph demonstrates reduction in the lumbar L2-3 disc space with mild endplate irregularity. An MRI of lumbar spine is carried out for further assessment. What feature on MRI is useful in differentiating discitis from modic type I endplate change?

A. Reduction in the disc height.
B. Low signal change in the endplate on T1WI.
C. High signal change in the endplate on T2WI.
D. Mild irregularity of the endplates.
E. High signal within the disc on T2WI.

32. You are discussing OA with a rheumatologist. He/she is curious to know what radiological findings seen in early disease are associated with progressive, as opposed to stable, arthritis. All of these are associated with OA, but which is least likely to indicate progressive disease?

A. Increased uptake on isotope bone scan.
B. Grade 1 osteophytosis in the knee.
C. Osteochondral defect.
D. A focal area of high signal on T2WI and STIR in the subchondral bone.
E. A serpiginous subchondral line that is low signal on T2WI and T1WI, with an adjacent T2WI high signal line.

33. You are asked to image the pelvis with MRI for someone who has a hip arthroplasty. Which of the following measures can be used to decrease the magnetic susceptibility artifact from the joint prosthesis?

A. Use fast spin echo (FSE) imaging rather than GE imaging.
B. Choose a higher field strength magnet, e.g. 3 T rather than 1.5 T.
C. Position the long axis of the prosthesis perpendicular to the main magnetic field strength (β0) direction if possible.
D. If fat saturation is to be employed, use spectral fat suppression rather than STIR imaging.
E. Increase the volume of the voxels (decrease spatial resolution).

34. A patient who is HIV positive presents with knee and ankle pain and swelling. Clinical examination is otherwise unremarkable. Initial radiographs reveal only a joint effusion. The complaint resolves after 4 weeks. What is the most likely diagnosis?

A. Septic arthritis.
B. Psoriatric arthritis.
C. HIV-associated arthritis.
D. Acute symmetric polyarthritis.
E. Hypertrophic pulmonary osteoarthropathy (HPOA).

35. A 26-year-old man presents to the A&E department with wrist pain and swelling after falling from a ladder on an outstretched hand. The lateral radiograph demonstrates posterior dislocation of the capitate relative to the lunate. What is the most commonly associated fracture with this injury?

A. Capitate.
B. Lunate.
C. Triquetral.
D. Scaphoid.
E. Radius.

36. A 55-year-old female with a history of pulmonary sarcoidosis presents with pain in both hands. Which of the following findings on plain radiograph of the hands is atypical of skeletal sarcoidosis?

A. Cyst-like radiolucencies.
B. Joint space narrowing.
C. Bone erosions.
D. Subcutaneous soft tissue nodules/mass.
E. Lace-like pattern of bone destruction.

37. A 55-year-old female presents to the rheumatologists with a history of episodic swollen red joints over the previous 2 years. She also complains of left hip pain. The patient's rheumatoid factor is not known at the time of requesting the radiographs. There is no other past medical history. The rheumatologists have requested bilateral hand and pelvis x-rays. The hand x-rays show bilateral asymmetric disease affecting the distal and proximal interphalangeal (IP) joints. In the affected distal IP joints there are central erosions, adjacent sclerosis, and marginal osteophytes. The first carpometacarpal joint in the left hand shows loss of joint space with osteophyte formation. The scaphoid-trapezium joint in the right hand also shows loss of joint space and adjacent sclerosis. In the left hip there is non-uniform loss of joint space, with associated subchondral cyst formation. What is the main differential?

A. RA.
B. Psoriatic arthritis.
C. Erosive OA.
D. Calcium pyrophosphate deposition (CPPD) arthropathy.
E. Ankylosing spondylitis.

38. A 39-year-old man presents with a gradually enlarging swelling in the upper lateral aspect of the right calf. He is also experiencing some numbness affecting the dorsum of his right foot. An ultrasound scan and subsequently an MRI scan demonstrate a well-defined, thinly septated cystic lesion intimately related to the proximal tibio-fibular joint and extending into the adjacent soft tissues. It measures approximately 4cm in maximum diameter. There is no enhancement of the soft tissue component post injection of gadolinium. What is the most likely diagnosis?

A. Parameniscal cyst.
B. Bursitis.
C. Focal tenosynovitis.
D. Ganglion cyst.
E. Chronic seroma.

39. A 30-year-old man presents with backache and morning stiffness. Examination reveals loss of spinal movement, uveitis, and upper zone end inspiratory fine crepitations on auscultation. Which of the following statements is most correct in relation to the radiological features of the underlying condition?

A. Romanus lesions (anterior or posterior spondylitis) are a late feature.
B. Syndesmophytes are better depicted on MRI than plain film.
C. Ankylosis involves the vertebral edges or centre.
D. Sacroiliac joint widening is not a feature.
E. Enthesitis appears as low signal within the ligaments on STIR imaging.

40. The case of a 22-year-old male with typical clinical and radiographic features of osteoid osteoma is discussed at the musculoskeletal multidisciplinary team meeting regarding treatment planning. A decision is made to offer radiofrequency ablation (RFA). You have been asked to consent the patient for the procedure. Which of the following statements is true?

A. Up to six repeat procedures may be required.
B. It is performed under local anaesthetic.
C. Biopsy is necessary to confirm diagnosis prior to treatment.
D. Complete symptom relief is seen in 90% after initial therapy.
E. RFA treatment of vertebral osteoid osteomas is contraindicated.

41. A 15-year-old boy presents with a history of knee pain. Plain radiographs demonstrate calcification at the patellar tendon attachment to the inferior pole of the patella. MRI of the knee demonstrates oedema at the patellar attachment of the patellar tendon. What is the diagnosis?

A. Osgood–Schlatter disease.
B. Patellar sleeve avulsion.
C. Sinding–Larsen–Johansson syndrome.
D. Complete rupture of patellar tendon.
E. Partial tear of quadriceps tendon.

42. An 81-year-old male diabetic is referred from the endocrinology team for an MRI of foot. This patient was seeing a podiatrist, who became concerned that the foot had become increasingly deformed and was acutely red and swollen around the tarso-metatarsal joints. The patient is asymptomatic as he has peripheral neuropathy. The clinical query is whether this patient has osteomyelitis/septic arthritis in this region, or neuropathic arthropathy. Which of these MRI features would be more typically associated with osteomyelitis than acute neuropathic arthropathy?

A. Focal involvement.
B. Predominant midfoot involvement.
C. Associated bony debris.
D. High T2WI and STIR, low T1WI. Enhancement present.
E. Bony changes are in a periarticular and subchondral location.

43. A 16-year-old boy presents with a slowly enlarging, painful swelling in his left lateral chest wall. A CXR shows an expansile lucent lesion arising from the lateral aspect of the left seventh rib. An MRI scan is performed for further evaluation and this demonstrates a lobulated, thin-walled multiseptated lesion with fluid–fluid levels, the dependent layer of which are hyperintense on T1WI. What is the most likely diagnosis?

A. Fibrous dysplasia.
B. Aneursymal bone cyst.
C. Enchondroma.
D. Chondroblastoma.
E. Cystic angiomatosis.

44. A 70-year-old man undergoes an x-ray of his right hand following trauma. There is no evidence of fracture, but incidental resorption of the middle portion of the distal phalanges is demonstrated. Which of the following would be the most likely underlying cause?

A. Scleroderma.
B. Frostbite.
C. Leprosy.
D. Polyvinyl chloride.
E. Psoriatic arthropathy.

45. A 56-year-old woman is referred for MR arthrography of her right shoulder for query rotator cuff tear. You are asked to explain the procedure to a group of medical students attached to the department. What is the advantage of using a fat-suppressed T1WI sequence?

A. Differentiating partial from full thickness tear.
B. Identify bursal fluid collections.
C. Differentiating inadvertent air injection from intra-articular loose body.
D. Diagnosing capsular laxity.
E. Detecting incidental bone marrow lesions.

46. A 40-year-old female presents with a small lump in her foot. An MRI of the foot demonstrates a small soft tissue mass, which has homogenous low signal on T1WI and T2WI. The mass enhances with gadolinium. What is the most likely diagnosis?

A. Morton's neuroma.
B. Lipoma.
C. Ganglion cyst.
D. Plantar fibromatosis.
E. Hemangioma.

47. A patient presents to their GP with a complex history of acute episodes of severe tender inflamed joints, in particular around the knee. At present the patient has joint stiffness which is most pronounced in the evenings and mild joint pain. The patient has a past medical history of hypothyroidism. A plain film is requested which shows chondrocalcinosis and moderate degenerative change in the lateral tibiofemoral compartment and the patellofemoral compartment. Regarding CPPD disease, which of the following statements is the most appropriate?

A. The presence of chondrocalcinosis indicates a radiological diagnosis of pseudogout.
B. Pseudogout syndrome is the most common means of presentation for this disease.
C. Disproportionate involvement of the patellofemoral joint is the most frequently seen radiographic finding.
D. The presence of crystals displaying positive birefringence at polarized light microscopy allows for the definitive diagnosis of pyrophosphate arthropathy.
E. The presence of hypothyroidism is associated with the diagnosis.

48. A 34-year-old woman has chronic right wrist pain, with no documented history of previous trauma. An x-ray of the right wrist shows sclerosis and irregularity of the scaphoid with early bony fragmentation. What is the most likely eponymous disease that has resulted in this abnormality?

A. Sever disease.
B. Freiberg disease.
C. Kohler disease.
D. Iselin disease.
E. Preiser disease.

49. A 76-year-old man presents with hip and pelvic pain. He has a past history of renal cell carcinoma treated by radiofrequency ablation, and has been treated on multiple occasions with heparin for thromboembolic disease. Plain films are non-contributory but a ^{99m}Tc bone scan reveals increased thoracic kyphosis and increased uptake in the body and bilateral alae of the sacrum in an H configuration. What is the most likely diagnosis?

A. Brown tumour.
B. Multiple myeloma.
C. Metastasis from renal cell carcinoma.
D. Chordoma.
E. Insufficiency fractures.

50. A 47-year-old man presents with a progressive history of pain, swelling, and reduced range of movement affecting his right knee. Symptoms have been ongoing for 2–3 years. Locking is noted on examination. Radiography of his knee reveals multiple intra-articular calcifications. A supra-patellar joint effusion is also present. The joint space is maintained. What is the most likely diagnosis?

A. Neuropathic arthropathy.
B. Osteochondritis dissecans.
C. Osteochondral fracture.
D. PVNS.
E. Synovial osteochondromatosis.

51. A 45-year-old female undergoes aggressive chemotherapy for bone metastases followed by bone marrow transplantation. Which of the following findings on MRI indicates recurrent metastatic disease instead of rebound hematopoietic marrow?

A. Intermediate signal on T1WI.
B. High signal on T2WI.
C. Loss of signal on out-of-phase GE images.
D. High signal on STIR images.
E. Increased conspicuity on prolonged time-to-echo (TE) images.

52. A 24-year-old male patient is referred from the rheumatologists with a history of back pain and hip pain. Plain films are carried out. These show bilateral sacroiliitis with erosive change on the iliac side on the left, but sacral and iliac erosions on the right. The imaging of the spine reveals large non-marginal syndesmophytes in the thoracolumbar spine with a relatively normal lower lumbar spine. The patient also complains of foot pain and plain films reveal evidence of a retrocalcaneal bursitis with erosion of the calcaneus. Hand x-rays reveal small erosions asymmetrically in the distal IP joints in both hands. What is the most likely diagnosis?

A. Ankylosing spondylitis.
B. Reactive arthritis.
C. Psoriatic arthritis.
D. Erosive OA.
E. Adult Stills disease.

53. A 34-year-old man has an MRI of the lumbar spine for lower back pain. This is normal apart from a focal lesion present in the L4 vertebral body. This is reported as a vertebral haemangioma. Which of the following MRI characteristics does this lesion most likely have?

A. ↓T1 ↓T2 ↓STIR
B. ↓T1 ↓T2 ↑STIR
C. ↓T1 ↑T2 ↓STIR
D. ↑T1 ↓T2 ↓STIR
E. ↑T1 ↓T2 ↑STIR
F. ↑T1 ↑T2 ↓STIR
G. ↑T1 ↑T2 ↑STIR

54. An 18-year-old male with fingernail dysplasia and a family history of renal failure is investigated for possible nail-patella syndrome. Which of the following radiographic findings is considered pathognomonic for this disorder?

A. Patellar hypoplasia.
B. Lateral elbow hypoplasia.
C. Posterior iliac horns.
D. Calcaneo-valgus feet.
E. Madelung deformity.

55. A 10-year-old male involved in an RTA is brought to the A&E department with a history of severe right thigh pain. Plain radiograph demonstrates a transverse fracture in the mid-diaphysis of the femur. Incidental note is made of bone osteopenia and undertubulation of the femur with metaphyseal flaring producing Erlenmeyer flask deformity and coxa magna related to previous avascular necrosis of the femoral head. What is the underlying bone disease?

A. Pyle's disease.
B. Osteopetrosis.
C. Gaucher's disease.
D. Fibrous dysplasia.
E. Ollier's disease.

56. A 45-year-old female is being investigated. She has a history of connective tissue disease. You are reviewing her imaging and trying to decide which connective tissue disease she has. Her hand x-rays reveal distal tuft resorption with cutaneous calcification. She also has erosion of the distal IP joints in the hands and the first carpometacarpal (CMC) joint. She has ulnar deviation deformity to the MCP joints in both hands on the Norgaard views, which corrects on the antero-posterior (AP) views. She also has an MRI scan of the pelvis which shows uniform high T2WI signal in the gluteal muscles bilaterally. From the list of connective tissues diseases below, select the one paired with a feature that is atypical for the disease but present in this patient?

A. Systemic sclerosis and high signal changes in muscles
B. SLE and deforming arthropathy
C. Systemic sclerosis and acro-osteolysis
D. Polymyositis and erosive arthropathy
E. Polymyositis and soft tissue calcification

57. A 34-year-old man has a 3-month history of right knee pain. There is a remote history of previous right leg trauma. He has an x-ray of the right knee performed, which demonstrates a densely ossified mass immediately adjacent to the posterior cortex of the distal femur. You determine that the differential diagnosis is between post-traumatic myositis ossificans or a parosteal osteosarcoma. Which of the following features on plain x-ray is likely to be most helpful in distinguishing between these diagnoses?

A. Periosteal reaction in the adjacent bone.
B. Presence of lucent areas in the lesion.
C. Pattern of ossification in the lesion.
D. Size of the lesion.
E. Presence of lucent cleft between the lesion and adjacent bone.

58. You are reviewing a plain film of pelvis of a 70-year-old woman with recent hip pain. She has a past medical history of bronchial carcinoid. You notice thick, coarsened trabeculae of the left iliac bone, but in comparison to a previous film there is an area of cortical destruction with 'ring-and-arc' calcification. There is no adjacent periosteal reaction. Which of the following is the most significant pathology present?

A. Paget's disease.
B. Chondrosarcoma.
C. Osteosarcoma.
D. Chondroblastoma.
E. Lung metastasis.

59. A 34-year-old man is admitted with sudden onset chest pain described as tearing in nature. Clinical examination reveals a diastolic murmur consistent with aortic regurgitation. Subsequent chest CT confirms ascending aortic dissection. He has a past medical history of spontaneous pneumothorax. Despite a negative family history, an underlying diagnosis of Marfan syndrome is suspected. Which of the following musculoskeletal manifestations is required for this diagnosis to be made?

A. Joint hypermobility.
B. Pectus excavatum of moderate severity.
C. Reduced upper-to-lower segment ratio.
D. High arched palate.
E. Malar hypoplasia.

60. A 25-year-old marathon runner presents with a history of right calf pain during exercise. Popliteal artery entrapment is suspected clinically. Which of the following statements regarding imaging of popliteal artery entrapment syndrome (PAES) is true?

A. In PAES, the popliteal artery is compressed with the ankle in the neutral position.
B. A normal Doppler ultrasound of the popliteal artery excludes the diagnosis.
C. In the normal popliteal fossa, the popliteal artery and vein pass lateral to the medial head of the gastrocnemius and are surrounded by fat.
D. The anatomical abnormality is invariably unilateral.
E. Catheter angiography is the gold standard for the diagnosis.

61. A patient is referred from the dialysis unit with a history of joint and muscular pain. In particular they complain of bilateral hand pain and hip pain. The plain films of both hands show a loss of distinction of the radial aspect of the phalanges of the index and middle fingers. There is an area of para-articular soft tissue calcification noted adjacent to the middle finger metacarpal of the right hand. The pelvic x-ray is distinctly abnormal. There is a large expansile lucent lesion in the right iliac bone, which has a narrow zone of transition and no evidence of internal matrix. The bony definition of the rest of the pelvic bone reveals a coarsened trabecular pattern, but no evidence of expansion of the bones. There are multiple small linear lucencies noted along the medial aspect of the femurs bilaterally, which demonstrate a periosteal reaction. What condition do you think this patient has?

A. Primary hyperparathyroidism.
B. Secondary hyperparathyroidism.
C. Paget's disease.
D. Osteomalacia.
E. Renal osteodystrophy.

62. A 55-year-old man is noted on a plain x-ray of pelvis to have a right hip prosthesis. There is a cemented acetabular component present with an uncemented stem. Of the following hip arthroplasties, which is the most likely procedure that he has undergone?

A. Unipolar hemiarthroplasty.
B. Bipolar hemiarthroplasty.
C. Hip resurfacing.
D. Hybrid total hip replacement.
E. Reverse hybrid total hip replacement.

63. A 62-year-old male with a known diagnosis of bronchogenic carcinoma presents with pain and swelling of his wrists. What radiographic features are consistent with hypertrophic pulmonary osteoarthropathy?

A. Metaphyseal lamellar periosteal reaction.
B. Irregular epiphyseal periosteal proliferation.
C. Asymmetrical, thick 'feathery' periosteal reaction.
D. Cortical thickening and trabecular coarsening.
E. Symmetrical, solid periosteal new bone formation.

64. A 57-year-old female patient with a history of multiple myeloma is referred for imaging due to a history of arthralgia primarily affecting the hands. The patient describes early morning stiffness that eases through the day. The clinicians report a finding of synovitis clinically. Blood results have revealed a raised ESR. Hand x-rays are carried out which reveal sharply defined intra-articular marginal erosions at the MCP joints of the index and middle fingers bilaterally. The joint spaces are well preserved. There are also well-marginated subchondral cysts noted in the carpal bones, again with joint space preservation. Soft tissue nodules are noted around the wrist joints, which are not calcified. There is no evidence of juxta-articular osteopenia. No osteophytes are noted. What diagnosis is most strongly suggested by these findings?

A. Gout.
B. CPPD.
C. RA.
D. Amyloidosis.
E. Wilson's disease.

65. A 24-year-old man undergoes acute trauma to his right knee playing football. He is unable to weight bear. An x-ray of the right knee is performed and this demonstrates a large joint effusion and a small, avulsed elliptical fragment of bone at the medial aspect of the proximal tibia at the joint margin. Which knee structure is likely to be deranged in association with this injury at a subsequent MRI?

A. Anterior cruciate ligament.
B. Posterior cruciate ligament.
C. Lateral collateral ligament.
D. Patellar tendon.
E. Lateral meniscus.

66. A 5-year-old boy presents with a history of walking difficulty. On examination he is noted to have an antalgic gait and lower limb length discrepancy, with the right limb being shorter than the left. Plain radiographs of the right leg show lobular ossific masses arising from the distal femoral epiphysis and the talus, which resemble osteochondromas. What is the most likely underlying diagnosis?

A. Dysplasia epiphysealis hemimelica (Trevor disease).
B. Multiple epiphyseal dysplasia.
C. Diaphyseal aclasis.
D. Dyschondrosteosis (Leri–Weil disease).
E. Klippel–Trenaunay–Weber syndrome.

67. A 22-year-old patient presents to casualty with a reduced GCS and hypotension. He is visiting the UK from abroad and fellow backpackers in a local youth hostel state that he was complaining of abdominal pain earlier that day. A CT abdomen reveals sclerosis in both femoral heads and H-shaped vertebrae. The spleen is small and calcified. What is the patient's most likely underlying diagnosis?

A. Scheuermann's disease.
B. Hereditary spherocytosis.
C. Gaucher disease.
D. Sickle-cell disease.
E. Primary bone lymphoma.

68. A 41-year-old male presents to the A&E department with knee pain following a fall at work. Plain radiography does not demonstrate any fracture, but note is made of continuous, irregular cortical hyperostosis along the lateral margin of the femur. What is the most likely diagnosis?

A. Osteopoikilosis.
B. Fibrous dysplasia.
C. Engelmann disease.
D. Melorheostosis.
E. Osteopathia striata.

69. A 30-year-old male presents with a history of painful heels after a fall from a height. Plain radiograph demonstrates calcaneal fractures. Which of the following statements regarding calcaneal fractures is true?

A. Extraarticular fractures represent 75% of all calcaneal fractures.
B. Calcaneal fracture classification is based on fracture line location at the posterior facet.
C. Bilateral fractures are present in 30% of cases.
D. The flexor hallucis longus tendon passes inferior to the sustentaculum tali on the lateral aspect of the calcaneus.
E. Normal Boehler's angle is less than 20°.

70. An orthopaedic surgeon in your hospital comes to your office to ask your advice on a 15-year-old girl he is about to see at his clinic. Although limited clinical information is available, he was able to find out that the patient has a congenital condition, which has resulted in her being confined to a wheelchair. As she was complaining of a sore knee, an x-ray was carried out. There is a long gracile femur and tibia, indicating undertubulation of the bone. What is the most likely cause for this appearance?

A. Dwarfism.
B. Gaucher's disease.
C. Cerebral palsy.
D. Arthrogryposis multiplex congenital.
E. Juvenile RA (JRA).

71. A patient is being assessed for a possible congenital foot deformity. Both AP and lateral weight-bearing views of the hind and fore foot have been taken. You are lucky to have an experienced radiographer working with you and she has carried out the standard measurements in assessing for foot deformities. The tibiocalcaneal angle measures 60° on the lateral foot image. On the AP hindfoot image, the talocalcaneal angle measures 30°. On the lateral foot image the metatarsals are superimposed, with the fifth metatarsal being in the most plantar position. What sort of deformity does this patient have?

A. None.
B. Clubfoot.
C. Rocker bottom foot.
D. Flexible flat foot deformity.
E. Pes cavus.

72. A 21-year-old patient attends the A&E department following a minor injury with a suspected fracture. The request form states that the patient has osteogenesis imperfecta. It is noted that the patient is of reduced stature and does not display any evidence of blue sclera, but that the colouration of his sclera has faded over time. He has normal hearing. What subtype of osteogenesis imperfecta does he likely have?

A. Type I.
B. Type II.
C. Type III.
D. Type IV.
E. Type V.

73. A radiologist is reporting a ^{99m}Tc bone scan and describes it as a 'superscan'. He can say this because of reduced uptake in the:

A. brain
B. skeleton
C. kidneys
D. bowel
E. myocardium.

74. You are reviewing the x-rays of a child that are stored in your department's museum. Sequential radiographs have been taken as the child has aged and the appearances have become more pronounced with time. The child has a form of dwarfism. On the CXR you notice 'oar-shaped' ribs. The metacarpals are short and wide, but narrow proximally, giving a fan-like appearance. The patient has a J-shaped sella turcica. The iliac wings are wide, but the iliac bones narrow inferiorly. On the lateral lumbar spine, the vertebra have central anterior beaks. A clinical vignette mentions that the patient was not intellectually impaired. What condition does the patient probably have?

A. Campomelic dysplasia.
B. Niemann–Pick disease.
C. Morquio syndrome.
D. Achondroplasia.
E. Hurler's syndrome.

75. A 35-year-old man presents with pain, swelling, and reduced movement of his knee. A plain film reveals a joint effusion, well-defined erosions with preservation of joint space, and normal bone mineralization. An MRI reveals, in addition, a mass in the region of the femoro-tibial joint space with low signal on T1WI and T2WI, and blooming artefact on GE imaging. What is the most likely diagnosis?

A. Synovial cell sarcoma.
B. Regional migratory osteoporosis.
C. Gout.
D. Synovial chondromatosis.
E. PVNS.

chapter 2

MUSCULOSKELETAL AND TRAUMA

ANSWERS

1. C. Chordoma.

Plain film is very insensitive for detecting sacral lesions. Metastatic disease is much more common in the sacrum than primary malignancy. Chordoma is the most common primary sacral lesion. It is derived from the embryonic remnants of the notochord and is thus almost always found in the midline or a paramedian location with respect to the spine. It is most commonly found in the sacrum (50%), clivus (35%), and vertebrae (15%). A chordoma manifests as a destructive, lytic lesion, commonly with internal calcifications, at both plain radiography and CT. A large presacral soft-tissue component is usually present, as are soft-tissue components within the sacrum and sacral canal. Symptoms can include pain, sciatica, and rectal bleeding as well as other bowel and bladder symptoms, reflecting compromise of sacral nerves. The tumours can extend across the adjacent disc space and sacroiliac joint.

On MRI, chordomas demonstrate low to intermediate signal intensity on T1WI and prominent increased signal intensity on T2WI. Enhancement of the soft-tissue components is variable, yet often moderate, on both CT and MR images. Chordomas demonstrate a prominent vascular stain at angiography. They are locally aggressive and develop in locations that do not permit easy surgical cure. There is an almost 100% recurrence rate; tumour seeding along biopsy tracts and surgical incisions can lead to multicentric local recurrences. Metastasis occurs in 5–43% to liver, lung, regional lymph nodes, peritoneum, skin, and heart. The 5-year survival rate is 66% for adults.

Osteomyelitis in the sacrum is most often due to contiguous spread from a suppurative focus and we are told this patient was previously well. Ewing sarcoma would occur at a younger age (peaking at 15 years, 90% manifest between the ages of 5 and 30). In the case of myeloma it would be atypical for the rest of the spine to be uninvolved. The sacrococcygeal region is the most common location of teratomas discovered in infancy. It is only rarely discovered in adulthood. Teratomas are composed of a mixture of cystic and solid components.

The other lesions to be included in the differential diagnosis of such a sacral mass are metastasis, sarcomas, GCT, chondrosarcoma, and ependymoma.

Diel J, Ortiz O, Losada RA, Price DB, Hayt MW, and Katz DS. The sacrum: pathologic spectrum, multimodality imaging, and subspecialty approach. *RadioGraphics* 2001; 21: 83–104.
Dähnert W. *Radiology Review Manual*, 5th edn, Lippincott Williams & Wilkins, 2003. p. 198.
Manaster BJ, May DA, and Disler DG. *Musculoskeletal Imaging: The Requisites*, 3rd edn, Mosby, 2007. p. 526.

2. A. Psoriatic arthropathy.

Bone involvement before skin changes is evident in up to 20% of cases. Nail pitting or discolouration is common and correlated with the severity of the arthropathy. Five distinct manifestations have been described: oligoarthritis, polyarthritis (predominately distal IP joints), symmetric type (resembling RA), arthritis mutilans, and spondyloarthropathy. The characteristic distribution involves the small joints of the hands and feet, with or without spondyloarthropathy. Involvement in the hands tends to include distal IP as well as MCP or PIP joints, with early tuft resorption and distal IP erosive disease. The erosions become so severe that a 'pencil-in-cup' deformity and telescoping of the joint may occur. Bone density can be normal and the joint distribution is asymmetric. Similarly, sacroiliitis is asymmetric, unlike ankylosing spondylitis and syndesmophtes, which are non-marginal and asymmetric; in ankylosing spondylitis they are marginal and asymmetric. The spondyloarthropathy of psoriatic arthropathy is indistinguishable from that of reactive arthritis, the clinical scenario (rash vs uveitis/urethritis) providing the diagnosis.

The arthropathies of CPPD disease and haemochromatosis are essentially identical radiographically. Chondrocalcinosis is commonly seen in the wrist (triangular fibrocartilage) and knee (menisci). The joints most affected are the knee, wrist and second and third MCPs of the hand: the IP joints tend to be spared. Early disease shows erosive change. More advanced disease demonstrates sclerosis, osteochondral fragments, and osteophytes. Subchondral cysts are common and large. RA is rarely found in the distal IP joints and periosteal reaction is not a feature. SLE is usually non-erosive and affects the MCP joints.

Manaster BJ, May DA, and Disler DG. *Musculoskeletal Imaging: The Requisites*, 3rd edn, Mosby, 2007. p. 321.

3. E. Bone oedema involving the medial facet of patella and lateral femoral condyle.

Transient dislocation of the patella typically occurs laterally as a result of a twisting injury in a fixed and flexed knee. The medial facet of the dislocated patella impacts against the lateral femoral condyle, resulting in the classic bone contusion pattern. Rarely oedema may also be seen in the adductor tubercle of the medial femoral condyle due to avulsion of the medial patello-femoral ligament.

Sanders TG, Medynski MA, Feller JF, and Lawhorn KW. Bone contusion patterns of the knee at MR imaging: footprint of the mechanism of injury. *RadioGraphics* 2003; 20: S135–S151.

4. E. Atlanto-axial impaction.

This is a more severe form of atlanto-axial subluxation where the C1-2 facets collapse and there is invagination of the dens of C2 into the foramen magnum. As such, the dens is not visible on the lateral radiograph. The key feature, apart from widening of the pre-dental space (which can also be caused by pannus eroding the dens or more commonly atlanto-axial subluxation), is that the anterior arch of C1 lies in front of the lower portion of C2, whereas it normally lies anterior to the dens.

Manaster B, May D, and Disler D. *Musculoskeletal Radiology: The Requisites*, 3rd edn, Mosby, 2007. pp. 296–298.

5. C. Osteoblastoma.

Osteoblastoma is similar both clinically and histologically to osteoid osteoma, but there are some differences that aid in distinguishing these two entities. Clinically osteoblastoma is typically less painful than osteoid osteoma and does not respond as well to salicylates. An osteoblastoma in the neural arch of the spine is more likely to cause neurological signs, as these lesions are typically larger and more expansile than osteoid osteoma. The lucent nidus seen in osteoid osteoma is usually less than 1.5–2 cm in size, whereas the nidus in osteoblastoma is usually larger than 2 cm at diagnosis and has less surrounding sclerosis. The nidus may or may not have a calcific focus within, in both these diagnoses. The appearance described in the question is the subgroup of osteoblastoma that has similar features to osteoid osteoma. Other appearances on imaging of osteoblastoma include an expansile lesion with multiple small calcifications and a peripheral sclerotic rim or, more rarely, an aggressive appearance with osseous expansion, bone destruction, infiltrating soft tissue, and intermixed matrix calcification.

An enostosis (or bone island) may be giant (greater than 2 cm), but should be well defined and densely sclerotic. It is possible a bone abscess could cause a lytic lesion with surrounding sclerosis, but the patient is systemically well, making infection less likely. A bone abscess is also unlikely to be as expansile as the lesion described. Intracortical haemangioma is a very rare diagnosis, usually within the cortex of a long bone, such as the tibia. On CT there is a hypoattenuating lesion, with spotty internal calcification or a 'wire-netting' appearance.

Chai JW, Hong SH, Choi J-Y, Koh YH, Lee JW, Choi J-A et al. Radiologic diagnosis of osteoid osteoma: from simple to challenging findings. *RadioGraphics* 2010; 30: 737–749.

6. B. Giant cell tumour (GCT).

This is the classical description and location of a GCT. They occur age 20–40 years, in the long bones and occasionally the sacrum and pelvis. They are lucent, eccentric, and expansile but do not usually produce sclerosis and produce a periosteal reaction in less than a third of patients. They may have a multiloculated appearance. They originate in the metaphysis but extend to the subchondral surface in the skeletally mature. MRI often reveals fluid–fluid levels and some low signal on T2WI due to haemosiderin or collagen deposition. The major differential diagnosis is an aneurysmal bone cyst (ABC), but this classically has a sclerotic margin and usually occurs under 30 years of age (75% occur before the age of 20 years). Fibrous dysplasia would usually present at a younger age in the metaphysis with extension into the diaphysis; a trabeculated/ground-glass appearance is typical with a thick sclerotic margin and endosteal scalloping. Metastasis would be relatively rare at this age and there is no mention of a primary tumour. Osteosarcoma would have a more aggressive appearance with a wide zone of transition, periosteal reaction, cortical destruction, and soft tissue extension.

Dähnert W. *Radiology Review Manual*, 5th edn, Lippincott Williams & Wilkins, 2003. p. 92.
Chapman S and Nakielny R. *Aids to Radiological Differential Diagnosis*, 4th edn, Elsevier, 2003. p. 552 (GCT), 534 (ABC).
Manaster BJ, May DA, and Disler DG. *Musculoskeletal Imaging: The Requisites*, 3rd edn, Mosby, 2007. p. 509.

7. C. Fracture of the proximal third.

Scaphoid fracture is the most common of all carpal bone fractures and also potentially serious due to the high rate of avascular necrosis. This fracture can be difficult to detect on initial radiographs. Wrist casting and repeat radiography after 1 week are typically advised if there is ongoing suspicion. Fractures of the proximal third account for 20% of injuries, but are associated with failure to unite in 90%. Middle third fractures make up the majority (70%), with up to 30% failing to reunite. Distal third fractures usually reunite. A vertical oblique fracture is more unstable than a horizontal oblique fracture. Fracture displacement of greater than 1mm is also a poor prognostic feature.

Dahnert W. *Radiology Review Manual*, 6th edn, Lippincott Williams & Wilkins, 2007. p. 86.

8. D. Bony ankylosis of the carpal bones.

Whilst fibrous ankylosis of the carpal and tarsal bones does occur, bony ankylosis is extremely rare in RA. It is, however, common in JRA. There are a number of unusual findings, which if present should indicate a diagnosis other than RA. Productive bone change (e.g. periostitis or enthesopathy) is extremely unusual. Osteophytes are also uncommon in the absence of advanced associated osteoarthritic change. The exception to this is the distal ulna, a feature known as ulnar capping. The other features are all typical of RA.

Sommer O, Kladosek A, Weiler V, Czembirek H, Boeck M, Stiskal M et al. Rheumatoid arthritis: a practical guide to state-of-the-art imaging, image interpretation and clinical implications. *RadioGraphics* 2005; 25: 381–398.
Manaster B, May D, and Disler D. *Musculoskeletal Radiology: The Requisites*, 3rd edn, Mosby, 2007. pp. 290–292.

9. D. GCT of the tendon sheath.

A GCT of the tendon sheath is a nodular form of PVNS. These tumours are intimately associated with a tendon sheath and are most commonly located in the hand. They usually manifest as a small slow-growing mass, with or without pain. Radiographs may show no abnormality or non-aggressive remodelling of the adjacent bone. These lesions are typically hypo- or iso-intense to muscle on T1WI and T2WI, owing to abundant collagen and haemosiderin, often with enhancement. This is similar to the findings of diffuse intra-articular PVNS, when the extent of haemosiderin deposition may cause hypointense nodules on T2WI and blooming artifact on gradient echo (GE) sequences. It must be stated that the degree of haemosiderin content may not always be enough to cause marked hypointensity on T2WI in GCT of the tendon sheath.

A ganglion cyst could occur in this location and be related to a tendon sheath, but on MRI it is typically hyperintense on T2WI secondary to its fluid component. There may be thin rim enhancement of the wall post administration of gadolinium. Peripheral nerve sheath tumours are typically hyperintense on T2WI with variable contrast enhancement. Lipomas are similar in signal characteristic to subcutaneous fat on MRI, i.e. hyperintense on both T1WI and T2WI. A soft-tissue haemangioma may contain phleboliths on plain radiographic imaging. On MRI, haemangiomas may be well circumscribed or have poorly defined margins, with varying amounts of increased T1WI signal owing to either reactive fat overgrowth or haemorrhage. Areas of slow flow are typically hyperintense on T2WI, while rapid flow can demonstrate a signal void on images obtained with a non-flow-sensitive sequence.

Wu JS and Hochman MG. Soft-tissue tumors and tumorlike lesions: a systematic imaging approach. *Radiology* 2009; 253: 297–316.

10. A. Ulnar collateral ligament.

The history and radiographic findings are typical of gamekeeper's thumb, which is an injury to the ulnar collateral ligament at its insertion site into the proximal phalanx of the thumb. This injury usually requires internal fixation to secure the ligament. Radial collateral ligament injuries of the thumb lead to painful deformity and articular degeneration. Rupture of flexor pollicis longus results in loss of active flexion of the thumb. The thumb remains in flexion with rupture of extensor pollicis longus. Thumb tendon injuries are typically seen in RA due to their susceptibility to synovitis.

Brant WE and Helms CA. *Fundamentals of Diagnostic Radiology*, 3rd edn, Lippincott Williams & Wilkins, 2007. p. 1113.

11. D. Myelofibrosis.

This is associated with collagen proliferation in the marrow, which may be primary or secondary/reactive following other myeloproliferative disorders. The highly structured collagen matrix has tightly bound protons that do not resonate or produce significant signal. As a result the marrow is of diffuse low signal intensity on all sequences. There is also no architectural distortion.

In contrast, myeloma, metastases, and lymphoma are generally associated with focal or multifocal signal abnormalities. Sickle-cell anaemia causes bone sclerosis secondary to bone infarcts, which have an irregular appearance.

In myelofibrosis, splenomegaly is secondary to extramedullary hematopoiesis. The presence of splenomegaly is helpful in limiting the differential diagnoses. Sickle-cell anaemia is associated with a small, sometimes calcified, spleen due to autoinfarction.

Cloran F and Banks KP. Diffuse osteosclerosis with hepatosplenomegaly. *American Journal of Roentgenology* 2007; 188: S18–S20.
Long SS, Yablon CM, and Eisenberg RL. Bone marrow signal alteration in the spine and sacrum. *American Journal of Roentgenology* 2010; 195: W178–W200.

12. C. Hypervascular pannus at the TFCC and RUJ, with joint effusion at DRUJ.

Hypervascular pannus is intermediate to high signal on T2WI and low signal on T1WI. It also enhances, retaining enhancement on delayed imaging. Joint effusions can be difficult to differentiate from hypervascular pannus on pre-contrast imaging. Following enhancement they show only delayed enhancement. Fibrous pannus is low signal on all sequences.

Narvaez JA, Narvaez J, Roca Y, and Aguilera C. MR imaging assessment of clinical problems in rheumatoid arthritis. *European Radiology* 2002; 12: 1819–1828.

13.C. Fast SE T2WI.

The parallel rim of hypo- and hyperintensity seen on T2WI refers to the 'double line' sign, which is almost pathognomic of osteonecrosis. It is most commonly associated with avascular necrosis of the femoral head, but can be seen in osteonecrosis at other sites on MRI. The 'double line' sign constitutes a hyperintense inner border (inflammatory response of bone with granulation tissue), with a hypointense periphery (reactive bone interface).

The characteristic plain radiographic pattern of metadiaphyseal osteonecrosis is that of a serpentine ring-like band of sclerosis that separates a central necrotic zone of variable lucency from surrounding normal marrow, although this pattern is a relatively late manifestation of osteonecrosis. Earlier in the course of the disease, osteonecrosis may result in a poorly defined region of lucency within the medullary space, a feature that may be indistinguishable from a lytic neoplastic process on x-ray. MRI is then very useful in these cases by showing the serpentine low signal rim of the lesion on T1WI. On T2WI, the rim of the lesion may have low signal, high signal or both (the 'double line' sign), the latter being the most specific sign for osteonecrosis.

Stacy GS and Dixon LB. Pitfalls in MR image interpretation prompting referrals to an orthopedic oncology clinic. *RadioGraphics* 2007; 27: 805–826.

14. E. A convex bulge involving the whole of the posterior cortex of the vertebral body.

The others are more in keeping with benign compression fractures. Retropulsion of a posterior fragment into the spinal canal is a highly specific (100%) finding of benign compression fracture, but has a sensitivity of only 16%. Other features in keeping with malignant compression fractures are complete replacement of normal marrow with low signal on T1WI, involvement of the pedicles, and the presence of an epidural and/or paraspinal soft-tissue mass. The presence of an epidural mass is said to have 80% sensitivity and 100% specificity for malignant fractures. Convex bulging of the posterior cortex of the vertebra and involvement of the pedicle have respective sensitivities and specificities of 70% and 94%, and 80% and 94%. Beware that compression fractures due to multiple myeloma only rarely show MRI features of malignant fracture and this diagnosis should be included in the differential of a non-traumatic, benign-appearing vertebral compression fracture.

Uetani M, Hashimi R, and Hayashi K. Malignant and benign compression fractures: differentiation and diagnostic pitfalls on MRI. *Clinical Radiology* 2004; 59: 124–131.

15. B. Coronoid process fracture.

Radial head fractures are common, accounting for approximately one-third of all elbow fractures and up to 5% of all fractures in adults. A recent retrospective study found that associated fracture of the upper extremity was seen in 10.2% of patients, with fractures of the coronoid process the most common (4.1%). Radial head fracture, coronoid fracture, and medial collateral ligament tear form the 'terrible triad' of the elbow, which requires operative fixation.

Kaas L, van Riet RP, Vroemen JPAM, and Eygendaal D. The incidence of associated fractures of the upper limb in fractures of the radial head. *Strategies in Trauma and Limb Reconstruction* 2008; 3: 71–74.

16. A. Mastocytosis.

This is a rare disorder characterized by proliferation of mast cells in the skin, bone marrow, liver, spleen, lymph nodes, and small bowel. Histamine released from mast cells is responsible for the associated symptoms of episodic flushing, pruritis, hypotension, and diarrhoea. The serum tryptase level is also elevated in mastocytosis.

Whilst the other conditions mentioned could also cause diffuse thickening of small bowel folds, the associated clinical laboratory findings and osteosclerosis are diagnostic of mastocytosis.

Levine MS, Rubesin SE, and Laufer I. Pattern approach for diseases of mesenteric small bowel on barium studies. *Radiology* 2008; 249: 445–460.

17. D. Haemophilia.

There are three salient features to this question. Firstly, widening of the intercondylar notch—this is typically caused by haemophilia and JRA, but can also be caused by tuberculous arthritis. Secondly, causes of arthritis with variable loss of joint space. This is seen in tuberculous arthritis, amyloid, and PVNS, and may be present in haemophilia, although this can also cause severe arthropathy. Thirdly, causes of blooming artefact on GE sequences. This is usually caused by haemosiderin and is found in PVNS and haemophilia. Thus, when the whole picture is considered, the diagnosis is haemophilia.

Manaster B, May D, and Disler D. *Musculoskeletal Radiology: The Requisites*, 3rd edn, Mosby, 2007. pp. 562–566.
Chapman S and Nakielny R. *Aids to Radiological Differential Diagnosis*, 4th edn, Saunders, 2003. p. 107.

18. A. Aggressive granulomatous disease.

Well-delineated, rounded, focal areas of lucency at the cement bone interface, which are progressive, are suggestive of either infection or aggressive granulomatous disease. It can occur with both cemented and non-cemented components. Its origin is thought to be multifactorial. Metal, cement, or polyethylene fragments may penetrate the cement bone interface and induce a focal inflammatory foreign-body reaction, leading to osteolysis.

Primary loosening usually manifests as a wide (>2 mm) radiolucent zone at the cement–bone or metal–bone interface or a progressive radiolucent zone at the metal–cement interface. The radiolucent zones are not typically rounded.

Cement fractures are thin linear lucent areas within the cement. They may be asymptomatic, but are important to identify as they may lead to component failure.

Metal bead shedding is defined as opaque microfragments separated from the porous-coated femoral stem. Metal beads can be seen on immediate postoperative radiographs, as a consequence of the stem insertion. Bead shedding might later occur with loose non-cemented components, reflecting micro-motion of the stem. These metal beads are seen in the soft tissue adjacent to the hip replacement and their increase in number on follow-up indicates loosening.

Pluot E, Davis ET, Revell M, Davies AM, and James SLJ. Hip arthroplasty. Part 2: Normal and abnormal radiographic findings. *Clinical Radiology* 2009; 64: 961–971.

19. B. Bruising at the anterior aspect of the tibia.

Such bruising occurs in a dashboard injury when a posteriorly directed force is applied to the anterior aspect of the proximal tibia with the knee in flexion, such as occurs in an RTA. Bruising is also occasionally found in the posterior patella in this situation. Associated soft-tissue injuries are disruption of the posterior capsule and posterior cruciate ligament (PCL).

The pattern of injury in option A is caused by the pivot shift injury (valgus load in flexion combined with external rotation of the tibia or internal rotation of the femur). This will result in anterior cruciate ligament (ACL) disruption and the resultant anterior subluxation of the tibia causes impaction of the lateral femoral condyle against the posterolateral margin of the lateral tibial plateau. Soft-tissue injuries that may occur are tears of the posterior capsule, the posterior horn of the lateral or medial meniscus, and the medial collateral ligament (MCL). The kissing contusions in option C are as a result of hyperextension injury; resulting injuries may be to the ACL, PCL, or menisci. Option D describes the pattern found in clip injury, which involves a pure valgus stress while the knee is in mild flexion. The second area of bruising in the medial femoral condyle in this situation is due to avulsive stress to the MCL. The findings in option E are in keeping with transient lateral patellar dislocation, as discussed elsewhere in this chapter.

Mandalia V, Fogg AJ, Chari R, Murray J, Beale A, and Henson JH. Bone bruising of the knee. *Clinical Radiology* 2005; 60: 627–636.
Sanders TG, Medynski MA, Feller JF, and Lawhorn KW. Bone contusion patterns of the knee at MR imaging: footprint of the mechanism of injury. *RadioGraphics* 2000; 20: S130–S151.

20. A. Pseudomeningocoele.

Imaging in brachial plexus injury via CT myelography and/or MRI helps to determine whether the injury is pre- or postganglionic, which has therapeutic implications. Signal intensity changes in the spinal cord are seen in only 20% of preganglionic injuries and lack specificity. Intradural nerve root enhancement suggests functional impairment of the nerve roots, despite morphological continuity. This is not a common finding. T2WI signal intensity changes within the paraspinal muscles are observed in nerve root avulsion, but this is less accurate than enhancement on T1WI post contrast. Abnormal enhancement within the multifidus muscle is the most accurate of all paraspinal muscle findings since it is innervated by a single nerve root. Thickening of the brachial plexus, secondary to oedema and fibrosis, is seen in postganglionic injury. Traumatic pseudomeningocoele, although not pathognomonic, is the most valuable sign of a preganglionic lesion.

Yoshikawa T, Hayashi N, Yamamoto S, Tajiri, Y, Yoshioka N, Masumoto T et al. Brachial plexus injury: clinical manifestations, conventional imaging findings and the latest imaging techniques. *RadioGraphics* 2006; 26: S133–S143.

21. F. Medial head of gastrocnemius and semimembranosis.

Identification of anechoic cysts communicating with fluid between the semimembranosis and gastrocnemius tendons confirms the diagnosis of Baker's cyst. It is important to perform further imaging if the mass in the posterior compartment lacks signs of communication with fluid between the semimembranosis and medial gastrocnemius tendons. If this is the case, there are other possibilities for the lesion, including meniscal cyst or even a myxoid sarcoma.

Paczesney L and Kruczynski J. Ultrasound of the knee. *Seminars in Ultrasound, CT and MRI* 2011; 32: 114–124.

22. B. SAPHO syndrome.

The most common presentation for this condition is acne and palmoplantarpustulosis with changes in the sternocostoclavicular region where hyperostosis is seen, often with some erosive change. The condition can also cause a number of manifestations in the spine, ranging from focal hyperostosis of one or more lumbar vertebrae, to a syndrome strikingly similar to psoriatic spondylarthropathy. In the appendicular skeleton hyperostosis is commonly seen. SAPHO can also give rise to manifestations identical to osteomyelitis, but with no causative organism. In this respect there is overlap with CRMO syndrome. Patients are frequently human leucocyte antigen (HLA) B27 positive and psoriasis frequently coexists, leading some authors to suggest that SAPHO is a variant of psoriatic arthropathy, although this is not widely accepted.

Cotton A, Flipo R, Mentre A, Delaporte E, Duquesnoy B, and Chastanet P. SAPHO syndrome. *RadioGraphics* 1995; 15: 1147–1154.

23. D. Chondroblastoma.

These are radiolucent lesions that typically occupy the epiphysis of long bones in younger people, usually before skeletal maturity. They tend to be less than 4 cm in size, with approximately three-quarters having a sclerotic border and one-third a calcified matrix seen on plain radiographs.

Chondromyxoid fibromas are rare benign tumours occurring in predominantly the second and third decades of life. They characteristically have sclerotic margins and appear lobulated or 'bubbly'. They usually arise in the metaphysis of long bones with occasional diaphyseal extension.

GCTs tend to occur in young adulthood following skeletal maturity. Patients usually present with pain. The lesion is purely lytic, typically with well-defined, but non-sclerotic, margins. When present in long bones, the lesions are typically metaphyseal, extending across a fused epiphysis to a subarticular location. Periosteal reaction is atypical, but expansile remodelling, cortical penetration, and soft-tissue extension may be seen.

Stacy GS, Peabody TD, and Dixon LB. Mimics on radiography of giant cell tumor of bone. *American Journal of Roentogenology* 2003; 181: 1583–1589.

24. B. 75% of patients will have positive radiographic findings on plain film.

The clinical vignette alludes to a diagnosis of multiple myeloma (MM) and 50% bone destruction must occur before a myelomatous lesion will be visible on plain film. Four distinct forms of bony involvement have been described in MM: (1) plasmacytoma, a solitary lytic lesion that predominately affects the spine, pelvis, skull, ribs, sternum, and proximal appendages, (2) diffuse skeletal involvement (myelomatosis), which classically manifests as osteolytic lesions with discrete margins and uniform size, (3) diffuse skeletal osteopenia, without well-defined lytic lesions, which predominately involves the spine (multiple compression fractures may be seen with this pattern), (4) sclerosing myeloma, which results in sclerotic bony lesions, and is associated with POEMS syndrome (polyneuropathy, organomegally, endocrinopathy, monoclonal gammopathy and skin changes).

As well as typically producing general hyperintensity on T2WI and hypointensity on T1WI in diffuse myelomatous involvement, plasmacytomas may produce focal areas of hypointensity on T1WI/hyperintensity on T2WI. STIR imaging allows better assessment of marrow involvement; fat-suppressed post contrast studies can demonstrate enhancement in focal or diffuse disease. These findings are not specific for MM and may be seen in spinal metastases. However, MM is suspected whenever MR images depict an expansile focal mass, multiple focal masses in the axial skeleton, diffuse marrow involvement, particularly at known sites of normal hematopoiesis, or multiple compression fractures in a patient with no known primary malignancy. ^{99m}Tc-based bone scanning under-appreciates the extent of disease. FDG-PET has been used to study relapsing patients in whom recurrent disease is not easily detectable with routine imaging. PET, in this instance, has been found to aid in the detection of unsuspected sites of medullary and extramedullary disease.

Angtuaco EJ, Fassas AB, Walker R, Sethi R, and Barlogie B. Multiple myeloma: clinical review and diagnostic imaging. *Radiology* 2004; 231: 11–23.

25. B. Wood.

Radiography is highly sensitive for foreign bodies considered radio-opaque. All glass material is radio-opaque to some degree on radiographs and does not need to contain lead. The role for ultrasound is limited to those foreign bodies that are radiolucent, such as wood and plastic. Wood appears hyperechoic with marked posterior acoustic shadowing. Ultrasound can detect wooden foreign bodies as small as 2.5 mm in length with 87% sensitivity and 97% specificity. Plastic is also radiolucent, but less echogenic than other foreign bodies on ultrasound.

Horton LK, Jacobson JA, Powell A, Fessell DP, and Hayes CW. Sonography and radiography of soft tissue foreign bodies. *American Journal of Roentgenology* 2001; 176: 1155–1159.

26. B. Shin splints.

Excessive exertion of tibialis and soleus muscles of the legs causes periostitis along the muscular attachments. This results in longitudinal linear uptake on delayed bone scan images. The angiogram and blood pool images are usually normal compared to stress fracture, which is associated with hyperperfusion and hyperaemia. On delayed images focal fusiform uptake is seen with stress fracture.

Infection is associated with hyperperfusion, hyperaemia, and focal increased uptake.

Osteoid osteoma demonstrates hyperperfusion, hyperaemia, and focal double density due to nidus and reactive osteosclerosis.

Paget's disease is associated with increased uptake in an enlarged and deformed bone. Age and clinical presentation are also against this diagnosis.

Hypertrophic osteoarthropathy is associated with irregular cortical uptake producing the 'tramline' sign.

Love C, Din AS, Tomas MB, Kalapparambath TP and Palestro CJ. Radionuclide bone imaging: an illustrative review. *RadioGraphics* 2003; 23: 341–358.

27. A. The MRI findings correlate well with the severity of findings on plain film radiography.

MRI has been shown to correlate well with the severity of OA as depicted on plain film radiography. Neither MRI nor plain film appearances are significantly associated with the patient's symptoms.

Link T, Steinbach L, Ghosh S, Ries M, Lu Y, Lane N et al. Osteoarthritis: MR imaging findings in different stages of disease and correlation with clinical findings. *Radiology* 2003; 226: 373–381.

28. D. Intraosseus lipoma.

This is usually asymptomatic and discovered as an incidental finding in adults between 30 and 60 years. The calcaneus is the most common site for intraosseus lipoma, accounting for approximately 32% of cases. The key radiographic features are as described. The central dystrophic calcification seen in approximately 62% of cases is considered pathognomic.

The major differential diagnosis of this lesion is a simple bone cyst, although this would not contain central calcification. Unlike bone cysts elsewhere, it is seen at this site into adulthood. Also within the differential diagnosis is a pseudolesion within the calcaneus, caused by a relative paucity of trabecular bone at the same location. Again, central calcification would not be a feature in this phenomenon.

Enchondroma is typically a well-defined osteolytic lesion with central calcification, but it usually has a predilection for tubular bones and would be exceedingly rare in the calcaneus. The described appearances are not typical for bone infarct.

Foo LF and Raby N. Tumours and tumour-like lesions in the foot and ankle. *Clinical Radiology* 2005; 60: 308–332.

29. C. Osteosarcoma.

The telangiectatic variety of osteosarcoma does show fluid–fluid levels, as does malignant fibrous histiocytoma or any necrotic bone tumour. Telangiectatic osteosarcoma is highly vascular and contains necrotic tissue and blood, with tumour located only along the periphery and septa. MRI will thus reveal enhancing nodularity in the latter locations; this finding will be absent in the case of ABC or GCT. In addition to those mentioned in the stem, the plain film findings include bone expansion and cortical breakthrough.

Unlike the other lesions, osteoblastoma does not demonstrate fluid–fluid levels on MRI; it is more common in the posterior elements of the spine than in the long bones. ABC, GCT, and chondroblastoma have a narrower zone of transition on plain film than telangiectatic osteosarcoma. GCT is subarticular. Chondroblastoma is epiphyseal.

Other benign causes of fluid–fluid levels include simple bone cysts and fibrous dysplasia.

Chapman S and Nakielny R. *Aids to Radiological Differential Diagnosis*, 4th edn, Elsevier, 2003. p. 62.
Manaster BJ, May DA, and Disler DG. *Musculoskeletal Imaging: The Requisites*, 3rd edn, Mosby, 2007. p. 429.

30. E. Posterior humeral head indentation.

Anterior dislocation occurs when the arm is forcibly externally rotated and abducted. Radiographically, the humeral head lies inferior and medial to the glenoid on the AP view. The Hill–Sachs deformity is an indentation on the posterosuperior portion of the humeral head and indicates a greater likelihood of recurrence. A Bankart deformity is a bony fragment off the inferior glenoid. Anterior humeral head indentation is a 'reverse Hill–Sachs' deformity seen in posterior dislocations.

Brant WE and Helms CA. *Fundamentals of Diagnostic Radiology*, 3rd edn, Lippincott Williams & Wilkins, 2007. pp. 1119–1123.

31. E. High signal within the disc on T2WI.

Degenerative disc disease with associated degenerative modic type 1 endplate change (endplate oedema) can mimic discitis. All the mentioned changes are seen in both conditions except high signal within the disc on T2WI, which is seen in infection/discitis. In contrast, the degenerated disc is of low signal due to loss of hydration.

In addition, disc enhancement and paravertebral inflammatory tissue, soft-tissue mass, and fluid collection are associated with infection.

Long SS, Yablon CM, and Eisenberg RL. Bone marrow signal alteration in the spine and sacrum. *American Journal of Roentgenology* 2010; 195: W178–W200.

32. B. Grade 1 osteophytosis in the knee.

While the Kellegren and Lawrence grading of OA is the most widely used scale for grading OA on plain films, early osteophyte formation is not definitively 'arthritic' change. Studies have shown that patients with this type of early change infrequently progress to developing more severe disease. Recent research in OA is focused on the impact of the subchondral bone on the disease, rather than hyaline cartilage. This is evidenced by increased uptake on bone scan being closely linked to progressive OA, even in patients with relatively normal joints on plain film. The foci of high signal on T2WI and STIR are bone marrow lesions that if persistent can indicate pathology in the subchondral bone, which can lead to arthritic change. The serpiginous line describes the classical finding of avascular necrosis. Both this and osteochondral defects lead to progressive OA change.

Watt I. Osteoarthritis revisited—again! *Skeletal Radiology* 2009; 38: 419–423.

33. A. Use fast spin echo (FSE) imaging rather than GE imaging.

Magnetization of the implant affects the local field gradient, proton dephasing, and spin frequency, resulting in signal void, spatial distortion, and spurious high signal. The lack of a 180° rephasing pulse in GE sequences, as opposed to SE/FSE sequences, means that T2* effects are not reversed and a greater dephasing of spins occurs in GE than in SE/FSE techniques. Thus GE techniques have a greater sensitivity to magnetic susceptibility effects. This is detrimental when imaging patients with metal prostheses, but can be used to advantage in certain clinical situations, e.g. when identifying subtle haemorrhage due to the magnetic susceptibility effects of iron in haemosiderin (a blood breakdown product).

Magnetic susceptibility artefacts are increased with higher field strengths. Positioning the long axis of the prosthesis parallel to the main magnetic field direction (β0) reduces susceptibility artefact.

Spectral fat suppression is particularly susceptible to metallic artefact and should be avoided in favour of STIR, where some of the dephasing of proton spins, due to magnetic field inhomogeneity, is refocused by the 180° inversion pulse.

Reducing the number of voxels (increasing spatial resolution) reduces diffusion-related signal intensity loss. It also reduces the spatial definition of the signal void and therefore leads to a reduction in the apparent size of the void.

Cahir JG, Toms AP, Marshall TJ, Wimhurst J, and Nolan J. CT and MRI of hip arthroplasty. *Clinical Radiology* 2007; 62: 1163–1171.

34. C. HIV-associated arthritis.

This is oligoarticular, asymmetric and peripheral. It primarily affects the knees and ankles. It has a short duration of 1–6 weeks; radiography may reveal a joint effusion. Acute symmetric polyarthritis also occurs in HIV. It behaves clinically like RA, but patients are negative for rheumatoid factor. Features that help differentiate it from RA are periostitis and proliferative new bone formation. Occasionally an erosive variety with little or no proliferative bone formation occurs. Psoriatric arthritis has a higher prevalence among AIDS patients than in the general population. HPOA is associated with *P carinii* pneumonia (PCP) in AIDS. Plain films reveal periosteal reaction.

Kaposi's sarcoma uncommonly affects the bone, but does so most commonly in Africa. Non-Hodgkin lymphoma (NHL) is the second most common tumour in HIV infection. It can produce lytic, sclerotic, or mixed lesions with a wide zone of transition; they are usually lytic. Other musculoskeletal complications in AIDS include infections (cellulitis, osteomyelitis, septic arthritis, pyomyositis, necrotising fasciitis), Reiter's syndrome, undifferentiated spondyloarthropathy, polymyositis, osteonecrosis (especially of the femoral head), osteoporosis, rhabdomyolysis, and anaemia.

Restrepo CS, Lemos DF, Gordillo H, Odero R, Varghese T, Tiemann W et al. Imaging findings in musculoskeletal complications of AIDS. *RadioGraphics* 2004; 24: 1029–1049.

35. D. Scaphoid.

The findings describe perilunate dislocation, which is the most common carpal dislocation. It can occur without fracture (lesser arc injury) or with fracture (greater arc injury). Greater arc injuries are twice as frequent as lesser arc injuries. When describing these injuries the fracture is named first with the prefix 'trans' followed by the dislocation. Trans-scaphoid perilunate dislocation is the most common type of perilunate injury. Fractures of the trapezium, capitate, hamate, and triquetrum are also part of the greater arc injuries. Other radiographic signs of this injury include disruption of the carpal (Gilula) arcs and a triangular lunate on the AP view. An early sign is widening of the scaphoid–lunate space (Terry-Thomas sign), which suggests scapholunate dissociation. Lunate dislocation is the final stage of perilunate injuries, and is associated with the highest degree of instability.

Kaewlai R, Avery LL, Asrani AV, Abujudeh HH, Sacknoff R, and Novelline RA. Multidetector CT of carpal injuries: anatomy, fractures and fracture-dislocations. *RadioGraphics* 2008; 28: 1771–1784.

36. B. Joint space narrowing.

Around 5–10% of patients with sarcoidosis demonstrate skeletal involvement. The phalanges in the hands and feet are most commonly affected.

Joint space narrowing is unusual in sarcoidosis, unless neuropathic changes develop. Typical radiographic changes include cyst-like radiolucencies, a 'lace-like' pattern of bone destruction, bone erosions, and subcutaneous soft-tissue mass. These changes occurring in combination are diagnostic of sarcoidosis.

Koyama T, Ueda H, Togashi K, Umeoka S, Kataoka M, Nagai S et al. Radiologic manifestations of sarcoidosis in various organs. *RadioGraphics* 2004; 24: 87–104.

37. C. Erosive OA.

If the presence of erosions is ignored the pattern of disease is typical of OA. Erosive, or inflammatory, OA shows typical OA distribution, but with central erosions in the affected joint spaces in the distal IP, and less commonly proximal IP, joints. These central erosions in combination with marginal osteophytes give the classical gull-wing appearance to affected joints. Whilst individual joint appearance can be identical to psoriatic arthropathy, which can precede the development of the skin disease, the overall pattern is atypical, making it less likely. Also, while the distribution of CPPD arthropathy is often identical to OA, it would not cause erosions, and would usually be associated with chondrocalcinosis.

Manaster B, May D, and Disler D. *Musculoskeletal Radiology: The Requisites*, 3rd edn, Mosby, 2007. pp. 304–311 and 325–326.

38. D. Ganglion cyst.

What is being described is a ganglion cyst adjacent to the proximal tibiofibular joint that is causing a common peroneal nerve palsy. This is a well-recognized entity. Ganglion cysts can be uni- or multilocular. They occur predominately in peri-articular locations and may arise from tendon sheaths, joint capsules, bursae, or ligaments.

Although parameniscal cysts can extend inferiorly from the lateral knee joint margin, they typically show a communication with a meniscal tear. This is not described in the radiological findings and they are not typically centred at the level of the proximal tibiofibular joint.

Bursal distension can cause a multiloculated fluid collection. It can occur in typical locations around the knee joint, but not usually adjacent to the proximal tibiofibular joint. Examples include pes anserine bursitis, semi-membranosis-tibial collateral ligament bursitis, and pre-, supra-, and infrapatellar bursitis.

Focal tenosynovitis and chronic seroma do not particularly fit with the clinical and radiological findings.

Crundwell N, O'Donnell P, and Saifuddin A. Non-neoplastic conditions presenting as soft tissue tumours. *Clinical Radiology* 2007; 62: 18–27.

39. C. Ankylosis involves the vertebral edges or centre.

The question refers to ankylosing spondyitis. Ankylosis involves the vertebral edges or centre, with bony extension through the disc. The former is thought to be secondary to a Romanus lesion, the latter an Andersson lesion. Romanus lesions are irregularities and erosions involving the anterior and posterior edges of the vertebral endplates and are the earliest changes of spondylitis depicted on conventional radiographs. On MRI an Andersson lesion is depicted as disc-related signal-intensity abnormalities of one or both vertebral halves of a discovertebral unit. They are often hemispherically shaped. MRI is better than conventional radiography at depicting Romanus lesions, Andersson lesions (spondylodiscitis), and most other abnormalities, although ankylosis is equally well detected by both modalities.

Syndesmophtyes are difficult to detect on MRI. Plain radiography is superior in this respect because of its superior spatial resolution; syndesmophtyes are seen as bony outgrowths of the anterior vertebral edges. They occur in 15% of the vertebrae of patients. Apical pulmonary fibrosis affects 1% of patients. Sacroiliac (SI) joint erosion and widening is an early feature, and this may initially be more prominent on the iliac side of the joint, as the cartilage on that side is normally thinner. Later in the disease, sclerosis and ankylosis occur and the SI joints become symmetrically fused. Enthesitis is most prominently seen when the interspinal ligaments, those that extend between the spinous processes, and the supraspinal ligaments are affected. Ligamentous involvement is characterized by an increased signal intensity on either STIR images or contrast-enhanced T1WI fat saturated sequences. It may be associated with osteitis of adjacent bone marrow in the spinous processes. Arthritis of the synovial joints (e.g. facet joints) and insufficiency fractures (often spontaneous or after minor trauma) are also features of the seronegative spondylarthritides.

Hermann KA, Althoff CE, Schneider U, Zühlsdorf S, Lembcke A, Hamm B et al. Spinal changes in patients with spondyloarthritis: comparison of MR imaging and radiographic appearances. *RadioGraphics* 2005; 25: 559–570.

40. D. Complete symptom relief is seen in 90% after initial therapy.

Osteoid osteoma is a benign, but painful, bone tumour typically found in the lower limbs of children and young adults. The use of CT-guided RFA is considered to be a safe and effective technique and is considered to be the treatment of choice over open surgical approaches. Complete relief of symptoms is observed in approximately 90% after initial therapy and is reported up to 100% for secondary procedures. The procedure is performed under general or spinal anaesthesia. A typical clinical history of night pain relieved by non-steroidal analgesia and radiographic features of the central nidus are considered sufficiently diagnostic to proceed with RFA. The procedure should not be performed if there are doubts regarding diagnosis. Osteomas within the spine are potentially treated by RFA if the nidus is >1 cm from the dura/neural structures. Since most spinal osteomas are located within the posterior elements, however, RFA is generally unsuitable.

Linder NJ, Ozaki T, Roedl R, Gosheger G, Winkelmann W, and Wortler K. Percutaneous radiofrequency ablation in osteoid osteoma. *Journal of Bone & Joint Surgery* 2001; 83: 391–396.
Rosenthal DI, Hornicek FJ, Torriani M, Gebhardt MC, and Mankin HJ. Osteoid osteoma: percutaneous treatment with radiofrequency energy. *Radiology* 2003; 229: 171–175.

41. C. Sinding–Larsen–Johansson syndrome.

This is a traction tendonitis occurring at the attachment of the patellar tendon to the inferior pole of the patella. Repetitive stress/microtrauma at the tendinous attachment results in calcification or ossification of the tendon on the plain film. MRI demonstrates oedema within the tendon and at the inferior pole of the patella.

Similar changes occurring at the tibial attachment of the patellar tendon is called Osgood–Schlatter disease.

Patellar sleeve fracture is a unique paediatric injury in which the cartilage at the inferior pole of the patella is avulsed along with a small bone fragment.

The quadriceps tendon inserts into the superior pole of the patella, therefore a partial tear produces oedema at the superior pole of the patella.

Dupuis CS, Westra SJ, Makris J, and Wallace EC. Injuries and conditions of the extensor mechanism of the pediatric knee. *RadioGraphics* 2009; 29: 877–886.

42. A. Focal involvement.

Whilst differentiating these conditions can be difficult and they frequently overlap, there are certain features that can be of value. Neuropathic arthropathy (NA) seldom affects a single bone/joint in the foot, and is most common in the midfoot region. As such a more focal abnormality, or abnormality affecting the metatarsal heads, or other points of pressure, should indicate osteomyelitis. Whilst high T2WI/STIR, low T1WI and enhancement are seen in osteomyelitis, it is also seen in acute NA and as such is not a good differentiating factor. The converse is not true, where low signal on T1WI and T2WI, typical of chronic NA, would make the presence of osteomyelitis unlikely.

Tan P and The J. MRI of the diabetic foot: differentiation of infection from neuropathic change. *British Journal of Radiology* 2007; 80: 939–948.

43. B. Aneurysmal bone cyst.

ABC accounts for approximately 5% of primary rib lesions, excluding myeloma. The radiological findings and age described in the question are classical for this lesion. Approximately 75% of patients are <20 years of age. The key findings on MRI are the fluid–fluid levels due to the settling of degraded blood products within the cysts. Fluid–fluid levels may also be a feature of other lesions, including GCT and chondroblastoma, but the thin, well-defined margins of an ABC should help to distinguish it from other lesions, particularly in this young age group.

Fibrous dysplasia is the most common benign rib lesion. The radiographic appearances are variable, but may show unilateral fusiform enlargement and deformity with cortical thickening and increased trabeculation of one or more ribs. The matrix may appear lytic, may demonstrate a ground-glass appearance, or rarely be sclerotic. Amorphous or irregular calcifications may be seen within the lesion on CT, and MRI shows low to intermediate signal on T1WI and variable T2WI signal.

Enchondromas more typically arise in the anterior cartilaginous portion of the rib. Radiographs reveal a lobulated, well-demarcated osteolytic lesion that demonstrates mild expansion and well-defined, sclerotic margins. There is typically matrix calcification and CT is more sensitive at detecting this when the calcification is subtle. MRI shows T2WI hyperintense foci that appear to coalesce with one another and reflect the high fluid content of hyaline cartilage.

Chondroblastoma of a rib is reported in the literature, but would be exceedingly rare and typically occurs in the epiphyses of long bones. Cystic haemangiomatosis is a rare disease of disseminated multifocal haemangiomatous or lymphangiomatous lesions in the skeleton and is usually an incidental asymptomatic finding.

Hughes EK, James SLJ, Butt S, Davies AM, and Saifuddin A. Benign primary tumours of the ribs. *Clinical Radiology* 2006; 61: 314–322.

44. D. Polyvinyl chloride.

This results in resorption of the middle portion of the terminal phalanx. The other answers cause resorption of the terminal tufts of the distal phalanges. Other causes of resorption of the terminal tuft include Raynaud's, diabetes, syringomyelia, burns, trauma, epidermolysis bullosa, congenital phenytoin toxicity (in infants of epileptic mothers), and snake and scorpion venom. Hyperparathyroidism can cause tuft, mid-portion, and periarticular resorption; psoriatic arthropathy can cause tuft and periarticular resorption.

Chapman S and Nakielny R. *Aids to Radiological Differential Diagnosis*, 4th edn, Elsevier, 2003. p. 60.

45. A. Differentiating partial from full thickness tear.

MR arthrography is most helpful for outlining labral-ligamentous abnormalities in the shoulder and distinguishing partial thickness from full thickness tears in the rotator cuff. The technique involves injection of diluted gadolinium mixed with iodinated contrast, which allows fluoroscopic confirmation of intra-articular needle placement. Partial and full thickness tears may not be distinguishable on standard T1WI because fat and gadolinium have similar signal intensities. This is especially the case when cuff tendons show contrast solution extending to the bursal surface but not definitively through it. This problem can be overcome with use of fat suppression. MR arthrography should include a T2WI sequence to identify bursal fluid collections and tears.

T2WI is also helpful in characterizing incidental bone marrow lesions. Inadvertent injection of gas may lead to a false-positive diagnosis of intra-articular loose bodies, but gas bubbles will rise to non-dependent regions, whereas loose bodies will gravitate to dependent locations. No accurate MR imaging criteria are recognized in the diagnosis of capsular laxity.

Steinbach LS, Palmer WE, and Schweitzer ME. Special Focus Session: MR arthrography. *RadioGraphics* 2002; 22: 1223–1246.

46. D. Plantar fibromatosis.

Fibrous masses containing mature collagen are homogenously low in signal on T1WI and T2WI sequences, and demonstrate enhancement with gadolinium. Common fibrous masses in the foot are plantar fibromatosis and fibroma of the tendon sheath.

Morton's neuroma is typically intermediate in signal on T1WI and low on T2WI with variable contrast enhancement. Lipomas follow fat signal intensity. They are high on T1WI and T2WI, and low on fat-suppressed sequences. A ganglion cyst follows fluid signal. Ganglion cysts are low on T1WI and high on T2WI with rim enhancement. Haemangiomas are of mixed signal on T1WI and T2WI due to the presence of vessels, fat, and fibrous tissue. The vascular portions of hemangiomas enhance homogenously.

Roberts CC, Morrison WB, and Liu PT. Imaging evaluation of foot and ankle pathology: self-assessment module. *American Journal of Roentgenology* 2008; 190: S18–S22.

47. E. The presence of hypothyroidism is associated with the diagnosis.

Disorders associated with CPPD are the four Hs: hyperparathyroidism, haemochromatosis, hypothyroidism, and hypomagnesaemia. Use of nomenclature in this disorder is confused. Pseudogout is the clinical presentation of an acutely inflamed joint due to calcium pyrophosphate crystal deposition, and as such is not a radiological diagnosis. Pseudogout syndrome is the dominant feature in only 10–20% of cases of CPPD. Another 10–20% of cases are asymptomatic, whilst most present with symptoms identical to OA, with occasional flares. Disproportionate involvement of the patellofemoral joint is a characteristic feature, but is only occasionally seen. Pyrophosphate arthropathy is a description of the pattern of disease present due to crystal deposition, and as such is not a diagnosis made by analysis of joint aspirate.

Steinbach L and Resnick D. Calcium pyrophosphate dehydrate crystal deposition disease revisited. *Radiology* 1996; 200: 1–9.

48. E. Preiser disease.

The x-ray appearances are typical for osteonecrosis within the scaphoid. This is usually post-traumatic in aetiology, but when idiopathic it is known as Preiser disease. Postulated mechanisms for the osteonecrosis are repetitive minor trauma or secondary to drug treatment (e.g. steroids).

The remaining wrong answers refer to osteochondroses affecting the foot. Freiberg disease affects the head of the second metatarsal, Kohler disease the tarsal navicular, Iselin disease the base of the fifth metatarsal and Sever disease the calcaneal apophysis.

Resnick D. *Diagnosis of Bone and Joint Disorders*, 3rd edn, Saunders, 1995. p. 3604.

49. E. Insufficiency fractures.

This patient has developed osteoporosis due to heparin administration (and with age). This has resulted in thoracic kyphosis and the 'H' sign of increased uptake within the sacral body and alae, which is classical of insufficiency fractures of the sacrum. Often there will have been relatively minor trauma that will not be reported by the patient, and there may be associated pubic rami fractures. Radiotherapy to the area (e.g. in gynaecological malignancy) is another predisposing factor.

Multiple myeloma, metastases from renal cell carcinoma, and chordoma are typically osteolytic and result in osteopenia at isotope bone scan (IBS), although the investigation has poor sensitivity for myeloma. Brown tumours do cause increased uptake on IBS, but we are not given a history of renal failure or hyperparathyroidism to explain their presence. There is no history given to suggest infection.

Bone metastases which cause an increased uptake on IBS are breast, prostate, lymphoma, pulmonary carcinoid, mucinous GI, and bladder tumours. Renal cell carcinoma, thyroid, and melanoma typically cause photopoenia.

Love C, Din A, Tomas M, Kalapparambath T, and Palestro C. Radionuclide bone imaging: an illustrative review. *RadioGraphics* 2003; 23: 341–358.

50. E. Synovial osteochondromatosis.

The primary form of this represents an uncommon benign neoplastic process with hyaline cartilage nodules in the subsynovial tissue of a joint, tendon sheath, or bursa. Secondary synovial chondromatosis is associated with joint abnormalities, such as mechanical or arthritic conditions, that cause intraarticular chondral bodies. The primary form of the disease predominantly affects men in the third to fifth decades. The knee is the most common site, but it is also seen in the hip, shoulder, elbow, and ankle; less commonly the MCP, IP, distal radioulnar, and acromioclavicular joints are involved. It can rarely involve extra-articular sites, the synovium about the tendons, or bursa. Clinical symptoms typically include pain, swelling, and restriction of the range of motion of the joint. Radiologic findings are frequently pathognomonic. Radiographs reveal multiple intraarticular calcifications (70–95% of cases) of similar size and shape distributed throughout the joint, with typical 'ring-and-arc' chondroid mineralization. Extrinsic erosion of bone is seen in 20–50% of cases. Juxtaarticular osteopenia is not typically apparent in synovial chondromatosis unless it is the result of disuse. CT is often diagnostic if the bodies are adequately mineralized and is particularly helpful for identifying characteristic ring-and-arc or punctate mineralization and the multiplicity of nodules in cases for which radiographic findings are normal or equivocal. Lack of mineralization of the bodies does occur in which cases MRI is very helpful to distinguish from, for example, PVNS or amyloid. The most common pattern on MRI (77% of cases) reveals low to intermediate signal intensity with T1WI and very high signal intensity with T2WI with hypointense calcifications.

Murphey MD, Vidal JA, Fanburg-Smith JC, and Gajewski DA. Imaging of synovial chondromatosis with radiologic–pathologic correlation. *RadioGraphics* 2007; 27: 1465–1488.
Manaster BJ, May DA, and Disler DG. *Musculoskeletal Imaging: The Requisites*, 3rd edn, Mosby, 2007. p. 355.

51. E. Increased conspicuity on prolonged TE images.

Distinguishing recurrent metastases from rebound hematopoietic marrow is difficult on standard T1WI and T2WI sequences because both have intermediate signal intensity on T1WI and high signal intensity on T2WI. They may also occur in same anatomic regions.

Out-of-phase GE imaging is useful in differentiating the two. Most neoplastic processes replace the marrow elements such as fat, osseous trabeculae, and hematopoietic elements, but hyperplastic red marrow does not. Out-of-phase imaging allows detection of intralesional fat by demonstrating a drop in signal intensity compared to in-phase images.

Lengthening of echo results in loss of signal of rebound red marrow due to T2* dephasing, while the water-laden metastatic foci become more conspicuous.

Andrews CL. Evaluation of the marrow space in the adult hip. *RadioGraphics* 2000; 20: S27–S42.

52. C. Psoriatic arthritis.

Ankylosing spondylitis causes a symmetrical sacroiliitis. The syndesmophytes associated with this are marginal and fine. It also typically progresses superiorly from the lumbar spine. Both reactive arthritis and psoriatic arthritis cause an asymmetric sacroiliitis and the syndesmophytes are usually centred on the thoracolumbar spine and are non-marginal and bulky. Retrocalcaneal bursitis and erosions, whilst more common in reactive arthritis, can occur in psoriatic arthritis, and reactive arthritis would uncommonly affect the hands. Also, with all other factors being equal, psoriatic arthritis is much more common than reactive arthritis, even without the skin manifestations, which are absent in up to 20% at presentation.

Manaster B, May D, and Disler D. *Musculoskeletal Radiology: The Requisites*, 3rd edn, Mosby, 2007. pp. 318–327.

53. F. ↑T1 ↑T2 ↓STIR

The variable proportions of vascular and fatty soft-tissue elements influence the MRI appearance of haemangiomas. Lesions with a predominantly fatty matrix show high signal intensity on T1WI, intermediate to high signal intensity on T2WI, and loss of signal on STIR or fat-suppressed T2WI. If the vascular elements predominate, the lesions appear hypointense on T1WI and extremely hyperintense on STIR and T2WI. If MRI is inconclusive, CT may be helpful in identifying the typical pattern of haemangiomatous bone replacement, such as the honeycomb, 'soap bubble' or 'sunburst' appearance.

Woertler K. Benign bone tumours and tumour-like lesions: value of cross-sectional imaging. *European Radiology* 2003;13: 1820–1835.

54. C. Posterior iliac horns.

Nail-patella syndrome (hereditary onycho-osteodysplasia) is an autosomal dominant condition characterized by nail dysplasia, patella hypoplasia, elbow hypoplasia, and iliac horns. Iliac horns are present in over 80% of patients and are considered pathognomonic. They arise at the site of gluteus medius and project posterolaterally. Patella hypoplasia results in chronic knee pain and recurrent dislocations. Elbow hypoplasia is typically towards the lateral side of the joint. Madelung deformity and calcaneo-valgus feet are other features described in nail-patella syndrome. The most important non-orthopaedic condition is an immune complex nephropathy, which can result in end-stage renal failure. These patients are also at risk of open-angle glaucoma.

Jones C, Diamond D, Amirfeyz R, and Gargan M. Nail-patella syndrome. *Orthopaedics & Trauma* 2009; 23: 362–364.

55. C. Gaucher's disease.

All these conditions cause Erlenmeyer flask deformity and are associated with pathological fractures. However, the history of previous avascular necrosis of femoral head suggests Gaucher's disease. Sickle-cell disease (SCD) may also cause all the above bone changes.

Gaucher's disease is a rare familial metabolic disorder caused by deficiency of the enzyme β-glucocerebrosidase. This leads to accumulation of glucocerebroside in reticuloendothelial cells (macrophages) of the liver, spleen, and bone marrow.

The imaging findings include delayed growth, osteopenia, Erlenmeyer flask deformity, metaphyseal notching of humeri, bone infarction/avascular necrosis, and pathological fractures. Diffuse marrow replacement with low signal on T1WI is noted on MRI. Visceral manifestations include hepato-splenomegaly and reticulonodular interstitial lung disease.

McHugh K, Olsen OE, and Vellodi A. Gaucher disease in children: radiology of non-central nervous system manifestations. *Clinical Radiology* 2004; 59: 117–123.

56. D. Polymyositis and erosive arthropathy.

There is a lot of overlap in the features of connective tissue diseases, with a number of patients labelled as mixed-connective tissue disease due to this. There are features of these conditions that can help differentiate them. SLE is a great mimic and can manifest in a myriad of ways. Erosive disease is not typically seen in SLE, but SLE does classically give a reducible deforming arthropathy of the hands, which is most pronounced on Norgaard views, but can appear completely normal on PA hand views. Avascular necrosis (AVN) and deforming arthropathy are not typically seen in systemic sclerosis. Acro-osteolysis and soft-tissue calcifications, especially in the fingertip pulps, are classical features of this disease. Polymyositis classically gives high T2WI signal in muscles due to myositis. It does not typically give erosions.

Boutry N, Hachulla E, Zanetti-Musielak E, Morel M, Demondion X, Cotten A et al. Imaging features of musculoskeletal involvement in systemic sclerosis. *European Radiology* 2007; 17: 1172–1180.

Manaster B, May D, and Disler D. *Musculoskeletal Radiology: The Requisites*, 3rd edn, Mosby, 2007. pp. 328–334.

57. C. Pattern of ossification in the lesion.

The pattern of ossification is likely to be the most helpful. In post-traumatic myositis ossificans, the ossification occurs classically first at the periphery, whereas in parosteal osteosarcoma, the ossification is diffuse, but predominantly central. Periosteal reaction is typically absent in both these lesions and both lesions may contain lucent areas on plain radiograph.

A lucent cleft between the mass and the bony cortex, representing periosteum, is characteristic in parosteal osteosarcoma, but frequently is not seen as the tumour envelops bone. A thick lucent zone separating myositis ossificans from an adjacent bony cortex is typical, but may not be seen on plain radiograph if the lesion is immediately juxta-cortical.

O'Donnell P. Evaluation of focal bone lesions: basic principles and clinical scenarios. *Imaging* 2003; 15: 298–323.

58. B. Chondrosarcoma.

The findings describe development of chondrosarcoma in an area of Paget's disease. While osteosarcoma is more common than either malignant fibrous histiocytoma or chondrosarcoma in Paget's disease, the 'ring-and-arc' calcification in the vignette indicates chondroid rather than osteoid calcification. Sarcomatous transformation in Paget's is rare, occurring in approximately 1% of cases, but should be suspected if there is new focal pain or swelling. Such lesions, even osteosarcomas, are usually lucent. Periosteal reaction is often absent due to the rapidity of bone destruction.

Other complications of Paget's disease include those related to osseous weakening (deformity and fracture), arthritis, neurological entrapment, and both benign and malignant GCT.

Chondroblastoma may have internal chondroid calcification (60%) but is a well-defined, benign, lucent lesion with a sclerotic rim occurring in the epiphyses of children and young adults. Bronchial carcinoid metastases are usually purely osteoblastic (i.e. sclerotic, not lucent).

Smith S, Murphey M, Motamedi K, Mulligan M, Resnik C, and Gannon F. Radiologic spectrum of Paget disease of bone and its complications with pathological correlation. *RadioGraphics* 2002; 22: 1191–1216.

59. C. Reduced upper-to-lower segment ratio.

Marfan syndrome is an autosomal dominant multisystem connective tissue disorder, but approximately 25% are sporadic mutations. Mutation of the fibrillin-1 gene is the underlying genetic abnormality. There is a broad phenotype expression, although diagnosis can be made clinically based on the presence of major and minor features as per the Ghent classification system. In the absence of a family history, the presence of two major criteria in two different organ systems and a minor criterion in a third system supports a diagnosis of Marfan syndrome.

In this case, dissection of the ascending aorta is a major cardiovascular criterion and spontaneous pneumothorax a minor pulmonary system criterion. Of the musculoskeletal manifestations, reduced upper-to-lower segment ratio is a major criterion, the remaining options are all minor criteria. Other musculoskeletal system major criteria include scoliosis with a curvature greater than 20°, pectus carinatum, pectus excavatum requiring surgery, acetabular protrusion, and medial displacement of the medial malleolus causing pes planus.

Ha HI, Seo JB, Lee SH, Kang J-W, Goo HW, Lim T-H et al. Imaging of Marfan syndrome: multisystemic manifestations. *RadioGraphics* 2007; 27: 989–1004.

60. C. In the normal popliteal fossa, the popliteal artery and vein pass lateral to the medial head of the gastrocnemius and are surrounded by fat.

Popliteal artery entrapment syndrome is a developmental abnormality resulting from an abnormal relationship between the popliteal artery and neighbouring muscles. It is commonly seen in healthy young adults and can present with symptoms of intermittent claudication or thromboembolism. The anatomical abnormality occurs bilaterally in 27–67%.

The popliteal vessels normally pass lateral to the medial head of gastrocnemius. An anomalous origin of the medial head or an anomalous course of the popliteal artery may result in extrinsic compression of the artery.

Doppler and digital subtraction angiography (DSA) findings may be non-specific with a wide spectrum of findings. A normal Doppler or DSA with neutral ankle position does not exclude the diagnosis. Provocative measures with ankle dorsiflexion and plantar flexion may be useful in confirming the diagnosis on Doppler and DSA, but they do not demonstrate the underlying anatomical cause. Non-invasive assessment with CT angiogram or MR angiogram is preferred as they also demonstrate the anatomical abnormality.

Hai Z, Guangrui S, Yuan Z, Zhoudong X Cheng L, Jingmin L et al. CT angiography and MRI in patients with popliteal artery entrapment syndrome. *American Journal of Roentgenology* 2008; 191: 1760–1766.

Chew FS and Bui-Mansfield LT. Imaging popliteal artery disease in young adults with claudication: self-assessment module. *American Journal of Roentgenology* 2007; 189: S13–S16.

61. E. Renal osteodystrophy.

The first important observation to note is the referral route. A patient from the dialysis unit is going to have renal failure, thereby excluding tertiary hyperparathyroidism and making primary less likely. This leaves Paget's disease, osteomalacia, and renal osteodystrophy. The patient clearly has features of both hyperparathyroidism (subperiosteal resorption, brown tumour in iliac bone) and osteomalacia (Looser's zones), giving the diagnosis of renal osteodystrophy, which has features of both. Another feature of renal osteodystrophy is the soft-tissue calcification noted in the hand. The Looser's zones are small stress fractures on the load-bearing aspect of a bone, caused by osteomalacia. This contrasts with the stress fractures seen on the tensile aspect of bones (i.e. lateral aspect of femur) seen in Paget's disease and fibrous dysplasia. Whilst Brown tumours are more closely associated with primary hyperparathyroidism, the majority actually occur in secondary hyperparathyroidism as this disease is much more prevalent.

Manaster B, May D, and Disler D. *Musculoskeletal Radiology: The Requisites*, 3rd edn, Mosby, 2007. pp. 373–385.

62. E. Reverse hybrid total hip replacement.

A combination of a cemented acetabular cup and an uncemented femoral stem is known as a reverse hybrid hip total hip replacement. A hybrid total hip replacement is a combination of a cemented femoral stem and an uncemented acetabular cup.

A unipolar hemiarthroplasty comprises a combination of a femoral component articulating directly with the native cartilage surface of the acetabulum.

A bipolar hemiarthroplasty comprises a combination of a femoral component articulating with a cup inserted into the native acetabulum without fixation. This cup is usually made of polyethylene with a metal backing and can normally move within the native acetabular cavity as a result of the absence of fixation.

Hip resurfacing consists of replacing the surface of the femoral head by a metallic 'cap' without removing the femoral neck or instrumenting the femoral diaphysis. The cap used on the femoral head is virtually the same size as the natural head and articulates with an acetabular prosthetic cup, usually made of metal. This type of procedure is favoured in younger active patients and may allow for easier revision to a total hip replacement in later years.

Pluot E, Davis ET, Revell M, Davies AM, and James SLJ. Hip arthroplasty. Part 1: Prosthesis terminology and classification. *Clinical Radiology* 2009; 64: 954–960.

63. A. Metaphyseal lamellar periosteal reaction.

Hypertrophic pulmonary osteoarthropathy is a paraneoplastic syndrome secondary to the release of vasodilators. It typically causes burning pain and swelling, with the ankles and wrists being most commonly affected. Pulmonary causes include bronchogenic carcinoma, mesothelioma, and pleural fibroma. Radiographs demonstrate cortical thickening and lamellar periosteal proliferation in a diametaphyseal location. Bone scintigraphy will demonstrate patchy linear increased uptake along the cortical margins. Option B describes pachydermoperiostosis, a self-limited condition in adolescents. Option C is typical of thyroid acropachy. Cortical thickening and trabecular coarsening is a feature of Paget's disease and symmetrical, solid periosteal new bone formation is described in hypervitaminosis A.

Dahnert W. *Radiology Review Manual*, 6th edn, Lippincott Williams & Wilkins, 2007. p. 106.

64. D. Amyloidosis.

There are a lot of conditions that are capable of mimicking RA. In these cases a few key features can help reach a diagnosis. The classic finding in gout is of non-marginal erosions, as opposed to those described. Nevertheless, marginal erosions can occur with gout. An RA-type picture in the presence of non-marginal erosions or calcified soft-tissue nodules (tophi) should suggest this diagnosis. CPPD gives a more productive pattern of arthritis, such as seen with OA, affecting the radio-carpal joint. Thus, it is often suspected when the appearance is of OA with a 'funny distribution'. Amyloidosis is suggested first by the history of MM. Involvement of the hands is more commonly seen in amyloid secondary to prolonged dialysis, but can be seen when the amyloid is secondary to MM, when the wrists are often affected. Amyloid can closely resemble RA in its distribution and the pattern of erosions. However, three important features can help differentiate: amyloidosis classically preserves the joint space, is not usually associated with periarticular osteopenia, and amyloidosis causes well-demarcated subchondral cyst formation in excess to that expected from the degree of joint disease.

Manaster B, May D, and Disler D. *Musculoskeletal Radiology: The Requisites*, 3rd edn, Mosby, 2007. pp. 335–345.

65. B. Posterior cruciate ligament.

The avulsion injury described is a reverse Segond fracture. This injury is known to be associated with both mid-substance tears of the posterior cruciate ligament and avulsions of the PCL from the posterior tibial plateau. They can also be associated with medial meniscus injuries. They are not to be confused with a Segond fracture, which is a small elliptical fragment of bone avulsed from the lateral tibial plateau at the lateral joint margin, best seen on the AP view of the knee. They have a strong association with tears of the anterior cruciate ligament and also meniscal tears.

Gottsegen CJ, Eyer BJ, White EA, Learch TJ, and Forrester D. Avulsion fractures of the knee: imaging findings and clinical significance. *RadioGraphics* 2008; 28: 1755–1770.

66. A. Dysplasia epihysealis hemimelica (Trevor disease).

This is an uncommon developmental disorder relating to the formation of an osteochondroma-type lesion at the epiphyses of usually a single lower extremity. The epiphyses most commonly involved are those on either side of the knee or ankle. Typically it is only the medial or lateral side of the epiphyses affected (medial:lateral 2:1). The disease is usually recognized at a young age because of an antalgic gait, palpable mass, varus or valgus deformity, or limb length discrepancy.

Murphey MD, Choi JJ, Kransdorf MJ, Flemming DJ, and Gannon FH. Imaging of osteochondromas: variants and complications with radiologic-pathologic correlation. *RadioGraphics* 2000; 20: 1407–1434.

67. D. Sickle-cell disease.

Gaucher disease and SCD can both cause H-shaped vertebrae and avascular necrosis of the humeral heads, but Gaucher disease causes splenomegaly, whereas by adulthood SCD will usually have caused splenic infarction, resulting in a small, calcified spleen. Films illustrating the complications of these diseases are beloved by examiners in the 2B exam: remember to look for the mediastinal mass (extramedullary haematopoiesis) and AVN of the proximal humeri on the chest film.

Other musculoskeletal manifestations of SCD include osteomyelitis (particularly *salmonella* species), septic arthritis, and medullary bone infarcts. Infarction in SCD is common throughout the body and is responsible for the acute pain crisis. Infarction can occur in the liver, spleen, and kidneys, and can result in stroke.

Scheuermann's disease is osteochondrosis of the apophyses of the thoracic vertebrae and results in end-plate irregularity, Schmorl's nodes, loss of disc space, and kyphosis. True H-shaped vertebrae are not a feature.

Hereditary spherocytosis is an autosomal dominant condition. It produces splenomegaly and, as with other haematological conditions, can result in widening of the diploic spaces of the skull.

Primary bone lymphoma typically appears as a solitary focal lesion with an aggressive appearance.

Lonergan GJ, Cline DB, and Abbondanzo SL. Sickle cell anemia. *RadioGraphics* 2001; 21: 971–994.

68. D. Melorheostosis.

The radiographic findings describe the 'flowing candle-wax' sign, which indicates melorheostosis, a non-hereditary sclerosing bone dysplasia of unknown aetiology. Patients are often asymptomatic, being discovered incidentally. It is most common in the long bones. The disease can overlap with other sclerosing bone dysplasias such as osteopoikilosis (multiple ovoid bone islands) and osteopathia striata (metaphyseal longitudinal striations). Engelmann disease presents in childhood with neuromuscular dystrophy. Diaphyseal fusiform enlargement with cortical thickening is seen in the long bones. Fibrous dysplasia causes bone thinning.

Bansal A. The dripping candle wax sign. *Radiology* 2008; 246: 638–640.

69. B. Calcaneal fracture classification is based on fracture location at the posterior facet.

Calcaneal fractures represent 60% of fractures involving the tarsal bones. Axial loading resulting from a fall from a height is the most common cause followed by motor vehicle accidents. Treatment is based on accurate evaluation and classification of calcaneal fractures using multidetector CT reformats.

Calcaneal fractures are classified into intra-articular and extra-articular based on the involvement of the posterior facet of the subtalar joint. Intra-articular fractures, accounting for 75% of all calcaneal fractures, are further classified into four types depending on the number of fracture lines and fragments. Extra-articular fractures are classified into three types depending on whether the fracture involves the anterior, middle, or posterior aspect of calcaneus.

Bilateral fractures are seen in less than 10% of cases. Approximately 10% of calcaneal fractures are associated with compression injuries of the spine, commonly at the thoracolumbar junction.

Boehler's angle is formed by the intersection of (a) a line from the highest point of the posterior calcaneal tuberosity to the highest point of the posterior facet and (b) a line from the latter point to the highest of the anterior process. Normal Boehler's angle is 20–40°. An angle less than 20° indicates collapse of the posterior facet.

The sustentaculum tali is an eminence on the medial aspect of the calcaneus bearing the middle facet of subtalar joint.

Badillo K, Pacheco J, Padua S, Gomez A, Colon E, and Vidal JA. Multidetector CT evaluation of calcaneal fractures. *RadioGraphics* 2011; 31: 81–92.

70. C. Cerebral palsy.

As a radiologist you would obviously have been able to correct your orthopaedic colleague, that long gracile bones are examples of overtubulation, not undertubulation. As such options A, B, and E are not diagnostic considerations as these result in undertubulation and may cause an Erlenmeyer flask abnormality. This phenomenon is further described elsewhere in this chapter, but causes of Erlenmeyer flask abnormality include anaemias (thalassaemia, SCD), storage disorders (Gaucher's, Niemann–Pick), and skeletal dysplasias (Pyle's disease, craniometaphyseal dysplasia, Melnick–Needles syndrome).

The most common cause of over-tubulation is in patients with diminished weight bearing (cerebral palsy, myelomeningocele, arthrogryposis), with cerebral palsy being the most common of these. JRA and Marfan syndrome can also cause this appearance.

Manaster B, May D, and Disler D. *Musculoskeletal Radiology: The Requisites*, 3rd edn, Mosby, 2007. pp. 577–581.
Chapman S and Nakielny R. *Aids to Radiological Differential Diagnosis*, 4th edn, Saunders, 2003. p. 49.

71. A. None.

This is a complicated question, but one that is frequently posed to musculoskeletal radiologists. A full description is beyond the remit of this section and the reader is referred to the excellent synopsis referenced below. Basically the foot is divided into the hind foot and fore foot when assessing for congenital abnormalities. The tibio-calcaneal angle (angle made by a line drawn along the length of both bones) should be between 60° and 90°. Less than this is due to abnormal dorsiflexion (e.g. as seen with congenital vertical talus, or rocker bottom foot) and more is due to equinus deformity. Secondly, degree of hindfoot varus or valgus is assessed. The talo-calcaneal angle (on an frontal hindfoot x-ray this is the angle between the lines drawn along the length of each bone) should be between 15° and 40°; less is varus deformity and more is valgus. On the lateral view, the fore foot can be roughly assessed with two observations. Normally the metatarsals overlap. However, if the first metatarsal is the most plantar, then forefoot valgus is present (as the foot is too flat). If the metatarsals are not superimposed, then varus is present. The final step is to remember the features of the common conditions. These are clubfoot (hindfoot equinus and varus), pes planovalgus (hind foot and fore foot valgus, not equinus), and pes cavus (hindfoot valgus).

Manaster B, May D, and Disler D. *Musculoskeletal Radiology: The Requisites*, 3rd edn, Mosby, 2007. pp. 610–621.

72. D. Type IV.

Osteogenesis imperfecta in an adult is almost always type I or IV. Type I is the most common. Patients have can have normal stature and the characteristic blue sclera are seen in 90%. Patients also often have hearing impairment. Type IV has variable bone fragility, from mild to severe. Hearing impairment is less common, as is reduced stature. Blue sclera are present in children, but are often absent after adolescence. Type II is universally fatal in the neonatal period. Type III is also severe and often associated with reduced lifespan. Stature is significantly reduced. In patients who survive to adolescence the blue sclera are also often absent. Type V is not universally recognized, but is similar to type IV.

Manaster B, May D, and Disler D. *Musculoskeletal Radiology: The Requisites*, 3rd edn, Mosby, 2007. pp. 622–625.
Chapman S and Nakielny R. *Aids to Radiological Differential Diagnosis*, 4th edn, Saunders, 2003. pp. 585–586.

73. C. Kidneys

A superscan refers to a ^{99m}Tc-labelled technetium IBS where there is diffuse increased osseous uptake with *apparent* reduced renal and soft tissue uptake. The appearance is commonly due to widespread osteoblastic bony metastases (e.g. prostate or breast carcinoma), but is also caused by non-malignant disease (e.g. renal osteodystrophy, hyperparathyroidism, osteomalacia, myelofibrosis, Paget's disease). In metastatic disease there is usually higher uptake in the axial than the appendicular skeleton.

In IBS uptake is normally seen in bone, kidneys, and bladder, soft tissues (low levels), breasts (particularly in young women), and epiphyses (skeletally immature patients). Uptake is seen in the myocardium (high), brain (high), and bowel (moderate) in FDG-PET scanning, not IBS; however myocardial uptake on IBS can be seen in cases of recent myocardial infarction and amyloidosis. Note that poor renal function can often demonstrate reduced or absent renal visualization producing an appearance similar to a superscan (false positive), whereas urinary tract obstruction in prostatic carcinoma can increase renal activity and lead to false negative scans.

Love C, Din A, Tomas M, Kalapparambath T, and Palestro C. Radionuclide bone imaging: an illustrative review. *RadioGraphics* 2003; 23: 341–358.

74. C. Morquio syndrome.

The constellation of skeletal manifestations describes the characteristic appearance of dyostosis multiplex. This pattern of skeletal abnormalities is seen with the mucopolysaccharidoses (MPS), although it can also be seen with other storage disorders. With the exception of Hurler's syndrome, where the manifestations are present at 1 year of age, the skeletal manifestations progress as the patients get older. Hurler's and Morquio's are the most common of the MPS conditions. Amongst the MPS conditions, Morquio's stands out as a favourite for single best answer (SBA) and viva questions as it is the only MPS where the patient is not intellectually impaired. It also displays a central anterior vertebral body beak, whereas the other conditions have an anterior beak in the lower third of the vertebral body.

The differences with achondroplasia are the progression with age and the pelvic shape. The pelvis in achondroplasia has widened iliac wings, with horizontal acetabular roofs and a narrow inlet, giving the classic 'champagne glass' appearance. The anterior beak in achondroplasia is also in the lower third of the vertebral body.

Manaster B, May D, and Disler D. *Musculoskeletal Radiology: The Requisites*, 3rd edn, Mosby, 2007. pp. 629–642.
Chapman S and Nakielny R. *Aids to Radiological Differential Diagnosis*, 4th edn, Saunders, 2003, p, 86.

75. E. PVNS.

This is a monoarticular tumour-like proliferation of synovium that occurs in joints, bursae, and tendon sheaths. It may be focal or diffuse. It occurs most frequently in the knee (80% of cases), then the hip, ankle, shoulder, and elbow. The abnormal synovium is prone to haemorrhage, thus producing blooming artefact on GE sequences, secondary to haemosiderin deposition. In general the classic MRI appearance is variable low signal intensity on all sequences (T2WI signal being more variable due to fat, oedema, and blood products). Early changes involve a focal mass and joint effusion. Subsequently large erosions, synovial hypertrophy, and subchondral cysts may occur. Joint space is preserved until advanced disease is present and bone density is normal. After IV contrast at CT, PVNS shows variable enhancement, which can be striking. The differential diagnosis includes diseases causing recurrent haemarthroses, e.g. haemophilia and haemochromatosis (PVNS is monoarticular) as well as gout, amyloid, synovial chondromatosis, and tuberculosis.

Some 90% of synovial cell sarcomas do not originate from a joint. They are usually isointense to muscle on T1WI, with heterogeneous high-signal intensity on T2WI. Regional migratory osteoporosis would obviously involve loss of bone mineralization, as well as marrow oedema. Gout demonstrates typically 'rat's bite' para-articular erosions and soft-tissue calcification; when it involves the knee it tends to affect the patello-femoral compartment.

Al-Nakshabandi NA, Ryan AG, Choudur H, Torreggiani W, Nicoloau S, Munk PL et al. Pigmented villonodular synovitis. *Clinical Radiology* 2004; 59: 414–420.
Manaster BJ, May DA, and Disler DG. *Musculoskeletal Imaging: The Requisites*, 3rd edn, Mosby, 2007. p. 50.

chapter 3

GASTROINTESTINAL

QUESTIONS

1. **A 63-year-old man is day 7 post operative following a Billroth II partial gastrectomy for a gastric carcinoma. The initial post-operative phase was uncomplicated, but the patient has begun complaining of increasing abdominal pain. Inflammatory markers have increased with white cell count (WCC), rising from 12 to 42, and CRP increased from 8 to 56. A CT scan carried out with oral and intravenous contrast demonstrates no evidence of contrast leakage into the peritoneum. A skiff of free air is noted in the abdomen. A fluid collection is noted in the right subhepatic space, which extends toward the peripancreatic area. What is the most likely diagnosis?**

   A. Leakage from the gastroduodenal anastomosis site.
   B. Leakage from the duodenal stump.
   C. Post-operative pancreatitis.
   D. Tumour recurrence.
   E. Pseudocyst formation following post-operative pancreatitis.

2. **A 32-year-old female patient attends for a barium swallow with a history of a sensation of food sticking in her throat. The barium swallow reveals uniform horizontally orientated folds in the lower oesophagus. There is a change in the texture of the mucosa 1 cm above the hiatus, which is sited 25 cm from the origin of the oesophagus. There is a slight smooth narrowing noted 2 cm above the hiatus, beyond which there is a slight dilatation of the oesophagus prior to it joining the stomach. Which of the following is an unusual finding?**

   A. The appearance of the oesophageal folds.
   B. The change in mucosal appearance 1 cm above the hiatus.
   C. The distance of the hiatus from the origin of the oesophagus.
   D. The slight narrowing 2 cm above the hiatus.
   E. The distal bulge just before the stomach.

3. A patient with a history of alcohol abuse presents to A&E with epigastric pain. His haemoglobin is 8 g/dl on admission. An oesophago-gastro-duodenoscopy (OGD) and ultrasound of abdomen are requested. The ultrasound of abdomen shows multiple hyperechoic lesions in the liver. There is no evidence of gallstones. Prior to the OGD the patient becomes acutely unwell and a CT scan is requested. This shows evidence of air and fluid in the subhepatic space. It also reveals a focal enhancing lesion causing prominence of the head of the pancreas. What is the most likely diagnosis?

A. Pancreatitis with associated peripancreatic abcscess.
B. Pancreatic carcinoma and liver metastases.
C. Pancreatitis and peptic ulcer perforation in an alcoholic patient.
D. Islet cell tumour with liver metastases.
E. Cholangiocarcinoma with liver metastases.

4. Which of the following is correct regarding carcinoid of the GI tract?

A. A minority are asyptomatic when discovered.
B. The appendix is the most common site of occurrence, representing 33% of all carcinoids.
C. Over 50% are multiple.
D. Although malignant change is uncommon in appendiceal carcinoid, as this is the most common site, it accounts for the majority of malignant carcinoids.
E. The size of the tumour at diagnosis is related to the risk of metastatic spread.

5. A 45-year-old male patient presents to A&E with an 8-hour history of epigastric pain. There is no history of alcohol intake. On examination he is tender in the epigastrium. The initial blood tests reveal that his amylase is 1024. His WCC is slightly elevated at 15. His glucose, calcium, PaO2, liver function tests (LFTs), lactate dehydrogenase (LDH) and serum electrolytes are all normal. Following an erect CXR, what is the next most appropriate radiological investigation?

A. Urgent CT scan to assess the pancreas.
B. CT within 24 hours.
C. Ultrasound scan within 24 hours.
D. Endoscopic retrograde cholangiopancreatography (ERCP) to look for ductal calculi.
E. MRCP on this admission to assess for ductal stones.

6. A patient presents to an outpatient barium meal list with a history of epigastric discomfort and weight loss of 8 kg over 6 months. The barium meal reveals an ulcer on the greater curve of the stomach, near the pylorus. This ulcer has a surrounding mound. It is demonstrated to project slightly beyond the lumen of the stomach. There is a thin line noted which crosses the base of the ulcer and a degree of retraction of the greater curve around the ulcer. What type of ulcer is this likely to be?

A. Benign due to the line noted crossing the base of the ulcer.
B. Benign due to the ulcer projecting beyond the lumen of the stomach.
C. Benign due to the surrounding mound.
D. Malignant due to the finding of scar retraction of the greater curve.
E. Malignant due to being found on the greater curve.

7. A 24-year-old male patient is brought into A&E following a high-speed RTA. His blood pressure was 90/60 mmHg and his heart rate was 112 on admission, but these observations respond well to intravenous fluids and the patient has remained stable since. He complains of left-sided abdominal pain. A pneumothorax is noted on CXR, with associated left-sided rib fractures. An urgent CT scan of chest and abdomen is carried out. This reveals fluid in the abdomen. A cresenteric area of low attenuation is noted around the spleen. There is a further area of hypoattenuation passing 4 cm into the splenic parenchyma, adjacent to the hilum. The rest of the splenic parenchyma is of uniform attenuation. The CT also shows a flail segment of chest and an area of lung contusion at the left base. Which of the following statements with regard to the spleen is true?

A. The appearances described represent subcapsular haematomas.
B. The appearances described represent a haematoma and a parenchymal laceration. The presence of free fluid represents acute haemorrhage and a laparotomy is indicated.
C. The appearances are consistent with a shattered spleen as the laceration extends to the hilum.
D. The appearances are consistent with a subcapsular haematoma and a splenic laceration. Conservative management is appropriate with serial CT scans.
E. Whilst the appearances are consistent with a laceration and subcapsular haematoma, radiological findings are not reliable in determining the need for a laparotomy.

8. A small bowel series is requested for a patient who has a history of systemic sclerosis. Which of the following is a feature of small bowel systemic sclerosis?

A. Stacked coin appearance due to infiltration of small bowel loops.
B. Pseudo-diverticula affecting the anti-mesenteric side of the bowel.
C. Decreased intestinal transit time.
D. Small bowel systemic sclerosis is only seen in 10% of patients with systemic sclerosis, but the disease is rapidly progressive when it is present.
E. Pneumatosis intestinalis.

9. A 26-year-old female presents with a 1-day history of right iliac fossa (RIF) pain. She is mid-cycle and prone to mittleschmerz-type pain, but reports that this pain is more severe than previously. Serum inflammatory markers are elevated. Clinical examination reveals tenderness in the RIF, but no rebound. Due to the compounding gynaecological history, a CT is requested. This reveals a thickened caecum and thickened appendix, which appears to have a defect in the wall on the multiplanar reformatted images. There is a calcified density present in the orifice of the appendix. There is a loculated fluid collection adjacent to the appendix, which has air bubbles within it. There is also fluid in the pelvis. A perforated appendix is removed at surgery. Which of the CT findings is most specific for detecting a perforated appendix?

A. Presence of a faecolith.
B. Identification of a wall defect.
C. Fluid in the pelvis.
D. Adjacent abscess formation.
E. Enlarged regional lymph nodes.

10. A 65-year-old man presents with weight loss and obstructive jaundice. An ultrasound reveals dilatation of the intra- and extrahepatic biliary system. MRCP reveals a stricture in the distal common bile duct (CBD). The patient becomes septic and biliary drainage is required. Which is the most appropriate method for this?

A. Percutaneous transhepatic cholangiography (PTC) and external drainage.
B. PTC with internal/external drainage.
C. ERCP with plastic stent insertion.
D. ERCP with metal stent insertion.
E. PTC/ERCP rendezvous procedure.

11. A lesion is noted in the liver on CT and ultrasound. It is inferior, anterior, and to the left of the right hepatic vein, but to the right of the middle hepatic vein. It is inferior of the confluence of the right and left portal veins. According to the Couinaud system, what segment of the liver is the lesion in?

A. Segment 4b.
B. Segment 5.
C. Segment 6.
D. Segment 7.
E. Segment 8.

12. A 56-year-old male patient is referred for an ultrasound of abdomen prior to undergoing an anterior resection for a proximal rectal carcinoma. The ultrasound reveals a 2cm lesion in the right lobe of the liver, which is hyperechoic centrally with a hypoechoic rim. Which one of the following cannot be considered in the differential for this lesion?

A. Metastases.
B. Haemangioma.
C. Sarcoid.
D. Candidiasis.
E. Lymphoma.

13. A patient is undergoing a barium meal. What is the best position to place the patient in to see an *en face* view of the lesser curve?

A. Left lateral.
B. Left anterior oblique (LAO).
C. Supine.
D. Right anterior oblique (RAO).
E. Right lateral.

14. Which one of the following is false regarding peritoneal and mesenteric structures?

A. The lesser sac communicates with the rest of the abdominal cavity through the foramen of Winslow.
B. The left paracolic gutter communicates with the left subphrenic space.
C. The falciform ligament connects to the left coronary lignament.
D. Part of the duodenum is suspended in the lesser omentum.
E. The right paracolic space communicates with the pouch of Douglas.

15. A patient is being worked up for a pancreatic neoplasm to assess potential resectability. Which one of the following does not rule out surgery?

A. Extension of the tumour beyond the margins of the pancreas into duodenum.
B. Tumour involvement of adjacent organs.
C. Enlarged peripancreatic lymph nodes (>15 mm).
D. Encasement or obstruction of superior mesenteric vessels.
E. Peritoneal carcinomatosis.

16. A 68-year-old male patient has a 20-year history of RA. During a recent flare he was commenced on steroid therapy, although this has now been discontinued. The patient is now complaining of mild abdominal discomfort, diarrhoea, and mild weight loss. A barium meal is performed, but is suboptimal, as the patient is poorly mobile. Within the limitations of the study, there is reduced peristalsis in the oesophagus and mild reflux. The antrum of the stomach is felt to be mildly narrowed and rigid. Thickened rugal folds are noted. A subsequent small bowel series is carried out. The jejunal folds measure 4 mm and the ileal folds appear more plentiful and measure 3 mm. Contrast is present in the caecum at 4 hours. Spot screening of the terminal ileum reveals the same findings as those described above. What is the most likely diagnosis?

A. Gastric erosions.
B. Whipple's disease.
C. Mastocytosis.
D. Amyloidosis.
E. Crohn's disease.

17. A 72-year-old male patient presents to the surgical team with a 3-week history of increasing painless jaundice. He has a past medical history of gallstones, prostatic carcinoma, and ischaemic heart disease. There is no history of alcohol abuse. The LFTs are abnormal. Serum bilirubin is 346. He is referred for an ultrasound scan of the abdomen, which identifies grossly dilated intrahepatic bile ducts, but no evidence of a dilated CBD. The common hepatic duct (CHD) is not clearly visible due to an isoechoic mass in the region of the porta hepatis at the ductal confluence. A triple phase CT scan of the liver is carried out. The lesion is iso- to hypo-attenuating. There is limited arterial enhancement, with some portal venous enhancement peripherally. On delayed images the lesion displays enhancement with mild peripheral washout. What is the most likely pathology?

A. Cholangiocarcinoma.
B. Portal metastasis.
C. Hepatocellular carcinoma.
D. Benign biliary stricture.
E. Cavernous haemangioma.

18. A patient is admitted with right upper quadrant (RUQ) pain to the surgical team and is referred for ultrasound. On the ultrasound there is a curvilinear echogenic line at the margin of the gallbladder and posterior acoustic shadowing in the gallbladder fossa. There is no evidence of peristalsis and the shadowing does not change on patient positioning. The sonographer states that the patient's pain has settled and they are otherwise well. What is the most likely cause of this appearance?

A. Bowel in the gallbladder fossa.
B. Porcelain gallbladder.
C. Gallstones.
D. Emphysematous cholecystitis.
E. Post-ERCP.

19. You are left in charge of a barium meal list. Due to an acute staff shortage there is only a student radiographer with you, who wants to know about which barium to use and why. Which one of the following statements regarding barium contrast media is correct?

A. Simethicone is added to reduce flocculation.
B. The weight/volume ratio of barium for barium meals is 150%.
C. The same weight/volume ratio is used for barium meals and follow-through examinations.
D. Uniform particle size improves mucosal coating.
E. Gastrografin can be added to improve transit time.

20. A patient presents to the surgical team with central abdominal pain and vomiting associated with abdominal distension. The abdominal x-ray (AXR) reveals numerous dilated loops of small bowel. A CT scan is carried out. Which of the following statements with regard to CT imaging in small bowel obstruction is accurate?

A. Small bowel mural hyperdensity is a feature and is due to vasodilatation seen in early ischaemia.
B. Oral contrast is mandatory for the investigation of small bowel obstruction.
C. Small bowel mural thickening is due to increased venous pressure.
D. Absence of small bowel mural enhancement is a feature of ischaemic gut secondary to emboli rather than small bowel obstruction.
E. Lack of small bowel pneumatosis excludes ischaemia of the gut.

21. A patient with a history of inflammatory bowel disease, treated with colonic resection and J pouch anastomosis, presents to the surgical team in your hospital. The operation was 3 months ago and the initial post-operative period was unremarkable. His post-operative pouchogram was reported as normal and he underwent a reversal of his defunctioning ileostomy 6 weeks ago. He now presents with central and lower abdominal pain associated with nausea and vomiting, but no diarrhoea. The surgeons request a pouchogram, which shows a small blind ending lumen at the superior aspect of the pouch. A follow-up CT scan shows dilated small bowel with a transition point in the ileum, beyond which the bowel is non-distended. The J pouch has mild inflammatory change in the surrounding fat. There is also a small amount of free fluid in the pelvis. The wall of the pouch is not thickened. What is the most likely diagnosis?

A. Small bowel obstruction, as can occur in up to 30% of these patients.
B. Pouchitis.
C. Pouch fistula.
D. Recurrence of Crohn's in the pouch and affected segment of bowel.
E. Pouch leak.

22. A 35-year-old male patient from the Indian subcontinent presents with a 2-month history of lower abdominal pain, per rectum (PR) bleeding, and weight loss. His haemoglobin is 9.4 and C-reactive protein (CRP) is 123. The patient is tender in the RIF. A CT scan is performed due the suspicion of appendiceal pathology, but unusual history. This shows bowel wall thickening of the terminal ileum with mild proximal bowel dilatation. The inner bowel wall is hypodense with enhancement of the outer bowel wall. There is stranding in the fat, which causes mass effect displacing other loops of bowel. Mild regional adenopathy is noted. The appendix is not visualized, but the caecum appears normal. There is a similar area of bowel wall thickening in the sigmoid colon. What is the most likely diagnosis?

A. Yersinia.
B. Tuberculosis.
C. Lymphoma.
D. Crohn's disease.
E. Carcinoid.

23. A 40-year-old female undergoes MRI of the liver, which demonstrates a 5-cm lesion that is isointense to liver on T1WI and slightly hyperintense on T2WI. It has a central scar that is hypointense on T1WI and hyperintense on T2WI. On contrast-enhanced dynamic MRI, the lesion is hyperintense in the arterial phase, and isointense to liver in the portal venous phase with delayed filling in of the central scar. What is the diagnosis?

A. Hepatic adenoma.
B. Fibrolamellar hepatoma.
C. Hypervascular metastasis.
D. Focal nodular hyperplasia (FNH).
E. Giant haemangioma.

24. A 50-year-old female patient is referred for an outpatient CT after an ultrasound carried out to look for gallstones revealed a cystic lesion within the pancreas. The CT shows a number of large cysts of over 2 cm in diameter, containing fluid measuring 3 HU in the head and body of the pancreas. These cysts have thin enhancing walls. The pancreatic duct is not significantly distended. On further questioning the patient denies a history of previous pancreatitis. An MRI does not extend the diagnostic process. An FNA reveals fluid low in amylase, but with high carcino-embryonic antigen (CEA) content. What is the most likely diagnosis?

A. Pancreatic pseudocyst.
B. Mucinous cystic neoplasm.
C. Microcystic pancreatic tumour.
D. Intraductal papillary mucinous tumour (main duct type).
E. Lymphangioma.

25. A 45-year-old female is suspected to have focal areas of fat infiltration on ultrasound of the liver. An MRI of the liver is requested for further assessment. What sequences are most useful in confirming the diagnosis of focal fat infiltration?

A. T1WI pre and post gadolinium.
B. T1WI and T2WI.
C. T1WI and fat-saturated T2WI.
D. Dual GE T1WI in phase and out of phase.
E. MR spectroscopy.

26. A 45-year-old male presents with a history of jaundice and RUQ pain. An ultrasound of the abdomen demonstrates an impacted calculus in the gallbladder neck with dilatation of the intrahepatic ducts. An MRCP is requested to exclude Mirizzi syndrome. What additional features on MRCP confirm the diagnosis of Mirizzi syndrome?

A. Dilated common hepatic duct.
B. Dilated common hepatic and common bile ducts.
C. Dilated common hepatic duct with normal common bile duct.
D. Double duct sign.
E. Normal ducts.

27. A 60-year-old diabetic male presents with a history of fever and right upper quadrant pain. Ultrasound of the abdomen demonstrates curvilinear high-amplitude echoes in the gallbladder wall with reverberation artefact and multiple high-amplitude echoes in the gallbladder lumen. What is the diagnosis?

A. Acute cholecystitis.
B. Emphysematous cholecystitis.
C. Adenomyomatosis.
D. Chronic cholecystitis.
E. Cholesterosis.

28. A 65-year-old male with a pancreatic head mass and obstructive jaundice undergoes percutaneous cholangiogram and external biliary drain insertion via the right lobe of the liver. The patient returns for a biliary stent insertion. On removing the external drain there is significant arterial bleed from the puncture site. A selective coeliac axis angiogram does not reveal any abnormality, but pulsatile bleeding persists. What would you do next?

A. Selective left gastric angiogram.
B. Selective superior mesenteric angiogram.
C. Selective inferior mesenteric angiogram.
D. Selective gastroduodenal artery angiogram.
E. Embolise coeliac axis.

29. A 55-year-old female with cirrhosis undergoes MRI of the liver, which demonstrates multiple small nodules that are hypointense on T2WI and enhance following administration of gadolinium in the arterial and portal venous phase. The nodules demonstrate uptake of hepatocellular agent and super paramagnetic iron oxide (SPIO) particles. What is your diagnosis?

A. Multifocal hepatocellular carcinoma (HCC).
B. Siderotic nodules.
C. Dysplastic nodules.
D. Regenerative nodules.
E. Multiple arterio-venous shunts.

30. A 62-year-old male with acute myocardial infarction develops abdominal discomfort and deranged liver function tests. A CT scan of the abdomen demonstrates heterogeneous liver enhancement, poor enhancement of the hepatic veins and inferior vena cava (IVC), ascites and bibasal pleural effusions. What additional feature would favour a diagnosis of passive hepatic congestion instead of acute Budd–Chiari syndrome?

A. Flip-flop enhancement pattern of the liver.
B. Absent flow in hepatic veins.
C. Dilated hepatic veins and IVC.
D. Enlarged caudate lobe.
E. Hepatomegaly.

31. A 47-year-old male patient undergoes an MRI examination for further characterization of an adrenal lesion. Axial gradient T1 in- and out-of-phase sequences confirm the benign nature of the adrenal lesion. Incidentally, the liver and pancreas demonstrate a signal drop on the in-phase images compared to out-of-phase images. What is your diagnosis and what additional sequence would confirm the diagnosis?

A. Diffuse fatty infiltration. GE T2WI.
B. Diffuse fatty infiltration. SE T2WI.
C. Haemochromatosis. SE T2WI.
D. Haemochromatosis. GE T2WI.
E. Haemosiderosis. GE T2WI.
F. Haemosiderosis. SE T2WI.

32. A 35-year-old female undergoes an MRI of abdomen that shows multiple cystic lesions in the pancreas. Each lesion consists of a cluster of small cysts with central scar. Multiple cysts and solid lesions are also noted in both kidneys. What further investigation/s would you recommend?

A. Ophthalmology referral.
B. MRI of the brain.
C. MRI of the spine.
D. Molecular genetic testing and genetic counselling.
E. All of the above.

33. A 55-year-old man presents with dysphagia. He gives no history of weight loss and investigations reveal a normal full blood picture. He is referred for a barium swallow, which reveals a long stricture (several centimetres) in the mid to distal oesophagus with a fine reticular pattern adjacent to the distal aspect of the stricture and distal oesophageal widening. What is the most likely diagnosis?

A. Reflux oesophagitis.
B. Candidiasis.
C. Barrett's oesophagus.
D. Oesophageal adenocarcinoma.
E. Hiatus hernia.

34. A patient presents to A&E with severe upper abdominal pain 4 days following a barium enema. There is no free air under the diaphragm on the erect CXR. There is mild elevation of the inflammatory markers, but the surgeon is concerned with the degree of peritonism and requests a CT scan of abdomen. On this, the small bowel is dilated to 5 cm, but is not thick walled. The vascular structures enhance normally. There is inflammatory change noted around the duodenum. Linear areas of low attenuation are noted extending from the porta hepatis into the liver parenchyma. These do not extend to the margin of the liver and are in general central in their location. The Hounsfield attenuation value of these areas is approximately –1500 HU. Barium in the rectum obscures the images of the pelvis. What is the most likely pathology?

A. Cholecystoduodenal fistula.
B. Mesenteric infarction.
C. Acute bowel obstruction.
D. Perforated duodenal ulcer.
E. Complication of barium enema.

35. A 74-year-old female patient undergoes a barium swallow and meal as part of investigation of anaemia, as she refuses endoscopy. She denies any weight loss, dysphagia, or odynophagia. The swallow reveals multiple rounded plaques and nodules in the mid oesophagus. What is the most likely diagnosis?

A. Oesophageal candidiasis.
B. Herpes oesophagitis.
C. HIV oesophagitis.
D. Glycogenic acanthosis.
E. Cytomegalovirus oesophagitis.

36. A 75-year-old woman presents with severe chest pain radiating to her back and some haematemesis. The surgical team have considered a differential diagnosis of aortic dissection or aorto-enteric fistula and requested a CT scan to assess the aorta. No aortic dissection is seen, but there is a long eccentric filling defect identified within the oesophageal wall, extending from the level of the carina to the gastro-oesophageal junction. This area did not enhance after contrast administration but did measure 75 HU on a pre-contrast scan. Barium swallow revealed a longitudinal impression on the oesophagus, which had resolved on a repeat swallow 6 weeks later. What is the most likely diagnosis?

A. Aorto-oesophageal fistula.
B. Mallory–Weiss tear.
C. Boerhaave syndrome.
D. Oesophageal varices.
E. Intramural haematoma of the oesophagus.

37. A 50-year-old male undergoes MRI of the liver for further characterization of a suspected haemangioma on ultrasound. In addition to the haemangioma, a peripheral wedge-shaped area of enhancement is seen in the arterial phase but no abnormality is seen in the corresponding area in the non-contrast or portal venous phases. What is the diagnosis?

A. Hepatocellular carcinoma.
B. Hepatic infarct.
C. Transient hepatic intensity difference (THID).
D. Hypervascular metastasis.
E. Haemangioma.

38. A patient with recently diagnosed oesophageal carcinoma is referred for endoscopic ultrasound (EUS) staging. This shows a hypoechoic area at 36 cm involving the mucosa extending into the submucosa, muscularis propria, and adventitia. It lies close to the aorta but there is no obvious invasion. There is a further hyperechoic lesion noted centrally within this area that only involves the mucosal layer. A subsequent staging CT scan shows an area of oesophageal thickening, which is in contact with 60% of the aorta and there is loss of fat plane between it and the pericardium. There is a lymph node noted adjacent to the oesophagus which measures 15 mm in diameter. Three 12-mm nodes are noted in the para-aortic region in the abdomen. There is a hypoattenuating lesion in segment six of the liver, which demonstrates nodular peripheral enhancement. A delayed scan shows that this lesion has filled in completely. For completion of staging, a PET-CT scan is performed and this shows increased uptake in the primary lesion. The lymph nodes in the abdomen have an SUV maximum of 3, and the para-oesophageal node has an SUV maximum of 13. There is mottled uptake in the liver. What is the radiological staging of this lesion?

A. T4, N1, M0.
B. T2, N1, M0.
C. T3, N1, M1.
D. T4, N2, M1.
E. T3, N1, M0.

39. A 45-year-old woman is referred by her GP for a barium swallow for investigation of dysphagia. Gastro-oesophageal reflux into the lower third of the oesophagus is demonstrated and delicate transverse striations in the lower oesophagus are observed as a transient phenomenon. What is the next appropriate action appropriate for the radiologist?

A. Recommend a staging CT of chest and abdomen.
B. Recommend oesophagoscopy and biopsy of the affected area.
C. Recommend to the GP that the study was unremarkable but for mild reflux.
D. Recommend referral for manometry.
E. Recommend endoscopic ultrasound.

40. A 50-year-old woman presents with dysphagia. At barium swallow, contrast passes sluggishly into the oropharynx. No peristaltic waves are seen in the upper oesophagus. After swallowing, the lumen of the hypopharynx and upper oesophagus remain patent and distended. The lower oesophagus outlines normally. What is the most likely diagnosis?

A. Achalasia.
B. Scleroderma.
C. Polymyositis.
D. Chagas disease.
E. SLE.

41. A 63-year-old male patient is admitted with acute pancreatitis. During his admission survey he is noted to have a Ranson score of 7 and he is transferred to the ICU. A CT scan is carried out prior to ICU admission and shows a homogeneously enhancing enlarged pancreas with a fluid collection in the tail. There are gallstones in the gallbladder, with a dilated duct. A further CT is carried out on day 3 and this shows two further fluid collections in the tail of the pancreas, with an area of poorly enhancing pancreas that involves over half of the gland. There is no evidence of abscess. Which of the following options is most useful in detecting the severity of this patient's pancreatitis?

A. Ranson score to indicate severity of pancreatitis. CT is of value in detecting complications.
B. CT within 24 hours to show presence of gland swelling and/or necrosis.
C. CT scan within 24 hours to indicate absence of complications and evidence that the causative factor has passed.
D. CT after 3 days showing necrosis and fluid collections.
E. CT scan after 3 days showing absence of abscess formation.

42. A 45-year-old man presents with acute abdominal pain. He has pyrexia and his inflammatory markers are raised. The surgical team request a CT scan of abdomen for '?perforation'. The CT reveals inflammatory change in the anterior pararenal space. Which of the following is least likely to be the underlying cause for the CT finding?

A. Acute pancreatitis.
B. Gastric ulceration.
C. Diverticulitis of the descending colon.
D. Duodenal perforation.
E. Perforation of ascending colon due to neoplasm.

43. A 73-year-old woman is referred from surgical outpatients for a barium enema. She has a 3-month history of weight loss and a microcytic anaemia. The procedure is unremarkable, and you leave the screening room to go and continue some plain film reporting. Ten minutes later you are contacted by one of the radiographers who was helping during the enema. She is distressed and tells you that she found the patient collapsed in the bathroom having what appeared to be a seizure. You immediately attend and assess the patient. She is drowsy, but heart rate, blood pressure, and SaO_2 are normal. What is the most likely complication to have caused her acute illness?

A. Cardiac arrhythmia secondary to rectal distension.
B. Venous intravasation.
C. Water intoxication.
D. Intramural barium.
E. Side-effect of hyoscine butyl bromide (*Buscopan*®).

44. A 67-year-old man presents to A&E with abdominal pain. Inflammatory markers are raised, but serum electrolytes, amylase, haemoglobin, and coagulation are normal. He takes no regular medication. On examination, there is a palpable mass in the right lower quadrant. CT reveals a lobulated, hypoattenuating mass with thick walls, septa, and curvilinear calcifications. It is located in the RIF, and displaces and distorts the adjacent psoas muscle. What is the most likely diagnosis?

A. Pancreatic pseudocyst.
B. Pseudomyxoma retroperitonei.
C. Urinoma.
D. Haematoma.
E. Retroperitoneal liposarcoma.

45. A 30-year-old man undergoes CT of the abdomen following a high-velocity collision during an RTA. The scan reveals peripancreatic fat stranding and a superficial laceration in the tail of the pancreas, which extends to less than 50% of the pancreatic thickness. What is the next most appropriate step?

A. Laparotomy.
B. ERCP.
C. Supportive therapy.
D. Ultrasound to assess the pancreatic duct.
E. Diagnostic peritoneal lavage.

46. An adolescent complains of chest and abdominal pain after suffering a handlebar injury whilst out riding his bicycle. He undergoes a CT scan of abdomen, as the surgical team fear he may have suffered a liver or splenic injury. In the recent past he has been complaining of loose motions and his mother has noticed he has failed to thrive. He has a long history of respiratory disease, which has been diagnosed as asthma. The CT scan shows low attenuation (–90 to –120 HU) in the region of the pancreas and air-trapping and cystic bronchiectasis in the upper lobes of both lungs. Which of the following is the most likely underlying pathological process explaining the appearance of the pancreas?

A. Chronic pancreatitis.
B. Congenital absence of the pancreas.
C. Lipomatous pseudohypertrophy of the pancreas.
D. Gluten enteropathy.
E. Shwachman–Diamond syndrome.

47. A 54-year-old man presents with persistent abdominal pain and fever. His amylase has been normal, and colonoscopy and small bowel series were unremarkable during previous investigation. He has a past medical history of thyroid disease. A CT of abdomen reveals ill-defined rounded areas in the root of the mesentery, with adjacent mild lymphadenopathy. There is some central calcification. A rim of preserved fat is seen surrounding the adjacent vessels. What is the most likely diagnosis?

A. Sclerosing mesenteritis.
B. Desmoid tumour.
C. Carcinoid tumour.
D. Lymphoma.
E. Metastatic disease.

48. A 58-year-old man with a history of alcohol abuse and diabetes presents with painless jaundice. Liver function tests reveal an obstructive picture and he undergoes an ultrasound of abdomen, which reveals dilatation of the CBD and a hypoechoic region in the head of the pancreas. He has a history of iodine allergy and undergoes MRI with dynamic gadolinium enhancement, as an alternative to contrast-enhanced CT. Which finding in the pancreatic head is most in keeping with the diagnosis of pancreatic adenocarcinoma?

A. Hypointensity on T1WI.
B. Hyperintensity on T2WI.
C. Hyperintensity on a STIR sequence.
D. Hypointensity during arterial phase enhancement.
E. Hypointensity during portal venous phase enhancement.

49. A 42-year-old man is referred for a CT scan by an upper GI surgeon. He has a long history of recurrent upper abdominal pain, with more recent episodic vomiting. CT shows excess soft-tissue thickening between the head of pancreas and duodenum. Small cystic lesions are seen along the medial wall of the duodenum. There is also mild dilatation of the common bile duct and distension of the stomach and proximal duodenum. What is the most likely diagnosis?

A. Autoimmune pancreatitis.
B. Groove pancreatitis.
C. Pancreatitis related to ectopic or heterotopic pancreatic tissue.
D. Hereditary pancreatitis.
E. Pancreas divisum associated pancreatitis.

50. An overweight 42-year-old man decides to join a gym as a New Year's resolution. During a vigorous work-out, he develops acute left lower quadrant pain and tenderness. An initial ultrasound demonstrates a small, 2-cm solid hyperechoic, non-compressible oval mass at the site of maximal tenderness. Further investigation via CT shows a pericolic pedunculated mass with fat attenuation and a hyperattenuating peripheral rim with adjacent fat-stranding abutting the anterior sigmoid colon. What is the most likely diagnosis?

A. Diverticulitis.
B. Appendicitis.
C. Epiploic appendagitis.
D. Omental infarction.
E. Sclerosing mesenteritis.

51. A 50-year-old male patient is admitted with congestive cardiac failure and undergoes a CT scan of the abdomen, which shows tortuous and prominent intrahepatic and extrahepatic arterial branches with early filling of dilated hepatic veins and IVC. The arterial phase scan shows mosaic perfusion with multiple enhancing foci. In the portal venous phase there is homogenous enhancement of the liver, with the prominent hepatic veins and IVC noted. What is the diagnosis?

A. Passive hepatic congestion.
B. Budd–Chiari syndrome.
C. Osler–Weber–Rendu syndrome.
D. Multifocal transient hepatic attenuation differences.
E. Von Meyerburg complex.

52. A 65-year-old man, being investigated for iron deficiency anaemia, altered bowel habit, and weight loss, is diagnosed with colon cancer. A staging CT demonstrates irregularity to the outer bowel wall at the site of tumour, a cluster of three lymph nodes with the largest individual node measuring 0.9cm, and no evidence of distant metastases. What is the most likely TNM stage?

A. T2, N0, M0.
B. T2, N1, M0.
C. T3, N0, M0.
D. T3, N1, M0.
E. T4, N1, M0.

53. A 41-year-old female with a background of arthralgia, chronic abdominal pain, and diarrhoea is investigated via a small bowel series. Findings include a prolonged transit time, and dilated loops of small bowel with normal appearing valvulae and pseudodiverticula. What is the most likely diagnosis?

A. GI scleroderma.
B. Behcet's disease.
C. Whipple disease.
D. Small bowel lymphoma.
E. Coeliac disease.

54. A 55-year-old man with a previous history of liver transplantation presents with a 1-week history of abdominal pain and distension. An AXR shows some distended small bowel loops centrally within the abdomen. You are asked to perform a CT scan of abdomen for further evaluation. This shows a cluster of non-encapsulated dilated small bowel loops adjacent to the anterior abdominal wall on the right side. There are adjacent crowded mesenteric vessels. What is the most likely diagnosis?

A. Small bowel adhesions.
B. Left paraduodenal hernia.
C. Right paraduodenal hernia.
D. Foramen of Winslow hernia.
E. Transmesenteric hernia.

55. A 64-year-old man presents to A&E with onset of severe watery diarrhoea and abdominal pain. An AXR is performed which shows dilated large bowel and nodular haustral fold thickening. The patient has a CT scan with oral and intravenous contrast. The CT scan shows large bowel dilatation with diffuse bowel wall thickening. Some of the oral contrast given has become trapped between the oedematous haustral folds, causing alternating bands of high and low attenuation. What is the most likely underlying diagnosis?

A. Ulcerative colitis.
B. Crohn's colitis.
C. Ischaemic colitis.
D. Pseudomembranous colitis.
E. Bacillary dysentery.

56. A 30-year-old man with a long history of dysphagia presents with food impaction. He has a past medical history of allergies but nothing else of note. The food bolus passes spontaneously, and a water-soluble followed by a barium swallow are requested prior to endoscopy, to ensure there has been no perforation due to chicken/fish bones. The barium study reveals a moderately long stricture in the lower oesophagus, with multiple distinct ring-like indentations. What is the most likely diagnosis?

A. Idiopathic eosinophilic oesophagitis (IEE).
B. Crohn's disease.
C. Oesophageal carcinoma.
D. Oesophageal perforation.
E. Peptic stricture.

57. A patient has an ultrasound scan carried out on a radiographer's ultrasound list. The radiographer notices an unusual finding and asks you to check the images. The liver, kidneys, and spleen appear unremarkable. There are gallstones in the gallbladder, but also in the fundus of the gallbladder, and there is a reverberation artefact that gives a comet tail appearance. This finding is pathogonomic of a condition. Which of the following statements is true regarding this condition?

A. Adenomyomatosis is caused by abnormal deposits of cholesterol esters in foam cells in the lamina propria.
B. Cholesterolosis is caused by the rupture of Rokitansky–Aschoff sinuses with subsequent intramural leak of bile causing an inflammatory reaction.
C. Xanthogranulomatous cholecystitis is characterized by an increase in the number and height of glandular elements in the gallbladder.
D. Xanthogranulomatous cholecystitis is associated with gallbladder carcinoma in around 10% of cases.
E. Adenomyomatosis is associated with cholesterolosis in up to a third of patients.

58. A 45-year-old man, with a history of AIDS, has a 3-month history of abdominal pain and weight loss. A CT scan of abdomen is performed which shows ascites with peritoneal thickening, several areas of mural thickening in the small bowel, and multiple low attenuation lymph nodes. Which one of the following infections is most likely?

A. CMV infection.
B. TB.
C. Cryptosporidiosis.
D. Amoebiasis.
E. Campylobacter.

59. A 44-year-old man presents with a vague history of central abdominal pain and mild weight loss. On further questioning, there are other features in the history suggestive of malabsorption. Amongst other investigations, a CT scan of abdomen is requested. This shows dilated fluid-filled small bowel loops and multiple enlarged mesenteric lymph nodes, encasing the mesenteric vessels. The lymph nodes are of homogeneous soft tissue density. What is the most likely cause of the CT findings?

A. Whipples disease.
B. Coeliac disease complicated by lymphoma.
C. Cavitating mesenteric lymph node syndrome.
D. Abdominal tuberculosis.
E. Castleman disease.

60. With regard to the use of glucagon in barium enema examinations, which of the following statements is correct?

A. 0.1mg of glucagon is an appropriate dose.
B. Diabetes is a contraindication to the use of glucagon.
C. Insulinoma is a contraindication to the use of glucagon.
D. Glucagon can be safely used in patients with phaeochromocytoma.
E. Smooth muscle relaxation is optimal at 5 minutes and lasts approximately 1 hour.

61. A 39-year-old male complains of severe, colicky left lower abdominal pain and rectal bleeding. He has experienced intermittent abdominal pain for the last 3–4 months. There is no previous history of medical problems. On examination he has left lower abdominal tenderness without signs of peritonism. A CT examination is performed which reveals a focal intraluminal abnormality, with the appearance of a mass within the sigmoid colon. There are concentric rings of soft tissue and fatty attenuation giving a 'target' like appearance. Mesenteric vessels are seen to course into the lesion. At the most distal point of the abnormality there is a more discrete low attenuation mass measuring approximately 3 cm in size of fatty attenuation. The large bowel distal to the sigmoid lesion is collapsed and proximal to the lesion there are multiple loops of small bowel and a dilated colon. What is the most likely underlying pathology for this condition?

A. Benign tumour.
B. Malignant tumour.
C. Inverted diverticulum.
D. Idiopathic.
E. Inflammatory bowel disease.

62. A patient with a known history of malignancy undergoes a CT scan of the chest, abdomen, and pelvis for staging purposes. This examination identifies a solitary hypodense lesion in the spleen measuring 4 cm in diameter, but no other evidence of metastatic disease. A PET-CT is considered as a possible mechanism for determining whether or not this is a metastasis, but is considered not likely to be helpful. Which malignancy is the patient most likely to have?

A. Melanoma.
B. Lung carcinoma.
C. Lymphoma.
D. Renal cell carcinoma.
E. Colon carcinoma.

63. A 54-year-old man has a CT scan of renal tracts for suspected right renal colic. The right renal tract is normal, but an incidental 6-cm well-defined cyst is noted within the spleen. There is no past medical history of note. What is the most likely aetiology of the splenic cyst?

A. Previous trauma.
B. Echinococcal infection.
C. Congenital cyst.
D. Liquefied infarct.
E. Unilocular lymphangioma.

64. A patient presents to the surgeons with a known history of gallstones, for which she underwent an ERCP 2 years earlier. She has had recurring pain and mildly elevated liver function tests. She underwent an MRCP/MRI liver prior to consideration for surgery. This showed a number of 8-mm filling defects in the CBD. Which of the following MRI sequences is likely to be the most helpful in trying to determine if these filling defects are due to pneumobilia, as opposed to retained calculi?

A. Axial T2 steady-state GE.
B. Coronal thick slab MRCP.
C. Three-dimensional volume coronal MRCP.
D. Two-dimensional coronal oblique thin (4mm) MRCP.
E. Axial T1 in phase and out of phase GE.

65. You have been asked to give a presentation on MRI of the liver to your radiological colleagues. One of the audience asks if any of the contrast agents used in MRI of the liver works best with any sequence other than a T1WI sequence. What do you respond?

A. Yes, gadopentate dimeglumine.
B. Yes, mangafodipir trisodium.
C. Yes, gadobenate dimeglumine (hepatocyte specific).
D. Yes, SPIO.
E. No, all liver contrast agents work best with T1WI.

66. A 55-year-old woman is admitted to hospital after several episodes of melaena. She has an upper GI endoscopy performed, which is normal. A CT scan of abdomen is requested and this demonstrates a large exophytic mass arising from the jejunum in the left upper quadrant. It is heterogeneous in density, and has some peripheral enhancement and central necrosis. There is no calcification, intestinal obstruction, or evidence of aneurysmal dilatation of the affected segment of jejunum. There is no adjacent lymphadenopathy or ascites. What is the most likely diagnosis?

A. Adenocarcinoma.
B. Lymphoma.
C. Carcinoid tumour.
D. Metastasis.
E. Gastrointestinal stromal tumour (GIST).

67. A 70-year-old woman presents with a history of high dysphagia. Barium swallow reveals a barium-filled sac extending postero-inferior from the C5/6 level to the left of the upper oesophagus. What is the most likely diagnosis?

A. Pulsion diverticulum.
B. Traction diverticulum.
C. Zenker diverticulum.
D. Early intramural diverticulosis.
E. Oesophageal perforation.

68. A 26-year-old man, with a previous history of a panprocto-colectomy for Gardner's syndrome, presents with vague abdominal discomfort and a CT scan is requested to ascertain the cause. He is found to have a well-defined mass of homogenous density, which you suspect may be a desmoid tumour, given the previous clinical history. Where in the abdomen is this most likely to be located?

A. Abdominal wall.
B. Retroperitoneum.
C. Small bowel mesentery.
D. Pelvis.
E. Duodenal wall.

69. A 75-year-old man is undergoing a CT colonography examination for investigation of a change in bowel habit. He has difficulty retaining the CO_2 for adequate bowel distension. Which of the following segments of colon is likely to be better distended on the prone scan?

A. Caecum.
B. Transverse colon.
C. Rectosigmoid.
D. Ascending colon.
E. Hepatic flexure.

70. A 55-year-old male liver transplant recipient undergoes Doppler ultrasound assessment at 1 year for deranged liver function tests. Colour Doppler imaging demonstrates a stenosis in the hepatic artery, at the presumed anastomosis. Which of the following statements with regard to the associated pulsed Doppler findings is likely to be false?

A. Tardus-parvus arterial waveform distal to the stenosis.
B. Resistive index of 0.9 distal to the stenosis.
C. Spectral broadening in the immediate post-stenotic portion.
D. Elevated peak systolic velocity at the stenosis.
E. Elevated end diastolic velocity at the stenosis.

71. A 50-year-old male with a 2.5-cm hepatocellular carcinoma undergoes RFA. Which of the following findings is uncommon in the immediate post-ablation period?

A. Transient peri-ablational hyperaemia.
B. Small number of tiny intra-lesional air bubbles.
C. Arterio-portal shunting.
D. Ablation zone larger than the primary lesion.
E. 'Mural nodule in cyst' pattern.

72. A 45-year-old man has a long history of intermittent diarrhoea, abdominal bloating, and cramps, but has neglected to seek medical advice until now. His GP is worried about undiagnosed Crohn's disease and sends him for a small bowel series. This shows some dilatation of the proximal small bowel, with segmentation and flocculation of the barium and an increased number of normal thickness folds seen in the ileum. There is no evidence of stricture formation or ulceration. What is the most likely underlying diagnosis?

A. Amyloidosis.
B. Chronic ischaemic enteritis.
C. Whipple's disease.
D. Coeliac disease.
E. Lymphoma.

73. A 40-year-old male with a 22-year history of Crohn's disease presents with abdominal pain, diarrhoea, and low-grade fever. To attempt to limit his lifetime radiation exposure he is investigated via MR enterography. Which of the following MRI findings is considered to be the earliest in active inflammation?

A. Increased mesenteric vascularity.
B. Small bowel wall thickening.
C. Mucosal hyperenhancement.
D. Perienteric inflammation.
E. Reactive adenopathy.

74. A 20-year-old male with a recent history of medulloblastoma now presents with vague abdominal pain, PR bleeding, and weight loss. Innumerable colonic polyps are demonstrated on colonoscopy. What is the most likely unifying diagnosis?

A. Familial adenomatous polyposis.
B. Turcot syndrome.
C. Gardner syndrome.
D. Lynch syndrome.
E. Chronic inflammatory bowel disease.

75. A 50-year-old male is admitted under the surgical team having presented with upper abdominal pain and raised inflammatory markers. Suspecting acute cholecystitis, an ultrasound is requested, but due to large body habitus there is poor visualization of his gallbladder. To further evaluate hepatobiliary scintigraphy using ^{99m}Tc-labelled iminodiacetic acid is arranged. Which of the following findings are consistent with acute cholecystitis?

A. Non-visualization of the gallbladder at 1 and 4 hours.
B. Non-visualization of the gallbladder at 1 hour but seen at 4 hours.
C. Visualization of the gallbladder at 1 hour.
D. Visualization of the gallbladder at 30 minutes after morphine administration.
E. Hepatobiliary scintigraphy is not appropriate for investigation of acute cholecystitis.

chapter 3

GASTROINTESTINAL

ANSWERS

1. B. Leakage from the duodenal stump.

There is no gastro-duodenal anastomosis in a Billroth II procedure. The amylase is not sufficiently elevated for pancreatitis in most cases and there is no described abnormality in the pancreas. It is too early for pseudocyst formation and tumour recurrence.

Kim KW, Choi BI, Han JK, Kim TK, Kim AY, Lee HJ et al. Postoperative anastomotic and pathologic findings at CT following gastrectomy. *RadioGraphics* 2002; 22: 323–336.

2. A. The appearance of the oesophageal folds.

The oesophageal folds are normally longitudinally orientated. Horizontally orientated folds are described as feline oesophagus. The change in mucosal appearance is the normal Z line – the squamo-columnar junction. The narrowing described is the A line at the origin of the vestibule of the distal oesophagus. The position of the hiatus is normally stated as being 40 cm. This is the distance from the teeth at gastroscopy – the distance from the origin of the oesophagus is 25 cm.

Grainger RG, Allison DJ, and Dixon AK. *Grainger & Allison's Diagnostic Radiology*, 4th edn, Churchill Livingstone, 2001.

3. D. Islet cell tumour with liver metastases.

Whilst this tumour is rare, the CT findings indicate a focal mass lesion in the head of the pancreas. Hyperechoic metastases in the liver are suggestive of islet cell tumour, rather than pancreatic carcinoma metastases, even though pancreatic carcinoma is more common. The islet cell tumour could be a gastrinoma, which is most commonly found in the head of the pancreas and is malignant in 60%. It is also associated with peptic ulcer disease and the finding of air and fluid in the subhepatic space suggests a perforated duodenal ulcer.

King C, Reznek R, Dacie J, and Wass J. Imaging islet cell tumours. *Clinical Radiology* 1994; 49: 295–303.

4. E. The size of tumour at diagnosis is related to the risk of metastatic spread.

Carcinoid is the 33% tumour, as 33% occur in the small bowel, 33% are multiple, 33% are malignant, and 33% are associated with a second malignancy. Appendiceal carcinoid accounts for 50% of all carcinoids and 67% are asymptomatic at presentation. Appendiceal carcinoid accounts for only 7% of metastatic disease, with small bowel carcinoid causing 75%. The size of the tumour at diagnosis is related to the risk of metastatic spread, which is 2% if the lesion is <1 cm, but 85% if the lesion is over 2 cm in size.

Dahnert W. *Radiology Review Manual*, 6th edn, Lippincott Williams & Wilkins, 2007. pp. 811–812.

5. C. Ultrasound scan within 24 hours.

CT is only indicated as an investigation in cases of pancreatitis with severe prognostic indicators. This patient's Ranson score is 1, which indicates a mild episode of pancreatitis and therefore CT is not indicated. ERCP was formerly contraindicated in pancreatitis, but is now recognized as a treatment for obstructing stones in the ampulla that are causing the pancreatitis. Ultimately further investigations can be directed based on the ultrasound findings.

Balthazar EJ. Acute pancreatitis: assessment of severity with clinical and CT evaluation. *Radiology* 2002; 223(3): 603–613.

6. A. Benign due to the line noted crossing the base of the ulcer.

This line—Hampton's line—represents undermining of the mucosa by the more vulnerable submucosa. It is not commonly seen, but is taken to be virtually diagnostic of a benign ulcer when present. Projection beyond the lumen and a symmetrical mound are features of a benign ulcer along with smooth radiating mucosal folds. Scar retraction can be seen with benign ulcers. Both benign and malignant ulcers are more commonly seen on the lesser curve.

Grainger RG, Allison DJ, and Dixon AK. *Grainger & Allison's Diagnostic Radiology*, 4th edn, Churchill Livingstone, 2001.

7. E. Whilst the appearances are consistent with a laceration and subcapsular haematoma, radiological findings are not reliable in determining the need for a laparotomy.

Splenic injuries can be graded 1–5 (American Association of Trauma Surgeons). Grade 1 is a subcapsular haematoma that involves <25% of the splenic surface or a laceration <1cm deep. Grade 2 is a haematoma that involves 25–50% of the surface or a laceration up to 3cm deep. Grade 3 is a haematoma involving >50% of splenic surface or 10 cm in length or a laceration greater than 3 cm into the parenchyma. Grade 4 is a laceration extending into the hilum that devascularizes up to 25% of the spleen. Grade 5 is a shattered spleen, with multiple lacerations or a spleen avulsed from its vascular bed. Radiological findings do not correlate well with requirement for laparotomy in the more minor splenic injuries. Clinical assessment is of more value, with surgery only indicated in unstable patients. The value of radiology is in detecting other injuries and in quantifying the amount of the haematoma due to the risk of delayed splenic rupture in more severe injuries.

Dahnert W. *Radiology Review Manual*, 6th edn, Lippincott Williams & Wilkins, 2007. pp. 807–808.

8. E. Pneumatosis intestinalis.

The stacked coin appearance is seen secondary to intramural haemorrhage—the appearances of systemic sclerosis are of tightly packed folds of normal thickness in a dilated portion of bowel, which has been given the title 'accordion' or 'hidebound' bowel. The pseudo-diverticula (10–40%) are seen on the mesenteric side of the bowel, unlike colonic diverticula. The transit time is prolonged, as there is reduced intestinal motility. Another classical feature is of a markedly dilated duodenum, due to the loss of the enteric innervations—mega duodenum. This classically terminates abruptly at the level of the superior mesenteric artery (SMA). Pneumatosis cystoides can occur in systemic sclerosis of the small bowel. Small bowel disease is seen in up to 40% of patients with systemic sclerosis and indicates rapidly progressing disease.

Dahnert W. *Radiology Review Manual*, 6th edn, Lippincott Williams & Wilkins, 2007. pp. 863–864.

9. D. Adjacent abscess formation.

Abscess formation has been found to be the most specific finding in appendiceal perforation, along with extraluminal gas and small bowel ileus. Abscess formation is also one of the least sensitive findings. Regional mesenteric lymph nodes are the most sensitive, but are reasonably non-specific. A focal wall defect, if seen, is reasonably sensitive and specific. Appendicolith is only found in 50% on CT and has a specificity of 70%.

Bixby SD, Lucey BC, Soto JA, Theysohn JM, Ozonoff A, and Varghese JC. Perforated versus nonperforated acute appendicitis: accuracy of multidetector CT detection. *Radiology* 2007; 243(1): 302.

10. C. ERCP with plastic stent insertion.

PTC is an appropriate approach, but biliary sepsis can cause bacteraemia during PTC and thus ERCP is preferable in this case, if possible. Contraindications to PTC include prothrombin time greater than 2 seconds higher than control, platelet count less than 100,000, ascites, hydatid disease, and lack of access to surgical facilities. If an ERCP were to fail, the other options would be viable alternatives. Metal stent insertion at the first instance is inappropriate unless it is known that the biliary dilatation is due to inoperable malignancy. This is because metal stents cannot be removed, whereas the plastic variety can be removed, if necessary.

Chapman S and Nakielny R. *A Guide to Radiological Procedures*. Saunders, 2001. p. 115.

11. B. Segment 5.

For a review of the segmental anatomy of the liver, please see the reference below.

Dahnert W. *Radiology Review Manual*, 6th edn, Lippincott Williams & Wilkins, 2007. p. 684.

12. B. Haemangioma.

The ultrasound findings describe a target lesion or bull's eye lesion. Cavernous haemangiomas can have unusual appearances, but a small lesion such as described will normally have a uniform hyperechoic appearance. Of all the other lesions described, metastasis would be top of the differential, although this appearance is not the most classical for a colonic metastasis.

Chapman S and Nakielny R. *Aids to Radiological Differential Diagnosis*, 4th edn, Saunders, 2003. pp. 288–289.

13. B. LAO.

The right lateral position is not routinely used. The RAO shows the body and antrum of the stomach. Supine positioning shows the greater curve and the antrum of the stomach. Left lateral position shows the fundus of the stomach.

Chapman S, Nakielny R. *A Guide to Radiological Procedures*, 4th edn, Saunders, 2001.

14. B. The left paracolic gutter communicates with the left subphrenic space.

There is no direct connection between these two spaces due to the phrenico-colic ligament. The rest of the statements are correct.

Brant WE and Helms CA. *Fundamentals of Diagnostic Radiology*, 3rd edn, Lippincott Williams & Wilkins, 2007. pp. 733–736.

15. C. Enlarged peripancreatic lymph nodes (>15mm).

Enlarged regional nodes are a sign of unresectability, but nodes adjacent to the pancreas are resected as part of Whipple's procedure. The other factors all indicate that a pancreatic lesion is unresectable. Other features of unresectable pancreatic carcinoma are liver metastases. Only 10–15% of pancreatic neoplasms are resectable at presentation.

Brant WE and Helms CA. *Fundamentals of Diagnostic Radiology*, 3rd edn, Lippincott Williams & Wilkins, 2007. pp. 786–787.

16. D. Amyloidosis.

This patient probably has amyloidosis secondary to prolonged RA. GI involvement is more common in primary (70%) than secondary (13%) amyloidosis. Nevertheless, the small bowel is involved in 74% of cases of GI amyloidosis and secondary amyloidosis is the most common type of amyloid disease. Amyloidosis is secondary to the deposition of insoluble amlyoid protein in soft tissues and organs. In primary amyloidosis the heart (90%), followed by the small bowel and the lungs (70%), are the most commonly affected organs. The kidneys are affected in 90% of cases of secondary amyloidosis. Amyloidosis classically causes a diffuse thickening of bowel folds. It may cause dilated bowel folds, if the myenteric plexus is involved. The main differential for amyloid is Whipple's disease and intestinal lymphangiectasia. Whipple's disease does not cause bowel dilatation or rigidity, as described in the antrum in this patient. Crohn's disease can also present with thickened folds, but it is more commonly focal with the most pronounced abnormality in the terminal ileum. Ulceration is also commonly seen in Crohn's, but 68 years old would be a late first presentation for Crohn's. Whilst option A is true, this is not what the question asked. Patients with mastocytosis most commonly present in infancy.

Dahnert W. *Radiology Review Manual*, 6th edn, Lippincott Williams & Wilkins, 2007. pp. 801–802.
Kobayashi H, Tada S, Fuchigami T, Okuda Y, Takasagi K, Matsumoto T et al. Secondary amyloidosis in patients with rheumatoid arthritis: diagnostic and prognostic value of gastroduodenal biopsy. *British Journal of Rheumatology* 1996; 35(1): 44–49.

17. A. Cholangiocarcinoma.

Specifically a Klatskin tumour, as it occurs at the porta hepatis. Cholangiocarcinoma can be iso- to hyperechoic on ultrasound. On CT and MRI, it shows delayed enhancement in 74%. Many conditions predispose to cholangiocarcinoma and gallstones are identified in 20–50% of patients with cholangiocarcinoma. Hepatocellular carcinoma would be the next most likely diagnosis. It can have a variable ultrasonographic appearance. Hepatocellular carcinoma usually demonstrates arterial phase enhancement (80%). Prostate does not commonly metastasize to the liver and would again demonstrate arterial phase enhancement classically. Whilst haemangiomas are classically hyperechoic on ultrasound, larger lesions can appear heterogeneously hypoechoic (40%).

Dahnert W. *Radiology Review Manual*, 6th edn, Lippincott Williams & Wilkins, 2007. pp. 696–698.

18. B. Porcelain gallbladder.

It can sometimes be difficult to see a cause for this appearance, and a number of the given options could result in it. However, peristalsis should be seen in a healthy patient if the abnormality is due to bowel. With gallstones, the appearance should change on positioning. There is no mention of an ERCP in the history, and whilst air in the biliary tree is common after sphincterotomy, it is often only seen in the gallbladder immediately after the procedure. Patients with emphysematous cholecystitis are usually clinically unwell and are unlikely to be asymptomatic. Porcelain gallbladder is associated with gallstones in 90% of cases. It is a relevant finding to make as 10–20% of patients develop carcinoma of the gallbladder.

Dahnert W. *Radiology Review Manual*, 6th edn, Lippincott Williams & Wilkins, 2007. p. 743.

19. E. Gastrografin can be added to improve transit time.

Simethicone is an antifoaming agent. While a uniform particle size helps reduce flocculation, a heterogeneous particle size improves mucosal coating. The barium densities used for different examinations are barium swallow 150%, barium meal 250%, barium follow-through 50%, barium small bowel enteroclysis 18%, double-contrast barium enema 125%, and single-contrast barium enema 70%.

Francis IS, Aviv RI, Dick EA, and Watkins AF. *Fundamental Aspects of Radiology*, Remedica Publishing, 1999.

20. A. Small bowel mural hyperdensity is a feature and is due to vasodilatation seen in early ischaemia.

Multi-detector CT (MDCT) has been found to correlate with pathological processes in small bowel obstruction. The earliest appearance is increased mural density due to hyperaemia. Wall thickening is due to increasing capillary permeability, which causes submucosal oedema. Dilatation is secondary to oedema that limits peristalsis. Lack of enhancement occurs when the bowel dilates and compresses the capillary bed. Pneumatosis is secondary to mucosal ischaemic change, which allows luminal air to track into the wall. Lack of enhancement is also seen in embolic ischaemia, but is not a specific sign of this process. Whilst oral contrast is preferred in many centres, as it can help define if complete obstruction is present, it is not mandatory. Some centres prefer the negative contrast provided by the fluid in the bowel lumen. Patients with small bowel obstruction are also often unable to tolerate oral contrast due to vomiting.

Qalbani A, Paushter D, and Dachman AH. Multidetector row CT of small bowel obstruction. *Radiological Clinics of North America* 2007; 45(3): 499–512.

21. A. Small bowel obstruction, as can occur in up to 30% of these patients.

Total colonic resection with J pouch anastomosis is carried out in patients with ulcerative colitis or familial adenomatous polyposis (FAP) in order to resect the entire colon, but retain anal defaecation. One of the main contraindications to total colectomy and J pouch formation is Crohn's disease and such a procedure is uncommonly carried out in this situation due to the high recurrence rate. Pouchitis and small bowel obstruction both occur in up to 30% of patients who undergo this procedure. The radiological features of pouchitis are non-specific, but include wall thickening and increased enhancement of the bowel wall, with peripouch fat-stranding. Fat-stranding on its own is common as a result of both the surgery and possible inflammatory change due to previous proctitis. Small bowel obstruction most commonly occurs in the region of the ileostomy. Free fluid is often seen in small bowel obstruction. The absence of fluid cavities or air pockets is against a leak from the pouch anastomosis and the clinical features are not consistent with fistula. The blind ending lumen described is the normal appearance seen on a pouchogram.

Crema MD, Richarme D, Azizi L, Hoeffel CC, Tubiana JM, and Arrive L. Pouchography, CT and MRI features of ileal J pouch-anal anastomosis. *American Journal of Roentgenology* 2006; 187: W594–W603.

22. D. Crohn's disease.

The findings described are classical for Crohn's disease and lymphadenopathy is seen in up to 30% of cases. Tuberculosis more typically involves the caecum. Lymphoma usually causes a nodular appearance to the bowel. It is not associated with stricturing of the affected segment and is more classically associated with dilatation of the affected segment due to destruction of the myenteric plexus.

Dahnert W. *Radiology Review Manual*, 6th edn, Lippincott Williams & Wilkins, 2007. pp. 818–820.

23. D. Focal nodular hyperplasia (FNH).

This is the second most common benign liver tumour. It is thought to represent a hyperplastic response of hepatocytes to an underlying vascular malformation. It is most common in young adult females and is usually an asymptomatic solitary lesion. On histology, FNH consists of hyperplastic hepatocytes and small bile ductules around a central scar. The bile ductules of FNH do not communicate with the adjacent biliary tree. At ultrasound, FNH is isoechoic or hypoechoic. Colour Doppler may show prominent central vascularity. At CT, FNH is typically slightly hyperattenuating or isoattenuating to surrounding liver on precontrast images. On post contrast images, FNH is hyperattenuating in the arterial phase and isoattenuating in the portal venous phase with hypoattenuating central scar. The scar shows delayed enhancement. At MRI, FNH is iso- to hypointense on T1WI and slightly hyper- to isointense on T2WI. The central scar is hypointense on T1WI and hyperintense on T2WI. The enhancement pattern is similar to that on CT. If the appearances are atypical, MRI with hepatocyte-specific contrast agent (gadobenate dimeglumine) may be useful in confirming the hepatocellular origin of the mass. With gadobenate dimeglumine, FNH is iso- to hyperintense on the 1–3 hour delayed images in over 96% of cases.

Silva AC, Evans JM, McCullough AE, Jatoi MA, Vargas HE, and Hara AK. MR imaging of hypervascular liver masses: a review of current techniques. *RadioGraphics* 2009; 29: 385–402.
Anderson SW, Kruskal JB, and Kane RA. Benign hepatic tumors and iatrogenic pseudotumors. *RadioGraphics* 2009; 29: 211–229.

24. B. Mucinous cystic neoplasm.

Mucin is detected in FNA fluid in these lesions. Pseudocysts are uncommon without a history of pancreatitis and the aspirated fluid is high in amylase. The cysts in microcystic lesions are usually smaller than 1cm, except in the oligocystic variant. They are also known as serous cystadenomas. Intraductal papillary mucinous tumours cause dilatation of the main pancreatic duct, side branch ducts or both. FNA, either percutaneous or via endoscopic ultrasound, has been described as a low-risk procedure for differentiating pancreatic cystic lesions.

Demos TC, Posniak HV, Harmath C, Olson MC, and Aranha G. Cystic lesions of the pancreas. *American Journal of Roentgenology* 2002; 179(6): 1375–1388.

25. D. Dual GE T1WI in phase and out of phase.

Three basic MRI techniques are available for fat detection, which work on the basis of the difference in precessional frequency between water and fat protons. These are chemical shift imaging, frequency-selective imaging, and MR spectroscopy. Dual GE T1WI is the most useful sequence in clinical practice. It is based on the phase interference effect or chemical shift imaging of the second kind. When the fat and water protons are in phase there is constructive interference and when they are out of phase there is destructive interference. By comparing the signal intensities on the in-phase and out-of-phase images, fat detection is possible.

Chemical shift imaging of the first kind, or chemical shift spatial misregistration, occurs at fat–water interfaces in the frequency-encoding direction, manifesting as alternating bands of high and low signal. It is present in all standard non-fat-saturated sequences, but it can be subtle and may be missed or mistaken for image noise. Frequency-selective imaging with selective excitation or saturation depends on the homogeneity of the magnetic field and the size of the lesion.

MR spectroscopy is too time-consuming for routine clinical use.

Cassidy FH, Yokoo T, Aganovic L, Hanna RF, Bydder M, Middleton MS et al. Fatty liver disease: MR imaging techniques for the detection and quantification of liver steatosis. *RadioGraphics* 2009; 29: 231–260.

26. C. Dilated common hepatic duct with normal common bile duct.

Mirizzi syndrome is a functional hepatic syndrome caused by extrinsic compression of the CHD by a calculus impacted in the gallbladder neck or cystic duct. Low insertion of the cystic duct into the CHD is a predisposing factor.

Typical features at imaging include extrinsic compression of the CHD, a gallstone in the gallbladder neck or cystic duct, dilatation of the intrahepatic ducts and CHD proximally, and a normal CBD. Rarely, inflammation around an impacted calculus leads to a stricture formation mimicking a periductal infiltrating cholangiocarcinoma.

Menias CO, Surabhi VR, Prasad, SR, Wang HL, Narra VR, and Chintapalli KN. Mimics of cholangiocarcinoma: spectrum of disease. *RadioGraphics* 2008; 28: 1115–1129.

27. B. Emphysematous cholecystitis.

This is a rare form of acute cholecystitis. The majority of patients are between 50 and 70 years of age. It is more common in men (male to female ratio of 2:1) and in those with diabetes and peripheral vascular disease. Emphysematous cholecystitis is a surgical emergency because there is an increased risk of gallbladder perforation and increased mortality rate. The definitive treatment is cholecystectomy, although in critically ill patients percutaneous cholecystostomy may be used as a temporary measure.

Grayson DE, Abbott, RM, Levy AD, and Sherman PM. Emphysematous infections of the abdomen and pelvis: A pictorial review. *RadioGraphics* 2002; 22: 543–561.

28. B. Selective superior mesenteric angiogram.

Variations in hepatic arterial anatomy are common. According to Michel classification, the classic hepatic arterial anatomy with the hepatic artery proper dividing into the right and left hepatic arteries is seen in only 55% of the population. A replaced right hepatic artery from the SMA is seen in 11% and an accessory right hepatic artery from the SMA is seen in 7% of the population. A selective SMA angiogram should therefore be performed in this case.

A selective left gastric angiogram is not required as it is a branch of the coeliac axis. The inferior mesenteric artery does not supply the liver.

The coeliac axis divides into the common hepatic, left gastric, and splenic arteries. Embolization of the coeliac axis is therefore not an option.

Catalano OA, Singh AH, Uppot RN, Hahn PF, Ferrano CR, and Sahani DV. Vascular and biliary variants in the liver: Implications for liver surgery. *RadioGraphics* 2008; 28: 359–378.

29. D. Regenerative nodules.

Regenerative nodules are formed in response to necrosis and altered circulation. They remain enhanced in the portal venous phase as opposed to HCC, which typically demonstrates contrast washout in the portal venous phase. Regenerative nodules have normal hepatocellular function and Kupffer cell density and therefore demonstrate uptake of both hepatocellular agents and SPIO particles. As dedifferentiation proceeds, the hepatocellular function and Kupffer cell density reduce.

Hanna RF, Aguirre DA, Kased N, Emery SC, Peterson MR, and Sirlin CB. Cirrhosis-associated Hepatocellular nodules: correlation of histopathologic and MR imaging features. *RadioGraphics* 2008; 28: 747–769.

30. C. Dilated hepatic veins and IVC.

Elevated right atrial/central venous pressure due to cardiac decompensation results in impaired venous drainage from the liver, producing passive hepatic congestion. If prolonged, passive hepatic congestion can result in cardiac cirrhosis. On CT imaging, retrograde enhancement of dilated IVC and hepatic veins is seen in the arterial phase. In the portal venous phase, there is delayed/reduced enhancement of the hepatic veins due to impaired venous drainage. There is heterogenous enhancement of the liver parenchyma due to venous stasis. Other features of cardiac failure may be evident.

Acute Budd–Chiari syndrome is characterized by narrowed hepatic veins and intrahepatic IVC (secondary to compression by the enlarged liver) and by flip-flop pattern of enhancement between the arterial and the portal venous phases.

Torabi M, Hosseinzadeh K, and Federle P. CT of Nonneoplastic hepatic vascular and perfusion disorders. *RadioGraphics* 2008; 28: 1967–1982.

31. D. Haemochromatosis. GE T2WI.

A dual GE T1 in- and out-of-phase sequence is routinely used in identifying lipid content within an adrenal lesion. It is based on the phase interference effect. When the fat and water signals are in-phase, there is constructive interference and when they are out-of-phase there is destructive interference. This results in signal drop-off on the out-of-phase sequence.

The reverse effect of decreased signal intensity on in-phase images compared to out-of-phase ones is seen in iron deposition diseases. This is because the echo time for the in-phase sequence is longer than for the out-of-phase sequence, therefore the in-phase sequence is more susceptible to the paramagnetic (dephasing) effects of iron.

Haemochromatosis is an autosomal recessive genetic disorder. There is abnormal deposition of iron in parenchymal organs such as the liver, pancreas, heart, etc.

In haemosiderosis or secondary haemochromatosis, iron deposition is seen in the reticuloendothelial system of the liver, spleen, and bone marrow. This type of deposition is not associated with tissue damage.

A GE T2 sequence demonstrates signal loss due to the magnetic field inhomogeneity produced by the paramagnetic effects of iron. GE sequences are more susceptible to the paramagnetic effects than SE sequences, as there is no 180° rephasing pulse in gradient sequences.

Cassidy FH, Yokoo T, Aganovic L, Hanna RF, Bydder M, Middleton MS et al. Fatty liver disease: MR imaging techniques for the detection and quantification of liver steatosis. *RadioGraphics* 2009; 29: 231–260.
Queiroz-Andrade M, Blasbalg R, Ortega CD, Rodstein MA, Baroni RH, Rocha MS et al. MR imaging findings of iron overload. *RadioGraphics* 2009; 29: 1575–1589.

32. E. All of the above.

All the findings are manifestations of von Hippel–Lindau (VHL) disease. VHL is a rare, inherited, multisystem disorder characterized by the development of multiple benign and malignant neoplasms. It is an autosomal dominant disorder caused by inactivation of a tumour suppressor gene located on chromosome 3p25.5.

The clinical manifestations are broad and include central nervous system (CNS) and retinal haemangioblastomas, renal cysts and tumours, pancreatic cysts and tumours, phaechromocytomas, endolymphatic sac tumours, and epididymal cystadenomas.

The diagnostic criteria for VHL include: (i) >1 CNS haemangioblastoma, (ii) one CNS haemangioblastoma + visceral manifestations of VHL, and (iii) any manifestation + known family history of VHL. The most common causes of death in VHL are renal cell carcinoma and neurologic complications of cerebellar haemangioblastomas. Genetic counselling and screening are important for early detection and treatment of VHL lesions.

Leung RS, Biswas SV, Duncan M, and Rankin S. Imaging features of von Hippel-Lindau disease. *RadioGraphics* 2008; 28: 65–79.

33. C. Barrett's oesophagus.

This represents progressive columnar metaplasia of the distal oesophagus secondary to reflux oesophagitis. It is a premalignant condition associated with an increased risk of adenocarcinoma, 40-fold that of the general population. Strictures are more common in the distal, then mid oesophagus, rather than the classically described proximal third. The typical finding is of 1-cm-long strictures or ulceration with associated gastro-oesophageal reflux and hiatus hernia. These findings are non-specific and may result from a variety of other causes such as corrosive ingestion, nasogastric intubation, Crohn's disease, or neoplasm (primary or secondary). However, the presence of a fine reticular pattern extending distally from the stricture appears to be specific for Barrett's. A reticulonodular pattern has been described in patients with a superficial spreading adenocarcinoma, but this is rare and not classically associated with a stricture.

Dahnert W. *Radiology Review Manual*, 6th edn, Lippincott Williams & Wilkins, 2007. pp. 805–806.
Levine MS, Kressel HY, Caroline DF, Laufer I, Herlinger H, and Thompson JJ. Barrett oesophagus: reticular pattern of the mucosa. *Radiology* 1983; 147: 663–667.

34. A. Cholecystoduodenal fistula.

The other answers are all causes of portal air, whereas the salient description is for air in the biliary tree.

Chapman S and Nakielny R. *Aids to Radiological Differential Diagnosis*, 4th edn, Saunders, 2003. p. 278.

35. D. Glycogenic acanthosis.

This is a common condition affecting elderly people. Cytoplasmic glycogen accumulates in the squamous epithelial lining of the oesophagus, producing the findings described in the question. Patients usually have no oesophageal symptoms, and the disease is not a precursor of malignancy (although extensive glycogenic acanthosis has been shown to be associated with Cowden's syndrome). The major differential diagnosis is candidiasis, but the plaques of candidiasis have a more linear, rather than rounded, appearance and it usually occurs in immunocompromised patients who complain of odynophagia. Options C, D, and E typically cause ulceration, not plaques.

Levine MS and Rubesin SE. Diseases of the esophagus: diagnosis with esophagography. *Radiology* 2005; 237: 414–427.

36. E. Intramural haematoma of the oesophagus.

Submucosal dissection of the oesophagus may be spontaneous or secondary to direct trauma or coagulopathy. Patients may present with chest pain, dysphagia, and nausea, often followed by haematemesis. The high attenuation in the wall of the oesophagus is the clue to the diagnosis. This feature and lack of enhancement are inconsistent with any alternative diagnosis. Follow-up with endoscopy is usually performed to exclude a predisposing pathological condition. The natural history is complete resolution without surgical intervention.

Herbetko J, Delany D, Ogilvie BC, and Blaquiere RM. Spontaneous intramural haematoma of the oesophagus: appearance on computed tomography. *Clinical Radiology* 1991; 44: 327–328.

37. C. Transient hepatic intensity difference (THID).

THID on MRI or transient hepatic attenuation difference (THAD) on CT is a pseudolesion caused by focal alteration in the haemodynamics of the liver due to either non-tumourous arterio-portal shunt or obstruction of distal portal venous flow. THID or THAD is seen as a focal area of enhancement in the arterial phase only, with no abnormality seen in the portal venous phase. Features suggestive of THID or THAD include peripheral location, wedge shape, straight margins, and normal vessels coursing through the area.

Silva AC, Evans JM, McCullough AE, Jatoi MA, Vargas HE, and .Hara AK. MR imaging of hypervascular liver masses: A review of current techniques. *RadioGraphics* 2009; 29: 385–402.
Lee JW, Kim S, Kwack SW, Kim CW, Moon TH, Lee SH et al. Hepatic capsular and subcapsular pathologic conditions: Demonstration with CT and MR imaging. *RadioGraphics* 2008; 28: 1307–1323.

38. E. T3, N1, M0.

The T staging of oesophageal tumours is most accurately carried out by EUS. The staging is T1 invading submucosa, T2 invading muscularis propria, T3 invading the adventitia, T4 invading adjacent structures. This is more accurate than the CT staging. Loss of fat planes on CT and the finding of tumour abutting the aorta—if it is in contact with less than 90% of the circumference—often does not preclude resectability, especially if these margins are clear on EUS. In the assessment of lymphatic spread, PET-CT has been shown to be more sensitive (81–99%) than CT alone (50–95%). Lymphatic spread is graded: N0, no spread; N1, loco-regional spread. There is no N2 grading of oesophageal carcinoma as further lymphatic spread is considered M1. Whilst the abdominal nodes may be involved, the low SUV max is reassuring. The para-oesophageal node is almost certainly involved. The finding described in the liver is classical of a haemangioma and a mottled uptake in the liver is a normal finding on PET-CT, thus there is no evidence of metastatic disease radiologically.

Dahnert W. *Radiology Review Manual*, 6th edn, Lippincott Williams & Wilkins, 2007. pp. 827–828.
Chowdhury FU, Bradley KM, and Gleeson FV. The role of FDG PET/CT in the evaluation of oesophageal carcinoma. *Clinical Radiology* 2008; 63(12): 1297–1309.

39. C. Recommend to the GP that the study was unremarkable but for mild reflux.

The findings described are in keeping with a 'feline' oesophagus. This is thought to be due to spasm in the muscularis mucosa. It is associated with gastro-oesophageal reflux, but is a benign entity.

Goherl VK, Edell SL, Laufer I, and Rhodes WH. Transverse folds in the human esophagus. *Radiology* 1978; 204: 303–330.

40. C. Polymyositis.

This condition and dermatomyositis affect skeletal muscle, which is found at the upper third of the oesophagus. These conditions begin in the upper oesophagus and extend caudally. Other findings at fluoroscopy include retention of barium in the valleculae and wide atonic pyriform fossae, regurgitation and nasal reflux, aspiration, and failure of contrast to progress in the upper oesophagus without the aid of gravity. Polymyositis and dermatomyositis are associated with underlying malignancy. The latter also involves a heliotrope rash and Gottrons papules on flexor surfaces.

The lower oesophagus is composed of smooth muscle and is affected by conditions such as scleroderma and SLE, which result in atony and lack of peristalsis in the lower two-thirds, beginning caudally and moving cranially. Achalasia and Chagas disease result in dilatation of the whole oesophagus, with a 'rat-tail' deformity at the lower end.

Grunebaum M and Salinger H. Radiological findings in polymyositis-dermatomyositis involving the pharynx and upper oesophagus. *Clinical Radiology* 1971; 22: 97–100.

41. D. CT scan after 3 days showing necrosis and fluid collections.

The Balthazar CT staging system grades pancreatitis based on the presence of gland enlargement and/or fluid collections, as well as the presence of necrosis involving <30%, 30–50% or >50% of the gland. This has been shown to be a more accurate predictor of severity of pancreatitis and morbidity than the Ranson or Acute Physiology and Chronic Health Evaluation II (APACHE II) criteria. This staging system is, however, most accurate when carried out after 48 hours, as the degree of pancreatic necrosis may not be apparent before this.

Balthazar EJ. Acute pancreatitis: assessment of severity with clinical and CT evaluation. *Radiology* 2002; 223(3): 603–613.

42. B. Gastric ulceration.

The anterior pararenal space extends between the posterior parietal peritoneum and the anterior renal fascia (Gerota's fascia). It is bounded laterally by the lateral conal fascia. The pancreas, second and third parts of the duodenum, and ascending and descending colon are located within the anterior pararenal space, and disease in this space usually arises in these organs. The stomach is intraperitoneal.

Brant WE and Helms CA. *Fundamentals of Diagnostic Radiology*, 3rd edn, Lippincott Williams & Wilkins, 2007. p. 734.

43. C. Water intoxication.

All five options are complications of barium enema. Additional potential complications include bowel perforation, barium impaction, and transient bacteraemia. Complications during barium enema are rare. Perforation of the bowel is the most frequent serious complication, occurring in approximately 0.02–0.04% of patients. Venous intravasation may result in a barium pulmonary embolus, which carries an 80% mortality. Water intoxication causes drowsiness and convulsions, as in this case. There is an increased risk in megacolon because of the large area of bowel mucosa available for the absorption of water. Water intoxication has also been attributed to the preparatory laxatives used. Buscopan® may cause cardiac arrhythmia and should be used with caution in those with cardiac disease; other relative contraindications include angle-closure glaucoma, myasthenia gravis, paralytic ileus, pyloric stenosis, and prostatic enlargement.

Chapman S and Nakielny R. *A Guide to Radiological Procedures*, Saunders, 2001. p. 72.

44. B. Pseudomyxoma retroperitonei.

The displacement of the psoas muscle indicates that this mass is most likely retroperitoneal. Pseudomyxoma peritonei is a rare condition that is characterized by intraperitoneal accumulation of gelatinous material owing to the rupture of a mucinous lesion of the appendix or ovary, e.g. mucinous cystadenoma/cystadenocarcinoma. It may occur in the retroperitoneum, where it is caused by the rupture of a mucinous lesion in the retrocaecal appendix and fixation of the lesion to the posterior abdominal wall. Clinically, it results in abdominal pain and a palpable mass. At CT, it appears as a multicystic mass with thick walls or septa that displace and distort adjacent structures. Curvilinear or punctuate mural calcifications may also occur and are highly suggestive.

Pancreatic pseudocysts usually occur in the peripancreatic space, but may occur in the abdomen, pelvis, or mediastinum. They are associated with the clinical findings of pancreatitis and elevation of serum amylase.

A urinoma is an encapsulated collection of chronically extravasated urine. There is usually a history of trauma and an associated hydronephrosis.

Haematomas are associated with trauma, coagulopathy/anticoagulants, or a ruptured abdominal aortic aneurysm. Chronic haematoma can result in low attenuation contents, but acutely the haematoma will have higher attenuation than pure fluid due to clot formation.

Retroperitoneal liposarcoma is most commonly of a density between water and muscle (myxoid type). It may have a solid, mixed, or pseudocystic pattern on CT. There may also be macroscopic areas of lipid in well-differentiated liposarcomas. Patients present with abdominal pain, weight loss, a palpable mass, and anaemia.

Yang DM, Jung DH, Kim H, Kang JH, Kim SH, Kim JH et al. Retroperitoneal cystic masses: CT, clinical and pathological findings and literature review. *RadioGraphics* 2004; 24: 1353–1365.

45. C. Supportive therapy.

Injury to the pancreas is relatively uncommon, occurring in less than 2% of blunt abdominal trauma patients. Direct signs of pancreatic injury at CT include laceration, transection, enlargement, and inhomogenous enhancement. Secondary signs include peripancreatic fat stranding and fluid collections, haemorrhage, and thickening of the anterior pararenal fascia. The management of pancreatic trauma depends on the integrity of the pancreatic duct. If it is intact, the treatment is supportive and expectant. If the duct is disrupted, surgery or stenting at ERCP is required. Although CT may not always directly demonstrate the pancreatic duct, the likelihood of ductal injury may be inferred from secondary signs. Wong et al. have devised a CT grading scheme, which is similar to the surgical classification of Moore. Grade A injuries comprise pancreatitis or superficial laceration (<50% pancreatic thickness), grade B1 is deep laceration

(>50% pancreatic thickness), grade B2 is transection of the pancreatic tail, grade C1 is deep laceration of the pancreatic head, and grade C2 is transection of the pancreatic head.

Grade A injuries spare the duct and are usually seen with an intact duct by surgical grading. Grade B and C injuries correlate with duct disruption. MR pancreatography is an alternative to ERCP to assess the integrity of the pancreatic duct. The duct integrity cannot be reliably assessed by ultrasound, particularly in the context of recent trauma.

Gupta A, Stuhlfaut JW, Fleming KW, Lucey BC, and Soto JA. Blunt trauma of the pancreas and biliary tract: a multimodality imaging approach to diagnosis. *RadioGraphics* 2004; 24: 1381–1395.
Wong YC, Wang LJ, Lin BC, Chen CJ, Lim KE, and Chen RJ. CT grading of blunt pancreatic injuries: prediction of ductal disruption and surgical correlation. *Journal of Computer Assisted Tomography* 1997; 21: 246–250.

46. C. Lipomatous pseudohypertrophy of the pancreas.

The history is one of undiagnosed cystic fibrosis (CF), with respiratory disease and pancreatic exocrine dysfunction. Pancreatic involvement in CF initially produces inhomogenous attenuation, then low attenuation, and then complete fatty infiltration and replacement. Microcysts may develop and some of these may become small macroscopic cysts demonstrable with CT. There may be scattered calcifications. On ultrasound, there is increased diffuse echogenicity in keeping with fatty infiltration and fibrosis. CF is a major cause of pancreatic exocrine failure in childhood. Pancreatic abnormalities are seen in 85–90% of CF patients. However, the disease progresses to pancreatitis in less than 1% of CF patients. It predisposes to pancreatic cancer.

Shwachman–Diamond syndrome is a rare congenital disorder characterized by pancreatic exocrine insufficiency, bone marrow dysfunction, and skeletal abnormalities. Patients usually present in infancy or early childhood with malabsorption and recurrent infections. Imaging reveals pancreatic lipomatosis.

Federle MP, Jeffrey RB, Desser TS, Anne VS, and Eraso A. *Diagnostic imaging: abdomen.* Amirsys, 2005, II-3: 18–19.

47. A. Sclerosing mesenteritis.

This is a rare condition of unknown cause characterized by chronic mesenteric inflammation. It is most frequently seen in the sixth decade and more commonly in males than females. It is often associated with other inflammatory disorders such as retroperitoneal fibrosis, Riedel thyroiditis, and sclerosing cholangitis. Symptoms include abdominal pain, nausea, fever, intestinal obstruction or ischaemia, a mass, or diarrhoea. The CT findings can range from subtle increased attenuation in the mesentery to a solid soft-tissue mass. The mass may envelop vessels, but there may be preservation of fat around the vessels, the 'fat halo' sign. This finding may help distinguish sclerosing mesenteritis from other mesenteric processes such as lymphoma, carcinomatosis, or carcinoid tumour. Calcification may be present, usually in the central necrotic portion. Enlarged mesenteric or retroperitoneal lymph nodes may also be present.

Lymphoma will not display calcification unless it has undergone treatment. Carcinoid can produce the appearance described, but the 'fat halo' sign favours sclerosing mesenteritis and the soft tissue in carcinoid usually has a surrounding desmoplastic reaction. Metastatic disease will not be confined to the root of the mesentery, but will also involve the omentum or the surfaces of the liver, spleen, or bowel. Ascites is also common with carcinomatosis, but is not associated with sclerosing mesenteritis. Mesenteric involvement in the case of desmoid tumours is more often seen in cases related to familial adenomatous polyposis syndrome or Gardner syndrome. They are usually large masses, measuring 15 cm or more at diagnosis. They do not typically contain calcification.

Horton KM, Lawler LP, and Fishman EK. CT findings in sclerosing mesenteritis (panniculitis): spectrum of disease. *RadioGraphics* 2003; 23: 1561–1567.
Lucey BC, Stuhlfaut JW, and Soto JA. Mesenteric lymph nodes seen at imaging: causes and significance. *RadioGraphics* 2005; 25: 351–365.

48. D. Hypointensity during arterial phase enhancement.

Pancreatic adenocarcinoma is generally a hypovascular tumour at CT as well as MRI. Dynamic contrast-enhanced CT has been the gold standard for the diagnosis of pancreatic adenocarcinoma, but MRI is of value in those with renal failure or sensitivity to iodine-based contrast media. Care should be taken in patients with a very low GFR (typically less than 30ml/min) because of the risk of nephrogenic systemic fibrosis. Contrast-enhanced MRI may have a lower false negative rate than CT, as approximately 10% of pancreatic adenocarcinomas have been shown to be iso- rather than hypoattenuating, on both the pancreatic and portal venous phases. Chandarana et al. have reported that 25 of 25 neoplasms showed hypointensity during arterial phase enhancement (and 20 remained hypointense in venous phase), whereas only 12 of 25 were hypointense on unenhanced T1WI, and only 11 of 25 were hyperintense on STIR/T2WI.

Chandarana H, Babb J, and Macari M. Signal characteristic and enhancement patterns of pancreatic adenocarcinoma: evaluation with dynamic gadolinium enhanced MRI. *Clinical Radiology* 2007; 62: 876–883.
Smith SL and Rajan PS. Imaging of pancreatic adenocarcinoma with emphasis on multidetector CT. *Clinical Radiology* 2004; 59: 26–38.

49. B. Groove pancreatitis.

This is a rare form of chronic pancreatitis. It occurs due to inflammation in the pancreatico-duodenal groove, the potential space between the pancreas, duodenum, and common bile duct. The clinical manifestations are primarily due to duodenal and biliary obstruction. The small cystic lesions in the duodenal wall refer to cystic dystrophy of the duodenum, which can be associated with groove pancreatitis.

Autoimmune pancreatitis generally shows a diffusely enlarged gland with loss of lobular architecture, a 'sausage' shape, and a peripheral 'rind' of hypoattenuation. There is usually a non-dilated or diffusely narrowed pancreatic duct and a distal biliary stricture.

Hereditary pancreatitis has a young age of onset of typical features of pancreatitis, with at least two acute attacks without an underlying cause.

Pancreas divisum associated pancreatitis is seen in young or middle-aged patients with recurrent acute pancreatitis or chronic relapsing pancreatitis. MRCP or ERCP are optimal for the diagnosis of the lack of communication between the ventral and dorsal pancreatic ducts.

Although ectopic pancreatic tissue is a proposed cause of groove pancreatitis, the ectopic or heterotopic tissue is most commonly seen in relation to the gastric wall.

Shanbhogue AKP, Fasih N, Surabhi VR, Doherty GP, Shanbhogue DKP, and Sethi SK. A clinical and radiological review of uncommon types and causes of pancreatitis. *RadioGraphics* 2009; 29: 1003–1026.

50. C. Epiploic appendagitis.

Acute epiploic appendagitis is a self-limiting inflammation of the appendices epiploicae, associated with obesity, hernia, and unaccustomed exercise. Omental infarction typically presents with pain of several days' duration. CT demonstrates a large non-enhancing omental mass with heterogenous attenuation, and is typically located towards the right lower quadrant. Sclerosing mesenteritis is commonly located at the root of the small bowel mesentery.

Singh AK, Gervais DA, Hahn PF, Sagar P, Mueller PM, and Novelline RA. Acute epiploic appendagitis and its mimics. *RadioGraphics* 2005; 25: 1521–1534.

51. C. Osler–Weber–Rendu syndrome.

Osler–Weber–Rendu syndrome or hereditary haemorrhagic telangiectasia (HHT) is a rare autosomal dominant multisystem vascular disorder characterized by angiodysplastic lesions in which there is communication between arteries and veins of varying sizes. It commonly affects the skin, lungs, and mucous membranes but any organ system may be involved.

The liver is the most common site of abdominal HHT. Lesions range from tiny telangiectases to transient perfusion abnormalities and large confluent vascular masses. Coronal maximum intensity projection (MIP) images are useful in appreciating telangiectases.

Liver involvement is associated with arterio-venous shunting, porto-venous shunting, or both, resulting in hyperdynamic circulation, which may lead to high-output cardiac failure.

Budd–Chiari syndrome is hepatic vein thrombosis and Von Meyerburg complex is multiple biliary hamartomas.

Torabi M, Hosseinzadeh K, and Federle MP. CT of nonneoplastic hepatic vascular and perfusion disorders. *Radiographics* 2008; 28: 1967–1982.
Siddiki H, Doherty MG, Fletcher JG, Stanson AW, Vrtiska JJ, Hough DM et al. Abdominal findings in hereditary hemorrhagic telangiectasia: pictorial essay on 2D and 3D findings with isotropic multiphase CT. *RadioGraphics* 2008; 28: 171–183.

52. D. T3, N1, M0.

T3 implies invasion beyond the muscularis propria into the pericolic fat. CT is quoted as 80% accurate in detecting extramural spread and nodal stage. T1 and T2 tumours are well-defined with no extension beyond the bowel contour. CT features of a T4 tumour include nodular penetration of the tumour through the peritonealized areas of the muscle coat or an advancing edge of the tumour penetrating adjacent organs. Nodal positivity is based on any node >1 cm or a group of three or more nodes.

Dighe S, Swift I, and Brown G. CT staging of colon cancer. *Clinical Radiology* 2008; 63: 1372–1379.

53. A. GI scleroderma.

Deeply penetrating ulcers are seen in Behcet's disease. Whipple disease is an extremely rare form of intestinal lipodystrophy. Thickening of jejuna folds is seen, but there is little or no small bowel dilatation and small bowel transit time is normal. Pseudodiverticula are not seen in coeliac disease. The valvulae are thickened in lymphoma.

Dahnert W. *Radiology Review Manual*, 6th edn, Lippincott Williams & Wilkins, 2007. pp. 863–864.

54. E. Transmesenteric hernia.

This is when small bowel herniates through a defect in the mesentery and is compressed against the abdominal wall, with little overlying omental fat at most levels of anatomic section through the herniated bowel. There will be some degree of compression, crowding, displacement, and obstruction of both the bowel and blood vessels. They are usually seen in association with previous abdominal surgery and the creation of a Roux-en-Y anastomosis, when the hernia occurs in a surgically created defect in the mesentery.

A left-sided paraduodenal hernia is via the paraduodenal (lateral to the fourth part) mesenteric fossa of Landzert, close to the ligament of Treitz. The characteristic features include a sac-like mass of dilated bowel lateral to the ligament of Treitz, which displaces and indents the adjacent stomach and transverse colon.

A right paraduodenal hernia occurs via the jejunal mesentericoparietal fossa of Waldeyer. A cluster of dilated small bowel loops is seen lateral and inferior to the descending duodenum.

Federle MP, Jeffrey RB, Desser TS, Anne VS, and Eraso A. *Diagnostic imaging: abdomen*. Amirsys, 2005, I-1: 40–42.

55. D. Pseudomembranous colitis.

The CT sign of oral contrast becoming trapped between thickened oedematous haustral folds is the 'accordion' sign, which is highly suggestive of pseudomembranous colitis. Bowel wall thickening, pericolonic stranding of fat, and ascites may be seen in all forms of colitis. Pseudomembranous colitis can be segmental, but is more commonly a pancolitis.

Kawamoto S, Horton KM, and Fishman EK. Pseudomembranous colitis: spectrum of imaging findings with clinical and pathological correlation. *RadioGraphics* 1999; 19: 887–897.

56. A. Idiopathic eosinophilic oesophagitis (IEE).

The cause of this condition is uncertain, but most authors believe it occurs as an inflammatory response to ingested food allergens. A history of allergies is more closely correlated in children with the condition than in adults. Only a minority of adults with IEE have peripheral blood eosinophilia or eosinophilic gastroenteritis. The condition is most common in males aged 20–40 who have a history of dysphagia and recurrent food impactions. The appearance of the stricture, with its distinctive ring-like indentations, has been termed a 'ringed' oesophagus. These indentations are characterized by multiple closely spaced concentric rings that traverse the stricture. A similar finding may be seen in congenital oesophageal stenosis, which typically occurs in the same demographic group, with similar symptoms. The 'ringed' oesophagus is thus relatively specific for IEE, but is not a necessary finding (in the study quoted, it was only present in 7 of the 14 patients, although these 7 all had strictures). In peptic strictures, the fixed transverse folds are incomplete and further apart, producing a characteristic step-ladder appearance as a result of trapping of barium between the folds.

Zimmerman SL, Levine MS, Rubesin SE, Mitre MS, Furth EE, Laufer I et al. Idiopathic eosinophilic esophagitis in adults: the ringed esophagus. *Radiology* 2005; 236: 159–165.

57. E. Adenomyomatosis is associated with cholesterolosis in up to a third of patients.

Option A describes the cause of cholesterolosis. Option B describes the features of xanthogranulomatous cholecystitis (XGC). Option C describes the features of adenomyomatosis. Option D is true, but the ultrasound features described are not those of XGC, so this is not true regarding the condition described in the clinical scenario. Adenomyomatosis and cholesterolosis are both classed as types of hyperplastic cholecystosis. Adenomyomatosis has two pathogonomic descriptions. Firstly, the 'pearl necklace' appearance on oral cholecystogram (OCG) (the same appearance can be seen on MRCP). Secondly, comet tail artefact seen on ultrasound, caused by reverberation artefact between cholesterol crystals in Rokitansky–Ashcoff sinuses.

Dahnert W. *Radiology Review Manual*, 6th edn, Lippincott Williams & Wilkins, 2007. pp. 726–727.

58. B. TB.

Cryptosporidiosis is the most common cause of enteritis in AIDS patients. It more commonly causes proximal small bowel thickening in the duodenum and jejunum, and CT may show small lymph nodes. CMV infection of the small bowel can show a terminal ileitis indistinguishable from Crohn's disease. The typical CT findings in amoebiasis are thickening of the right colonic wall and a rounded abscess in the right lobe of liver with a peripheral zone of oedema. TB usually shows ileocaecal involvement, low attenuation mesenteric nodes, and ascites with peritoneal thickening. Mycobacterium avium intracellulare may also occur with low attenuation mesenteric nodes and thickening of small bowel folds.

Federle MP, Jeffrey RB, Desser TS, Anne VS, and Eraso A. *Diagnostic imaging: abdomen*. Amirsys, 2005, I-4: 26, 75.

59. B. Coeliac disease complicated by lymphoma.

Whipples disease, cavitating mesenteric lymph node syndrome, and abdominal TB more typically have mesenteric lymph node enlargement that has central low attenuation, rather than being of homogeneous soft-tissue density. Whipple disease is a systemic bacterial infection caused by *Tropheryma whippelii*. Lymph nodes affected by Whipple disease typically have a high fat content, causing the low attenuation, usually between 10 and 20 HU.

Cavitating mesenteric lymph node syndrome is associated with coeliac disease. The lymph nodes are truly cavitating and usually regress following a gluten-free diet.

The lymph nodes in abdominal tuberculosis typically have caseous necrosis and thus central low density on CT.

Castleman disease causes benign masses of lymphoid tissue of unknown aetiology. It can cause mesenteric lymphadenopathy, which is homogeneous, but the disease itself is rare and mesenteric involvement is much less common than mediastinal involvement.

Lucey BC, Stuhlfaut JW, and Soto JA. Mesenteric lymph nodes seen at imaging: causes and significance. *RadioGraphics* 2005; 25: 351–365.

60. C. Insulinoma is a contraindication to the use of glucagon.

Glucagon is a potent hypotonic agent. If 1mg of glucagon is injected intravenously it takes approximately 1 minute to work and lasts about 10–20 minutes. Intravenously administered glucagon decreases discomfort during barium enema examinations. Glucagon administration is generally safe, but is contraindicated in patients with insulinoma and phaeochromocytoma. Diabetes is not a recognized contraindication.

Rubesin SE, Levine MS, Laufer I, and Herlinger H. Double-contrast barium enema examination technique. *Radiology* 2000; 215: 642–650.

61. A. Benign tumour.

The patient has presented with a colo-colic intussusception secondary to a lipoma of the colonic wall. The intussusception has been complicated by large bowel obstruction.

Intussusception is caused by prolapse of a portion of the bowel into the lumen of the adjoining bowel lumen segment. Intussusception is most commonly a disease of young children and most commonly occurs in an ileocolic location. In children, over 90% of intussusceptions are idiopathic and no lead point is identified. In adult patients approximately 80% of intussusceptions are caused by lead point lesions.

The CT appearances described are typical of an intussusception. The low attenuation distal lead point represents the lipoma. Ultrasound is often used to diagnose intussusception in children and will show a mass with echogenic rings representing the fat in the invaginated mesentery.

Kim YH, Blake MA, Harisinghani MG, Archer-Arroyo K, Hahn PF, Pitman MB et al. Adult intussusception: CT appearances and identification of a causative lead point. *RadioGraphics* 2006; 26: 733–744.

62. D. Renal cell carcinoma.

All the other tumours are more likely to be FDG avid than renal cell carcinoma.

Ahmed S, Horton KM, and Fishman EK. Splenic incidentalomas. *Radiological Clinics of North America* 2011; 49: 323–347.

63. A. Previous trauma.

Splenic cysts are classified into two major subtypes: true cysts and false cysts (post-traumatic pseudocysts). This differentiation is based on the presence or absence of an epithelial lining.

They cannot be distinguished on imaging. On CT as both usually appear well-defined and of fluid density.

True cysts, which constitute approximately 20% of all splenic cysts and show an epithelial lining, are further divided into non-parasitic cysts and parasitic subtypes. Non-parasitic, true cysts, primarily known as epidermoid cysts, are congenitally derived from peritoneal mesothelium and represent only 2.5% of all splenic cysts. The majority of true cysts are related to parasitic infection, usually hydatid disease.

False cysts, also known as post-traumatic pseudocysts, lack an epithelial lining and are considered to represent the end stage of a previous intrasplenic hematoma. They account for up to 80% of all splenic cysts. Patients may report a history of trauma to the left upper quadrant, but up to 30% of patients do not recall any association with such an event. More rarely they may be the result of previous infarction or infection.

True cysts are more likely to have slight wall trabeculation and thin peripheral septation (up to 86%), whereas false cysts are more likely to have mural calcification (up to 50%).

Isolated splenic lymphangioma is uncommon in adults, usually being diagnosed in childhood. It usually appears as thin-walled, well-defined masses of low attenuation, without enhancement. They may have curvilinear peripheral mural calcification.

Ahmed S, Horton KM, and Fishman EK. Splenic incidentalomas. *Radiological Clinics of North America* 2011; 49: 323–347.

64. A. Axial T2 steady-state GE.

Axial imaging is generally going to be better than coronal imaging when trying to distinguish between pneumobilia and calculi within the CBD. The biliary air causes an air/fluid level of air lying on top of fluid in a non-dependent position in the CBD and this is more easily appreciated on an axial image. Calculi tend to lie dependently within the CBD. As fluid is hyperintense on T2WI and hypointense on T1WI, and both air and calculi are hypointense on both these sequences, then both will stand out as being more conspicuous on T2WI.

Irie H, Honda H, Kuroiwa T, Yoshimitsu K, Aibe H, Shinozaki K et al. Pitfalls in MR Cholangiopancreatographic interpretation. *RadioGraphics* 2001; 21: 23–37.

65. D. Yes, SPIO.

Gadolinium chelates are extracellular agents. Gadolinium shortens the T1 relaxation time of adjacent water protons, resulting in signal enhancement on T1WI. It can be used for lesion detection, characterization, and liver vasculature assessment. Gadopentate dimeglumine (Magnevist®) is a commonly used extracellular agent.

SPIO particles are reticulo-endothelial agents that are phagocytosed by Kupffer cells. SPIO causes local magnetic field inhomogeneity and T2 and T2* shortening, resulting in signal loss on T2WI and T2*WI. Most liver tumours, including HCC, are deficient in Kupffer cells (cf. focal nodular hyperplasia) therefore after administration of SPIO the tumour appears hyperintense relative to the background liver.

Mangafodipir trisodium (Teslascan®) is a manganese-based hepatocyte specific agent that increases the signal intensity of the liver, bile ducts, and some hepatocyte-containing lesions (e.g. FNH) at T1WI. Similarly, gadobenate dimeglumine (Multihance®) is a gadolinium-based hepatocyte specific agent, which also works best with T1WI due to the T1 shortening effects of gadolinium.

Gandhi SN, Brown, MA, Wong JG, Aguirre DA, and Sirlin CB. MR contrast agents for liver imaging: what, when, how. *RadioGraphics* 2006; 26: 1621–1636.

66. E. Gastrointestinal stromal tumour (GIST).

At contrast-enhanced CT, GISTs appear as large exophytic masses with peripheral enhancement. They usually have an attenuation similar to that of muscle, but they may have heterogeneous attenuation, depending on their level of aggressiveness. More aggressive GISTs may also contain a central area of necrosis.

Adenocarcinoma of the jejunum is rare, more commonly occurring in the duodenum. They also tend to be stricturing lesions, rather than exophytic masses and may present with obstruction.

Carcinoid is also rare in the proximal small bowel, the distal ileum being a more usual location. The primary lesion is often quite small, with the nodal metastatic lesion in the small bowel mesentery being more conspicuous on CT. This is often spiculated (surrounding desmoplastic reaction) and may contain calcification.

Lymphoma can have a number of manifestations in the small bowel, from nodular thickening of the mucosal folds to large masses with aneurysmal dilatation of the small bowel in the affected segment. Associated lymphadenopathy is typical.

Horwitz BM, Zamora GE, and Gallegos MP. Gastrointestinal stromal tumor of the small bowel. *RadioGraphics* 2011; 31: 429–434.

67. C. Zenker diverticulum.

The findings are classical of a Zenker diverticulum or pharyngeal pouch, a pseudo-diverticulum of the posterior hypopharyngeal wall between the fibres of cricopharyngeus. 50% of cases occur in the seventh and eighth decades. Other symptoms can include halitosis, regurgitation of undigested food, aspiration pneumonia, oesophageal perforation, and carcinoma. It is associated with hiatus hernia, achalasia, and gastroduodenal ulcer. Treatment options include surgical excision, laser therapy, and endoscopy with stapling.

Traction diverticula classically occur in the mid-oesophageal region and in the past were most often a secondary manifestation of mediastinal fibrosis associated with TB. True oesophageal pulsion divertcula are most commonly in the epiphrenic region (last 10 cm of the oesophagus).

Oesophageal perforation is more commonly iatrogenic, being rarely spontaneous (Boerhaave syndrome).

Boxerman JL. Zenker's diverticulum: reappraisal. *Radiology* 1997; 204: 118.
Watemberg S, Landau O, and Avrahami R. Zenker's diverticulum: reappraisal. *American Journal of Gastroenterology* 1996; 91(8): 1494–1498.
Thomas ML, Anthony AA, Fosh BG, Finch JG, and Maddern GJ. Oesophageal diverticula. *British Journal of Surgery* 2001; 88: 629–642.

68. C. Small bowel mesentery.

Desmoid tumours are non-malignant fibrous tumours that have a particular association with FAP/Gardner syndrome. They may be locally infiltrative. On CT they are usually of homogeneous density, but can have well-defined or irregular margins. On MRI, the signal intensity on T1WI is similar to muscle and on T2WI their signal can be variable. Lower signal tumours on T2WI probably have a denser fibrous component. Desmoid tumours in association with FAP/Gardner syndrome are most commonly seen in the small bowel mesentery, followed by the abdominal wall. Intra-abdominal desmoid tumours can also occur in the retroperitoneum and pelvis, but these locations are more common in isolated desmoids.

Kawashima A, Goldman SM, Fishman EK, Kuhlman JE, Onitsuka H, Fukuya T et al. CT of intraabdominal desmoid tumors: is the tumor different in patients with Gardner's disease? *American Journal of Radiology* 1994; 162: 339–342.

69. C. Rectosigmoid.

On a prone scan during a CT colonography examination, the rectosigmoid is generally better distended than on the supine scan because it is a more posteriorly placed structure and air gets displaced to the non-dependent position. The other segments named are usually better distended on the supine scan, particularly the caecum and transverse colon, as these are more anteriorly placed within the abdomen.

Yee J, Kumar NN, Hung RK, Akekar GA, Kumar PR, Wall SD et al. Comparison of supine and prone scanning separately and in combination at CT colonography. *Radiology* 2003; 226: 653–661.

70. B. Resistive index of 0.9 distal to the stenosis.

Knowledge of the vessel 'waveform signature' and stenosis flow dynamics is essential in interpreting the Doppler findings. The hepatic artery is a low resistance vessel with continuous antegrade flow during systole and diastole. Generally, low-resistance arteries have a resistive index (RI) of 0.55–0.7. RIs higher or lower than this range are abnormal. RI is calculated by using the formula RI = (peak systolic velocity – end diastolic velocity)/peak systolic velocity. Most modern ultrasound machines calculate this automatically.

A stenosis results in increased arterial resistance to the blood flow proximal to the stenosis. This causes a reduction in the end diastolic velocity disproportionately more than the peak systolic velocity, producing a high-resistance waveform and high RI (due to a greater difference between the peak systolic and end diastolic velocities). This finding is not specific to stenosis and may be seen in the postprandial state, and in patients of advanced age and diffuse peripheral microvascular disease or compression (cirrhosis, hepatic venous congestion, cold ischaemia, and any stage of transplant rejection).

At and immediately distal to the stenosis there is turbulent flow and a jet phenomenon resulting in an increase in the peak systolic and end diastolic velocity and spectral broadening. Depending on the severity of the stenosis, the artery distal to the stenosis demonstrates the following findings: tardus-parvus waveform that refers to the late and low systolic peak (i.e. increased acceleration time and reduced peak systolic velocity). Low RI due to a greater reduction in peak systolic velocity compared to the end diastolic velocity.

Low RI may also be seen with distal vascular shunts (trauma, iatrogenic, cirrhosis, Osler–Weber–Rendu syndrome).

McNaughton DA and Abu-Yousef MM. Doppler US of the liver made simple. *RadioGraphics* 2011; 31: 161–188.

71. E. 'Mural nodule in cyst' pattern.

RFA produces thermally-induced coagulation necrosis, which manifests usually as an oval or round defect on contrast-enhanced CT. The ablation zone is slightly larger than the actual lesion to achieve curative treatment and prevent local recurrence, which is usually seen at the margins of the ablation zone. The following findings are common in the immediate post ablation period: transient peri-ablational hyperaemia, tiny air bubbles, and arterio-portal shunting.

A 'mural nodule in cyst' indicates the development of a biloma as a complication of RFA. This is usually seen several months after treatment. It is associated with interval enlargement of the RFA zone.

Kim Y, Rhim H, Lim HK, Choi D, Lee MW, and Park MJ. Coagulation necrosis induced by radiofrequency ablation in the liver: histopathologic and radiologic review of usual to extremely rare changes. *RadioGraphics* 2011; 31: 377–390.

72. D. Coeliac disease.

The segmentation and flocculation of barium are findings on a small bowel series that are typical of malabsorption and therefore the most likely diagnosis is coeliac disease. Other findings in coeliac disease include dilatation, a granular appearance to the barium secondary to hypersecretion, jejunization of the ileum, and the 'moulage' sign. The latter refers to a smooth, tubular appearance to the jejunum in longstanding coeliac disease, secondary to atrophy and effacement of the jejunal mucosal folds.

Lymphoma can be a complication of coeliac disease and generally causes shallow, ulcerated masses or the development of thickened, nodular small bowel folds.

Whipple's disease, amyloidosis, and chronic ischaemic enteritis all cause thickening of the small bowel folds.

Eisenberg RL. *Gastrointestinal Radiology: a pattern approach*, 4th edn, Lippincott Williams & Wilkins, 2003. pp. 441–444.

73. C. Mucosal hyperenhancement.

The lack of ionizing radiation is a major advantage to MRI for patients with Crohn's disease given the chronic nature of this condition necessitating frequent investigation. MRI can be performed via enterography or enteroclysis. In enterography, large volumes of fluid (or a fluid-inducing laxative) are ingested. Enteroclysis involves administration of enteric contrast material via a nasoenteric tube. Sequence acquistion involves fat suppression and intravenous contrast. Increased mucosal hyperenhancement (compared with that seen in normal surrounding loops) may be the earliest sign of active inflammation, even in the absence of wall thickening. Increased vascularity, perienteric inflammation, and reactive adenopathy are other signs of active Crohn's disease. In severe Crohn's disease mucosal hyperenhancement combined with submucosal oedema gives a 'stratified' appearance. Serosal hyperenhancement may also be seen, giving a 'target' appearance. Mural thickening is defined as greater than 3mm, although an underdistended bowel may mimic this finding.

Fidler JL, Guimaraes L, and Einstein DM. MR imaging of the small bowel. *RadioGraphics* 2009; 29: 1811–1825.

74. B. Turcot syndrome.

FAP is a rare autosomal dominant condition resulting in the growth of hundreds of adenomatous polyps in the large bowel. Clinical symptoms commence from the third decade and include abdominal pain and PR bleeding. Colorectal cancer develops in almost all before the age of 40 years. Turcot syndrome is characterized by the association of colonic polyps similar to FAP and central nervous system tumours, typically medulloblastoma and glioblastoma multiforme. The combination of intestinal polyposis (identical to FAP) and numerous osteomas and epidermal cysts is typical of Gardner syndrome. Lynch syndrome is hereditray non-polyposis colorectal cancer. Colorectal carcinoma occurs earlier than in the average population. There is also an association with ovarian and endometrial malignancy. Chronic inflammatory bowel disease is not associated with CNS malignancy.

Neri E, Faggioni L, Cini L, and Bartolozzi C. Colonic polyps: inheritance, susceptibility, risk evaluation and diagnostic management. *Cancer Management & Research* 2011; 3: 17–24.

75. A. Non-visualization of the gallbladder at 1 and 4 hours.

Hepatobiliary scintigraphy is most commonly used to evaluate suspected acute cholecystitis. A minimum of 2 hours fasting is required. Following prompt uptake by the liver, the radiotracer is excreted into the biliary system and drains into the small bowel. Activity should be demonstrated within the gallbladder by 1 hour. Morphine can be used during the scan to relax the sphincter of

Oddi, thus pushing radiolabelled bile into the gallbladder. Acute cholecystitis is characterized by non-visualization of the gallbladder at both 1 and 4 hours or at 30 minutes following morphine administration. Non-visualization of the gallbladder at 1 hour, but seen at 4 hours, is indicative of chronic cholecystitis. A false-positive diagnosis of acute cholecystitis can occur with previous cholecystectomy, gallbladder agenesis, and tumour obstructing the cystic duct.

Brant WE and Helms CA. *Fundamentals of Diagnostic Radiology*, 3rd edn, Lippincott Williams & Wilkins, 2007, pp. 1423–1425.

chapter

4

GENITO-URINARY, ADRENAL, OBSTETRICS AND GYNAECOLOGY, AND BREAST

QUESTIONS

1. *E. coli*, with or without an underlying diagnosis of diabetes mellitus, is the most common pathogen behind many urological conditions. All of the following conditions are most commonly due to *E. coli* infection except one, which one?

A. Xanthogranulomatous pyelonephritis (XGP).
B. Emphysematous pyelonephritis.
C. Pyonephrosis.
D. Pyeloureteritis cystica.
E. Malakoplakia.

2. A 45-year-old women presents with menorrhagia and dysmenorrhea. She has had three successful pregnancies and one therapeutic abortion in the past. She undergoes an MRI of the pelvis 14 days after the start of her last menstrual period. It reveals a junctional zone which measures 13 mm throughout, with hyperintense T2WI foci within it. With what conditions are these findings most consistent?

A. Endometrial hyperplasia.
B. Endometrial carcinoma stage 1A.
C. Pseudothickening.
D. Adenomyosis.
E. Myometrial contraction.

3. A 50-year-old male patient on long-term analgesia presents with a history of macroscopic haematuria. An intravenous urogram is requested. The preliminary film is unremarkable. Following intravenous contrast administration, there is a delay in excretion on the right side. Subsequent images demonstrate a filling defect in the distal ureter with proximal dilatation. The ureter immediately distal to the filling defect is also mildly dilated, but normal in calibre further down. What is the diagnosis?

A. Non-radioopaque calculus.
B. Transitional cell carcinoma (TCC).
C. Blood clot.
D. Sloughed papilla.
E. Pyeloureteritis cystica.

4. **A 60-year-old male with a history of prostate cancer is referred to the symptomatic breast clinic complaining of a palpable breast lump which has been present for several months. Clinical examination reveals a palpable firm mass towards the left subareolar region. A nodular, fan-shaped subareolar lesion is seen on mammography. The mass is hypoechoic on ultrasound and surrounded by normal fatty tissue. Hypervascular flow within the mass is noted on Doppler ultrasound. Which of the following is the most likely diagnosis?**

    A. Invasive ductal carcinoma.
    B. Lipoma.
    C. Gynaecomastia.
    D. Lymphoma.
    E. Dermatofibrosarcoma.

5. **A 62-year-old woman presents with recurrent urinary tract infections (UTIs) and a pelvic/renal tract ultrasound is performed. This demonstrates normal kidneys and bladder, but there is a 5-cm solid, hypoechoic mass seen arising from the right ovary. There is acoustic shadowing caused by the mass, but a subsequent CT scan does not show any calcification within the mass or any metastatic disease. What is the most likely cause of the ovarian mass?**

    A. Sertoli–Leydig cell tumour of the ovary.
    B. Cystadenocarcinoma of the ovary.
    C. Fibrothecoma of the ovary.
    D. Granulosa cell tumour of the ovary.
    E. Embryonal cell carcinoma of the ovary.

6. **A 32-year-old male has been referred from urology for assessment. The patient was involved in an RTA 2 years ago, during which he sustained a urethral injury. The patient had failed to attend urology outpatients for follow-up in the interim, but has re-attended with recurrent UTIs. An attempted cystoscopy identified a tight proximal urethral stricture. The urologists have requested an ultrasound and voiding cystourethrogram (VCUG) to investigate the degree of bladder outlet obstruction. The ultrasound demonstrates a mild degree of renal pelvic dilatation bilaterally. The bladder has a residual volume of 500 ml on post-void imaging. The VCUG reveals reflux into the renal pelvis bilaterally with mild ureteric and pelvic dilatation, but no calyceal dilatation and preserved forniceal angles. What grade of reflux does this patient have?**

    A. Grade 1.
    B. Grade 2.
    C. Grade 3.
    D. Grade 4.
    E. Grade 5.

7. A 43-year-old female presents with pelvic pain. On examination she is tender in the left iliac fossa and midline. Inflammatory markers are normal. A trans-abdominal ultrasound reveals a normal right ovary and uterus, but a 5.5-cm simple appearing cyst arising from the left ovary. As the reporting radiologist you:

A. refer to gynaecology for clinical assessment and serum Ca-125 measurement.
B. recommend trans-vaginal ultrasound.
C. recommend a repeat trans-abdominal ultrasound in 6 weeks' time.
D. recommend MRI of pelvis.
E. issue a report stating that a benign simple cyst is seen to arise from the left ovary.

8. A 25-year-old female undergoes a hysterosalpingogram (HSG) that reveals a unicornuate uterus. This is confirmed on MRI, which also demonstrates a non-functioning rudimentary contra-lateral horn. What further investigation is indicated?

A. Laparoscopy.
B. Renal imaging.
C. Pelvic ultrasound.
D. Laparotomy and resection of rudimentary horn.
E. Speculum examination.

9. A 56-year-old asymptomatic woman undergoes routine screening mammography. Which of the following forms of calcification raises greatest suspicion of ductal carcinoma *in situ* (DCIS)?

A. Egg-shell.
B. Sedimented.
C. Tubular.
D. Dot-dash.
E. Coarse.

10. A 46-year-old woman has an incidentally discovered large mixed echogenicity mass in the left flank on an ultrasound examination. A follow-up CT examination is performed and this shows a predominantly fatty lesion exophytic to the left kidney, measuring approximately 12 cm in maximum diameter. Which of the following findings would make the diagnosis of large renal angiomyolipoma more likely than a perirenal well-differentiated retroperitoneal liposarcoma?

A. The presence of mass effect with displacement of the left kidney.
B. The presence of aneurysmal blood vessels within the lesion.
C. The presence of soft-tissue density areas within the lesion.
D. The presence of ill-defined margins.
E. The presence of fluid density components.

11. A 64-year-old female patient presents with a 3-month history of right-sided loin pain, microscopic haematuria, and low-grade pyrexia. Her GP had been treating the patient as a presumptive UTI, given the background history of diabetes, but is concerned that the symptoms are not resolving. On clinical examination the urologists have felt a right-sided ballotable loin mass. They have requested a CT scan of abdomen. This reveals a large irregular mass replacing most of the parenchyma of the right kidney, which measures 10 × 11 cm in axial diameter and does not demonstrate significant enhancement. There are a number of focal masses noted within the dominant mass that have attenuation values of between –15 and –5 HU. The renal outline is poorly defined, with involvement of the perirenal fascia. A large staghorn calculus is also present. There is no evidence of invasion of the renal vein. What is the primary diagnosis?

A. Renal cell carcinoma.
B. Renal oncocytoma.
C. Renal lymphoma.
D. XGP.
E. Renal angiomyolipoma.

12. A 2-day-old male infant with cryptorchidism and an antenatal diagnosis of dilated bladder and ureters is referred for a micturating cystourethrogram (MCUG). MCUG reveals a dilated bladder, tortuous and dilated ureters, dilated posterior urethra, and renal cortical thinning. Note is also made of bulging flanks. What is the diagnosis?

A. Posterior urethral valve.
B. Congenital megacystis and megaureter.
C. Bilateral vesicoureteric reflex.
D. Eagle Barrett syndrome.
E. Meatal stenosis.

13. A previously well 70-year-old woman is investigated via CTPA for acute left-sided chest pain and hypoxia. The test is negative for PE, but an incidental 1.7 × 1.2 cm retro-areolar lesion is noted in the right breast by the reporting registrar. Which of the following features, if any, would be suggestive of breast malignancy?

A. Ill-defined margin.
B. Spiculated margin.
C. Calcification.
D. Multiple lesions.
E. CT is not reliably predictive of breast malignancy.

14. A 67-year-old male patient presents with an 8-week history of left loin pain. A renal CT is obtained and this shows a 6-cm enhancing left renal lesion that has a fibrotic central scar. What is the most likely diagnosis?

A. Renal leiomyoma.
B. Renal oncocytoma.
C. Renal metanephic adenoma.
D. Renal haemangioma (giant).
E. Renal juxta-glomerular cell neoplasm.

15. A 54-year-old female patient with diabetes presents with a history of left loin pain, pyrexia, and pyuria over the past 24 hours. The patient develops sepsis soon after admission and is brought for a CT scan following appropriate resuscitation. The CT shows a mildly dilated left renal pelvis, which contains small pockets of air extending into the calyces. A small wedge-shaped area of poor enhancement in the lower pole is the only parenchymal abnormality. The clinical diagnosis is of pyelonephritis, but what subtype of pyelonephritis is best represented by these imaging features?

A. Acute pyelonephritis.
B. Emphysematous pyelitis.
C. Emphysematous pyelonephritis.
D. Acute pyonephrosis.
E. XGP.

16. A 36-year-old woman undergoes MRI of the pelvis for assessment of pelvic pain. She had a previous hysterectomy due to post-partum haemorrhage and thus transvaginal ultrasound (TVUS) is not an option. Abdominal ultrasound is technically difficult due to body habitus and the ovaries cannot be visualized. MRI reveals a 7-cm left adnexal lesion of predominantly intermediate and high signal on T2WI, but with low-signal components within. On T1WI, there is layering of low and high signal, with suppression of the high signal on the T1WI with fat saturation. What do you advise in your report?

A. Referral for chemoradiotherapy.
B. Referral for laparoscopy for staging.
C. Follow up in 3 months' time.
D. Referral for surgery.
E. No follow-up required.

17. A 40-year-old female with uterine fibroids is referred for uterine artery embolization. Which of the following statements regarding the relevant arterial anatomy is incorrect?

A. Uterine artery is the first or second branch of the anterior division of internal iliac artery in 51% of cases.
B. The ipsilateral ovarian artery often replaces an absent uterine artery.
C. The ovarian artery has a characteristic corkscrew appearance on angiogram.
D. Utero-ovarian anastomosis is identified in less than 5% of cases.
E. Ovarian artery supply to fibroids is more frequently found in women with a history of previous pelvic surgery.

18. A 48-year-old woman who had bilateral breast augmentation with single-lumen silicone gel implants 20 years ago presents with pain in her left breast and distorted breast shape. Which of the following radiological findings on T2WI MRI are in keeping with intracapsular implant rupture?

A. Thickened T2WI hypointense capsular margin.
B. T2WI hyperintense globules surrounding the implant.
C. Multiple curvilinear lines of low T2WI signal within the implant.
D. Inferior extension of the implant beyond the inframammary fold.
E. Marginal low T2WI signal radial folds within the implant.

19. A 72-year-old man presents with a 4-month history of painless enlargement of the right testis. He undergoes scrotal ultrasound, which demonstrates a uniformly hypoechoic lesion that is enlarging and almost replacing all the normal parenchyma of the right testis. It has also caused enlargement of the right epididymis and adjacent spermatic cord. Review of the left testis shows a 2.5-cm hypoechoic lesion with normal spermatic cord and epididymis. What is the most likely diagnosis?

A. Lymphoma.
B. Leukaemia.
C. Testicular metastases.
D. Bilateral seminoma.
E. Granulomatous epididymo-orchitis.

20. A 56-year-old female diabetic patient presents to urology with a history of microscopic haematuria. There is a past history of multiple UTIs. The standard urology investigative process in your hospital consists of ultrasound, intravenous urogram (IVU) and cystoscopy. Ultrasound is normal. Cystoscopy has found a number of yellowish raised lesions in the bladder. You are reviewing the IVU with this information. The IVU shows multiple small filling defects in the distal left ureter and bladder which are 3–8 mm in size. What is the diagnosis?

A. Malakoplakia.
B. Leukoplakia.
C. Pyeloureteritis cystica.
D. Multifocal TCC.
E. Cystitis with distal ureteric reflux.

21. A 45-year-old male presents with severe epigastric pain radiating to the back. Blood tests reveal elevated serum amylase and calcium. A CT scan of abdomen demonstrates peripancreatic inflammatory stranding, renal medullary nephrocalcinosis, and sacro-iliac joint erosions. What further investigation(s) would you recommend?

A. Serum parathyroid hormone assay and ^{99m}Tc sestamibi scan.
B. Serum parathyroid hormone assay and ^{111}In pentetreotide scan.
C. Serum parathyroid hormone assay and meta-iodobenzyl-guanidine (MIBG) scan.
D. Serum parathyroid hormone and ^{99m}Tc pertechnetate scan.
E. Serum parathyroid hormone assay and ^{201}Tl scan.

22. A 32-year-old asymptomatic woman who is BRCA1 positive undergoes breast cancer surveillance via MRI. A lesion within the left breast is identified. Which of the following MRI features is the most predictive for malignancy?

A. Irregular margin.
B. T2WI signal hyperintensity.
C. Progressive enhancement curve on dynamic T1WI post contrast.
D. Plateau enhancement curve on dynamic T1WI post contrast.
E. Washout enhancement curve on dynamic T1WI post contrast.

23. A 72-year-old man presents with a palpable mass adjacent to the right testis. An ultrasound scan is performed and this demonstrates a large epididymal cyst. In addition there is an abnormal area within the postero-lateral aspect of the right testis, which is rounded in shape on transverse scanning, but more elongated on longitudinal scanning. It is hypoechoic, with multiple small cystic areas giving a 'sponge-like' consistency. There is no flow within this on colour Doppler imaging. What is the most likely cause of this?

A. Thrombosed intra-testicular varicocele.
B. Cystic degeneration in a testicular infarct.
C. Chronic testicular abscess.
D. Tubular ectasia of the rete testis.
E. Epidermoid cyst.

24. A 73-year-old male diabetic patient, with poorly controlled hypertension, is referred for renal Doppler ultrasound due to an episode of flash pulmonary oedema. He has a history of stage 3 chronic kidney disease. The ultrasound shows a small left kidney, which measures 5 cm in bipolar diameter. The right kidney is also small, measuring 6 cm. The resistive indices measure 0.9 on both sides. The peak systolic velocity is 130 cm/s on the left and 150 cm/s on the right. Which interventional treatment would be recommended for this patient?

A. Renal artery angioplasty on left side.
B. Renal artery stenting on left side.
C. Renal artery stenting on right side.
D. Bilateral renal artery stenting.
E. No intervention.

25. A 23-year-old woman is referred for an MRI of pelvis because of dyspareunia and pelvic pain. The ovaries are normal, but a 6-mm rounded area of high signal on T1WI and T2WI sequences is demonstrated in the left postero-lateral aspect of the distal vagina. What is the most likely diagnosis?

A. Squamous cell carcinoma of the vagina.
B. Urethral diverticulum.
C. Nabothian cyst.
D. Bartholin's gland cyst.
E. Vaginal septum.

26. A 50-year-old male with thyroid swelling undergoes ultrasound of the thyroid that shows a solitary hypoechoic nodule with punctate calcification and increased vascularity. An ultrasound guided fine needle aspiration is carried out and is reported as benign. What would you do next?

A. Repeat fine needle aspiration.
B. Follow-up ultrasound in 6 months.
C. No further follow-up.
D. Staging CT.
E. ^{99m}Tc sestamibi scan.

27. A 50-year-old female colleague asks you for information and advice regarding breast screening. Which of the following statements regarding breast screening in the UK is correct?

A. She will not be eligible for screening until she is 55.
B. Screening occurs every 2 years.
C. Compression is not required for screening mammography.
D. There is a 70% reduction in mortality from breast cancer among screened women.
E. Two lives are saved for every over-diagnosed case.

28. You are asked to perform an antenatal ultrasound examination and note that the placenta has an unusual morphology. You see an additional lobule, which is separate from the main bulk of the placenta. What is this variant of placental morphology known as?

A. Circumvallate placenta.
B. Bilobed placenta.
C. Placenta membranacea.
D. Succenturiate placenta.
E. Placenta accreta.

29. You are the interventional radiology fellow in your hospital. A nephrologist has asked you for an opinion on four patients they feel require renal arterial intervention. Patient A is a 68-year-old male who has had a catheter angiogram which showed a 60% narrowing in the right renal artery. This patient has refractory hypertension. Patient B is a 42-year-old female, also with refractory hypertension. She has had an MR angiogram, which has shown a number of stenoses, with intervening mild aneurysm formation, in the proximal right renal artery. Patient C is a 72-year-old female with impaired renal function, who underwent captopril renal scintigraphy. On the baseline study, there was a similar appearance of the kidneys. On the captopril study, there was a differential split of renal function of 15% between the right and left kidney, with a decrease of time to peak activity of 320 seconds. The final patient D had a renal Doppler ultrasound, which showed a biphasic flow pattern in the segmental arteries, with a slow upstroke. Which of these patients has significant atherosclerotic renal artery stenosis?

A. Patients A and B.
B. Patients C and D.
C. Patients A, C, and D.
D. Patients B, C, and D.
E. All of them.

30. A 36-year-old male patient presents with abdominal pain. He has a history of hypertension and obesity. A CT of abdomen reveals a 6-cm right adrenal mass, which shows heterogenous but peripheral enhancement, necrosis, and some calcification. There is early invasion of the IVC. The left adrenal gland is atrophied. What is the most likely diagnosis?

A. Neuroblastoma.
B. Adrenal cortical carcinoma.
C. Myelolipoma.
D. Adrenal adenoma.
E. Phaeochromocytoma.

31. A 30-year-old male with a thyroid nodule is referred for an ultrasound guided FNA. The FNA cytology reveals medullary thyroid carcinoma, which is treated by total thyroidectomy. The following year he undergoes a CTPA examination, which shows a small nodule in the thyroid region. Which of the following serum markers is useful in assessing recurrence?

A. CA 19-9.
B. Calcitonin.
C. CA 125.
D. Thyroglobulin.
E. Calcium.

32. A 24-year-old woman presents to the symptomatic breast clinic with a palpable left-sided breast lesion. There is no family history of breast cancer. Clinical examination reveals a smooth, relatively mobile 2-cm lesion within the left upper quadrant. Ultrasound depicts a well-defined oval hypoechoic lesion with an echogenic capsule following the tissue planes. No malignant features are present. The patient states that she has a phobia of needles. What should be the next step in this patient's management?

A. Reassurance and discharge with advice.
B. Correlation with mammography.
C. Ultrasound guided core biopsy.
D. Ultrasound guided FNA.
E. Referral for MRI.

33. A 40-year-old man has an ultrasound examination of the abdomen for epigastric pain. The examination is normal apart for an isoechoic 'mass' at the midpole of the left kidney. You suspect this may be a normal variant, such as a prominent column of Bertin. You recommend a CT scan of kidneys to confirm this. Which phase of a CT renal tract examination would best show this variant?

A. Unenhanced scan.
B. Cortico-medullary phase.
C. Nephrographic phase.
D. Early excretory (3-minute) phase.
E. Late excretory (10-minute) phase.

34. You are consulted about a 24-year-old male patient who is day 3 following a blind right-sided renal biopsy, which diagnosed glomerulonephritis. He has been well until today, when he developed acute right flank pain and haematuria. The urologists asked for an IVU prior to assessing the patient. They feel this showed an absent kidney, but on the 15- and 20-minute images, you feel you can detect a faint nephrogram that is slightly more pronounced on the 20-minute image. Given your suspicions about the cause, which of the following would be the least likely to contribute to the diagnosis?

A. Ultrasound.
B. MRI with GE sequences of the right kidney.
C. MRI with SE sequences of the right kidney.
D. Arterial phase CT abdomen.
E. Portal venous phase CT abdomen.

35. A 58-year-old smoker presents with haemoptysis and chest pain. A CT of chest confirms a lung carcinoma. While reporting the CT you notice that there is enlargement of the right adrenal gland. The patient has already left the department, but by chance is due to have an MRI scan of lumbar spine at a nearby institution the following morning. Due to time constraints, they can only fit in one sequence to image the adrenal glands. Which one sequence is of most use in further characterizing the adrenal abnormalities?

A. T2WI.
B. STIR.
C. Axial T1WI with fat saturation.
D. In- and out-of-phase T1WI.
E. DWI.

36. A 40-year-old male with a history of haematuria undergoes CT urography. Initial non-contrast scan demonstrates right-sided medullary nephrocalcinosis. Following intravenous contrast administration, a striated 'paintbrush' appearance of the renal medulla is noted. The left kidney is unremarkable. What is the diagnosis?

A. Hyperparathyroidism.
B. Renal tubular acidosis.
C. Medullary sponge kidney.
D. Sarcoidosis.
E. Multiple myeloma.

37. A 49-year-old woman presents with a rapidly enlarging left-sided breast mass. A large, firm, non-tender discrete mass is noted on clinical examination with overlying skin ulceration. Mammography reveals a 7-cm multilobulated soft tissue density mass in the left upper quadrant. On ultrasound the mass is solid with cystic areas. Posterior acoustic enhancement is demonstrated. What is the most likely diagnosis?

A. Adenoid cystic carcinoma.
B. Fibromatosis.
C. Granular cell tumour.
D. Phyllodes tumour.
E. Melanoma metastasis.

38. A 50-year-old man attends his GP feeling generally lethargic. The GP organizes blood tests and these reveal renal impairment. A subsequent ultrasound examination shows bilateral hydronephrosis without obvious cause. A CT scan of the abdomen then demonstrates that the hydronephrosis is secondary to bilateral ureteric obstruction from abnormal retroperitoneal soft tissue, intimately related to the aorta and IVC. Which of the following features on CT would suggest that the soft tissue is more likely due to retroperitoneal fibrosis, rather than a malignant cause?

A. Nodular contour to the soft tissue.
B. Contrast enhancement of the soft tissue.
C. More severe hydronephrosis in the kidneys.
D. Close application of the soft tissue to the adjacent vertebrae.
E. Soft-tissue extension above and below the level of the renal hila.

39. A 73-year-old male patient is referred from the urologists with a new diagnosis of prostate cancer. He is having an MRI scan to help stage the tumour. The patient reports that he has had a trans-rectal ultrasound (TRUS) biopsy done, but cannot remember when and the date is not on the form. The following information is present on the request form: 'The tumour is not palpable on digital rectal examination (DRE). The prostate specific antigen (PSA) is 2.4. One of four biopsies was positive and the Gleason score from this was 5.' When you do the MRI scan there is low signal in the peripheral zone on the left. There is also low signal on the right, which extends into the seminal vesicles. The images of the pelvis and para-aortic region do not show any evidence of lymphadenopathy. Which of these options would you choose for your report?

A. Repeat scan in 4 weeks.
B. T1 disease.
C. T2a disease.
D. T2c disease.
E. T3b disease.

40. A 45-year-old woman presents with anorexia and loss of weight. A CT of abdomen reveals bilateral non-calcified ovarian masses, but no ascites and no significant pelvic lymphadenopathy or peritoneal disease. Serum alpha fetoprotein, beta human chorionic gonadotrophin (β-HCG), and CA-125 are normal. The gynaecology team request an MRI of pelvis. This reveals that both ovaries are enlarged, the left more than the right. Bilateral cystic masses with low signal on T2WI/intermediate signal T1WI with solid portions are demonstrated. Gadolinium-enhanced T1WI with fat saturation reveals marked enhancement of these solid components and septa. What is the most likely diagnosis?

A. Krukenberg tumours.
B. Sertoli–Leydig tumours.
C. Dysgerminomas.
D. Fibromas.
E. Endodermal sinus tumours.

41. A 54-year-old female patient presents with anaemia and haematuria. A CT of abdomen confirms renal cell carcinoma of the right kidney, but there is also enlargement of the right adrenal gland. Which of the following CT characteristics is most consistent with a benign adrenal adenoma?

A. A pre-contrast attenuation of 50.
B. An immediate post-contrast attenuation of 50.
C. A relative percentage washout (RPW) of 60%.
D. Lesion size of 50 mm.
E. Heterogeneity of the lesion.

42. A 35-year-old female presents with a history of menorrhagia. MRI of pelvis demonstrates a fibroid uterus for which treatment with high-intensity focused ultrasound (HIFU) is proposed. What is the principle mechanism of action of HIFU?

A. Coagulation necrosis.
B. Apoptosis.
C. Cavitation.
D. Microstreaming.
E. Radiation forces.

43. A 60-year-old woman presents with a palpable lump in her right breast. Her recent screening mammogram 6 months previously was negative. Clinical examination reveals a subtle mass in the right lower quadrant. Which of the following mammographic findings is the most common in invasive lobular carcinoma (ILC)?

A. Spiculated mass.
B. Architectural distortion.
C. Microcalcification.
D. Nipple retraction.
E. Skin thickening.

44. You are asked to assess a 24-year-old woman with TVUS. The patient presents with lower abdominal cramps and is approximately 5 weeks post last menstrual period (LMP). Her pulse and blood pressure are normal. β-HCG levels suggest that the patient is pregnant. On TVUS, no adnexal mass or free fluid is seen. Which of the following findings would you expect to see in the uterus to confirm that the patient does not have an ectopic pregnancy?

A. Pseudogestational sac.
B. Normal endometrium.
C. Trilaminar endometrium.
D. Double decidual sac sign.
E. Thin-walled decidual cyst.

45. A 56-year-old male patient has presented to the urologists with a PSA of 17 ng/ml. He does not have a mass palpable on DRE. Two separate TRUS investigations, with a total of eight biopsies, have failed to yield a tissue diagnosis. The urologists have asked you to carry out an MRI to help guide their future biopsies. As is routine in these difficult cases, magnetic resonance spectroscopy (MRS) is carried out on suspicious areas to provide extra information. The MRI identifies an area of low signal in the anterior peripheral zone. This reveals an elevated choline and creatine peak, and a reduced citrate peak. Which of these features is suggestive of carcinoma?

A. Elevated choline.
B. Reduced polyamine peak.
C. Reduced citrate peak.
D. None of them, MRS is only sensitive in the transition zone.
E. All of them.

46. A 64-year-old patient is referred for a CT of abdomen 10 days post laparotomy for a right hemicolectomy for colonic adenocarcinoma. His post-operative course is initially uneventful, but the request form states that over the last 2 days he has developed pyrexia and today his inflammatory markers are markedly raised, he is 'septic' and unwell. The surgeons suspect a perforation or anastomotic leak, but you find no significant free fluid or air. There is marked bilateral enhancement of the adrenal glands, which are normal in size. The remainder of the abdominal viscera are unremarkable and the IVC and aorta are normal in calibre. There is marked consolidation at both lung bases. What is the significance of the appearance of the adrenal glands?

A. Hypovolaemic shock.
B. Phaeochromocytoma.
C. Hypervascular metastases.
D. Addisonian crisis secondary to tuberculous adrenalitis.
E. Adrenal hyperplasia as a response to the recent surgery.

47. A 46-year-old female with pressure symptoms related to uterine fibroids is referred for fibroid embolization. Which of the following complications is the patient at increased risk of?

A. Uterine sepsis.
B. Fibroid passage.
C. Fibroid regrowth.
D. Ovarian dysfunction.
E. Hysterectomy.

48. A 28-year-old primiparous woman has been breastfeeding for the past 3 months. She is admitted surgically complaining of warmth and pain in her right breast associated with swinging fever. A 3 × 2 cm inhomogenous, hypoechoic abscess within the right lower inner quadrant is identified on ultrasound. How should this patient be managed?

A. 6 weeks' antibiotic therapy followed by repeat ultrasound.
B. Ultrasound guided needle aspiration.
C. Ultrasound guided catheter drainage.
D. Surgical incision and drainage.
E. Analgesia and advice to stop breastfeeding.

49. A 60-year-old man has an unenhanced CT scan of renal tracts for suspected right renal colic. The examination is normal apart from an exophytic rounded lesion at the midpole of the left kidney, which is denser than adjacent renal parenchyma. You elect to perform an intravenous contrast-enhanced examination in the nephrographic phase to further evaluate this lesion. Which of the following Hounsfield attenuation values would be most appropriate if this lesion is benign?

A. 20 pre-contrast attenuation, 30 post-contrast attenuation.
B. 30 pre-contrast attenuation, 60 post-contrast attenuation.
C. 40 pre-contrast attenuation, 50 post-contrast attenuation.
D. 50 pre-contrast attenuation, 80 post-contrast attenuation.
E. 60 pre-contrast attenuation, 70 post-contrast attenuation.
F. 70 pre-contrast attenuation, 100 post-contrast attenuation.

50. A 24-year-old male patient presents to the A&E department with a history of severe episodic right-sided loin pain, radiating to the groin. He has no history of previous renal calculi. A low-dose non-contrast CT of the renal tracts shows a calculus in the distal right ureter, adjacent to the vesico-ureteric junction. The calculus measures 7 mm in diameter. The patient has a horseshoe kidney. There is stranding in the peri-nephric fat and around the right ureter. The density of the calculus is measured to be 1500 HU. Which of these observations is least likely to have relevance to this patient's treatment?

A. Site of the calculus.
B. Size of the calculus.
C. Perinephric and periureteric stranding.
D. Density of the calculus.
E. Horseshoe kidney.

51. A 60-year-old woman presents with pelvic pain. An MRI reveals multiple large areas of well-circumscribed, predominantly homogenous low T2WI and low/intermediate T1WI signal within the myometrium. There are also a number of peritoneal nodules demonstrated. What is the most likely diagnosis?

A. Endometriosis.
B. Adenomyosis.
C. Uterine leiomyomas.
D. Endometrial carcinoma.
E. Metastases to the uterus.

52. A 2-day-old male neonate with a right-sided abdominal mass is referred for ultrasound of abdomen. Ultrasound demonstrates an enlarged right kidney containing multiple non-communicating cysts of varying size with little normal parenchyma. What is the most common associated abnormality of the contra-lateral kidney?

A. Ectopic ureter.
B. Pelvi-ureteric junction obstruction.
C. Vesico-ureteric reflux.
D. Renal hypoplasia.
E. Renal aplasia.

53. A 36-year-old labourer working on a building site falls 15 feet from scaffolding on his back onto a wheelbarrow. He is catheterized in the resuscitation room and is noted to have gross haematuria. Which of the following CT findings are consistent with a grade 4 renal injury?

A. Renal artery avulsion.
B. Shattered kidney.
C. Deep laceration to the collecting system.
D. Subcapsular haematoma.
E. Parenchymal contusion.

54. A 54-year-old woman with no history of major illness is incidentally discovered to have a small, solid enhancing lesion on CT at the lower pole of the right kidney. The CT has been performed pre and post intravenous contrast. The lesion measures 9 mm in size. What is the most appropriate management for this lesion?

A. Nephron sparing surgery.
B. Percutaneous biopsy.
C. Repeat CT in 3–6 months.
D. Right nephrectomy.
E. Lesion ablation.

55. A 55-year-old female patient presents to your hospital with a history of recurrent UTIs and gross haematuria. Repeated urine cultures are negative, but analysis reveals copious white and red cells in the urine. The patient fails to improve with antibiotics. A CT scan of renal tracts is carried out, which shows an atrophic right kidney containing calcification. There is also an area of increased density on the unenhanced portion of the scan noted in the upper pole of the kidney, with overlying cortical thinning. There are multiple strictures noted in the ureter, with intervening areas of dilatation, giving a corkscrew appearance. There is extensive coarse calcification noted in the wall of the bladder. A CXR is carried out and is normal. Early morning urine collections finally identify mycobacterium tuberculosis in the urine, confirming the suspicion of renal and urinary tract TB. Which of these features is atypical of renal TB?

A. High-density material in the calyceal system.
B. Bladder calcification.
C. Renal calcification.
D. Normal CXR.
E. Corkscrew appearance to the ureter.

56. A 26-year-old female patient is referred to the gynaecology team with a history of primary infertility and oligomenorrhoea. On examination she is hirsute and has a body mass index (BMI) of 31. Which of the following MRI findings are most consistent with her diagnosis?

A. High T2WI signal C-shaped cystic masses with thin, longitudinally oriented folds along their interior in both adnexae.
B. Multiple small peripheral rounded high T2WI signal areas with hypointense central stroma in both ovaries.
C. Normal ovaries.
D. A small 'banana'-shaped uterus with a single fallopian tube.
E. A junctional zone of 14 mm with multiple hyperintense T2WI foci.

57. A 12-month-old infant with a history of aniridia and nephroblastomatosis undergoes a follow-up CT of abdomen that demonstrates bilateral enlarged kidneys with a thick rind of homogenous, non-enhancing, hypodense tissue bilaterally. A focal heterogenous enhancing mass with cystic change is noted on one side. What is the diagnosis?

A. Neuroblastoma.
B. Wilms tumour.
C. Lymphoma.
D. Renal cell carcinoma.
E. Cystic nephroma.

58. An 18-year-old mountain bike enthusiast is suspected of sustaining a renal injury after attempting a front wheel touch-up manoeuvre. A laceration to the right kidney is noted on CT, which demonstrates contrast enhancement during the pyelographic phase of the examination. What is the significance of this finding?

A. Pre-existing angiomyolipoma.
B. Active haemorrhage.
C. Devascularization.
D. Renal infarction.
E. Urine leak.

59. A 45-year-old man has a complex cyst identified in the right kidney on an ultrasound scan performed to assess non-specific epigastric pain. He subsequently has a CT scan of kidneys carried out pre and post administration of intravenous contrast. You classify the complex cyst as IIF (II requiring follow-up) according to the Bosniak classification. Which of the following features is most likely seen at CT imaging?

A. Presence of calcification.
B. Thickened smooth wall with enhancement.
C. Multiple thin non-enhancing septa.
D. Hyperattenuating cyst <3 cm in size.
E. Thickened irregular wall.

60. A 25-year-old male patient presents to A&E with left renal angle pain, radiating to the groin and significant haematuria on dipstick urinalysis. His kidneys, ureters, and bladder (KUB) x-ray is normal. He has a CT KUB, which shows no evidence of a calculus, but a mildly dilated left renal system as far as the mid ureter with peri-ureteric stranding to this point. Given the classical history, the patient undergoes an MR urogram, which shows a filling defect in the mid left ureter and a diagnosis of an obstructing ureteric calculus is made. The patient is observed and this diagnosis is confirmed when the patient passes a calculus the following day. The patient has a relevant past medical history, which led you to suspect a calculus in spite of the CT findings. Which of these clinical histories would lead you to suspect this?

A. Recurrent proteus infection.
B. HIV-positive patient on antiretroviral therapy.
C. Dehydrated patient.
D. Familial history of xanthine calculi.
E. Gout.

61. A 43-year-old woman with a history of breast carcinoma undergoes a CT of abdomen for abdominal pain and menorrhagia. This reveals an enlarged uterus and she proceeds to MRI. The normal T2WI zonal anatomy of the uterus is preserved. The endometrial stripe is of high T2WI signal and measures 14 mm in diameter, and the myometrium is thickened. Lattice-like enhancement of the high-signal T2WI endometrial area is demonstrated on T1WI post contrast administration. There is no evidence of myometrial invasion. What is the diagnosis most consistent with these findings?

A. Intrauterine contraceptive device (IUCD).
B. Tamoxifen therapy.
C. Lymphoma of the uterus.
D. Endometrial stromal sarcoma.
E. Pelvic congestion syndrome.

62. A 28-year-old male with a history of von Hippel Lindau disease and a 3-cm renal cell carcinoma undergoes cryo-ablation. Which of the following is suggestive of incomplete treatment/recurrence?

A. Hypodense ablation zone larger than the original tumour.
B. Lack of enhancement in the ablation zone.
C. Ablation zone unchanged in size over time.
D. Peripheral ring enhancement.
E. Perinephric fat-stranding post procedure.

63. A 22-year-old male front seat passenger is admitted following a RTA. On examination in A&E, blood is noted at the external urethral meatus and there is swelling of the penis. An urethrogram is performed which demonstrates contrast extravasation below the urogenital diaphragm only. What type of urethral injury does this represent?

A. Anterior urethral injury.
B. Disruption of the membranous urethra.
C. Bladder neck injury extending into the proximal urethra.
D. Bladder base injury.
E. Penile fracture.

64. A 46-year-old man presents with a 6-week history of painless haematuria. A CT urogram is performed and this demonstrates a 4-cm left renal mass, which is centrally placed involving both cortex and medulla. Which of the following findings will be most helpful when determining if this is a TCC invading the cortex, rather than a renal cell carcinoma invading the collecting system?

A. Presence of calcification.
B. Necrosis within the mass.
C. Renal vein invasion.
D. Maintenance of reniform shape.
E. Hypovascularity of lesion to renal parenchyma.

65. A 38-year-old patient is referred for an urgent IVU and ultrasound by their GP, who has picked up mild renal impairment on recent blood tests. The ultrasound shows two normal-sized kidneys with no evidence of cortical loss. The IVU shows a normally enhancing renal outline, but the pelvi-calyceal system is abnormal. Some calyces show a non-specific clubbed or blunted appearance. Thin tracks are noted extending from other calyces. In a number of calyces there is a filling defect noted within a rounded, blunted calyx. From these appearances you are able to make a diagnosis. The patient has a classical history for this condition. From the given options, what is the most typical history?

A. Recent history of acute hypotension on a background of dehydration.
B. Pyrexia, renal angle pain, and urine culture positive for *E. coli*.
C. Chronic non-steroidal anti-inflammatory drug (NSAID) analgesic overuse.
D. Previously diagnosed reflux nephropathy.
E. History of TCC within bladder.

66. A 37-year-old woman presents with a watery vaginal discharge and attends for an MRI of pelvis. She becomes quite claustrophobic at the end of the scan and you are called to assess her as she has been hyperventilating and the radiographers have become concerned. As you reassure her, you notice some peri-oral pigmentation. The MRI reveals a multicystic lesion (high T2WI and low T1WI signal) in the uterine cervix with a solid (low signal T1WI and T2WI) component in the deep cervical stroma. You note from the picture archiving and communication system (PACS) system that a barium enema previously revealed several colonic polyps. What is the likely cause for the MRI findings?

A. Malignant melanoma of the cervix.
B. Carcinoid tumour of the cervix.
C. Cervical pregnancy.
D. Minimal deviation adenocarcinoma of the cervix.
E. Invasive cervical squamous cell carcinoma.

67. A 48-year-old women presents with shortness of breath and undergoes an HRCT of the chest to assess interstitial changes seen on plain film. She has emigrated from Eastern Europe and knows that she had a gynaecological cancer that was treated there, but is unsure of her treatment. The HRCT reveals unilateral thickened interlobular septa, perilymphatic nodules, and ipsilateral hilar adenopathy. What is the most likely underlying diagnosis?

A. Cervical carcinoma.
B. Ovarian epithelial carcinoma.
C. Endometrial carcinoma.
D. Leiomyosarcoma of the uterus.
E. Vaginal carcinoma.

68. A 30-year-old female patient with a history of infertility is referred for an HSG. She has a past history of pelvic inflammatory disease. HSG reveals multiple small outpouchings from the uterine cavity. What is the diagnosis?

A. Salpingitis isthmica nodosa.
B. Asherman syndrome.
C. Adenomyosis.
D. Endometritis.
E. Multiple endometrial polyps.

69. A 14-year-old female presents with a history of cyclic pelvic pain. Speculum vaginal examination reveals a bulging vaginal mass. An MRI of the pelvis demonstrates divergent uterine horns with a deep midline fundal cleft, two separate uterine cavities, two separate cervices, and a unilateral hemivaginal septum causing hematometrocolpos. There is associated renal agenesis on the side of the hemivaginal septum. What is the primary uterine anomaly?

A. Uterus didelphys.
B. Uterine bicornuate bicollis.
C. Septate uterus.
D. Arcuate uterus.
E. Imperforate hymen.

70. An 18-year-old male fractures his pelvis following a motorcycle accident. He is suspected of sustaining a bladder injury and undergoes CT cystography. This reveals ill-defined contrast medium within the peri-vesical space with a 'molar-tooth' appearance. What is the significance of this finding?

A. Interstitial bladder injury.
B. Intraperitoneal rupture.
C. Extraperitoneal rupture.
D. Combined intra- and extraperitoneal rupture.
E. Bladder contusion.

71. A 54-year-old woman is noted to be hypercalcaemic after complaining of lethargy and abdominal pain. Subsequent biochemical testing reveals an elevated parathyroid hormone. She is referred for scintigraphy with ^{99m}Tc sestamibi. Which of the following radiological findings would suggest a diagnosis of parathyroid adenoma?

A. Focus of decreased radionuclide activity within the lower pole of the right lobe of thyroid on initial and delayed images.
B. Focus of decreased radionuclide activity within the lower pole of the right lobe of thyroid on delayed images only.
C. Focus of increased radionuclide activity within the lower pole of the right lobe of thyroid on initial and delayed images.
D. Focus of increased radionuclide activity within the lower pole of the right lobe of thyroid on initial images only.
E. Focus of increased radionuclide activity within the lower pole of the right lobe of thyroid on delayed images only.

72. A 50-year-old man is discovered to have a cystic abnormality at the lower pole of the left kidney during an ultrasound scan performed for right upper quadrant pain. You think this might be a complex cystic lesion and therefore recommend a CT scan of renal tracts. This shows a conglomeration of variable sized cysts at the lower pole of the left kidney, but no capsule or mural irregularities of the cysts. What is the most likely diagnosis?

A. Localized cystic renal disease.
B. Multilocular cystic nephroma.
C. Renal lymphangiomatosis.
D. Cystic clear cell carcinoma.
E. Multicystic dysplastic kidney.

73. A 32-year-old patient with a history of renal failure has undergone a renal transplant in your centre. You are carrying out serial ultrasound investigations over the weekend to assess the success of the transplant. The graft was a cadaveric transplant. The initial ultrasound scan showed no evidence of perigraft collection, but did show mild renal pelvic dilatation. The pulsatility index (PI) was 2.0 and the resistive index was 0.9. The patient was oliguric. Due to the fears of acute rejection, the patient was commenced on cyclosporine and steroids. The patient, now day 4, is currently anuric and has developed pain over the graft site. You have done an ultrasound. The arterial flow in the kidney has changed. Proximally you notice reversal of diastolic flow evident on spectral waveforms, but in other areas there is no flow evident in the interlobar arteries. Flow is still present in the main renal artery. The RI is now 0.95 and the PI is unchanged. There is still mild renal pelvic dilatation, but you notice a tubular structure of intermediate echogenicity in the renal hilum. There is no evidence of perigraft collection. What do you think the most appropriate next investigative/ therapeutic step is?

A. Continue immunosuppression and further observation, with appropriate fluid administration.
B. Continue immunosuppression and renal biopsy.
C. Refer for immediate arterial intervention.
D. Refer for immediate venous intervention.
E. Nephrostomy.

74. You are asked to assess a renal transplant kidney in the early post-operative period for any abnormality and to serve as a baseline study. Which of the following findings on colour Doppler ultrasound with regard to the PI, RI and B mode ultrasound imaging, with regard to renal morphology, would be considered within normal limits?

A. PI < 1.5, RI < 0.7, loss of cortico-medullary differentiation.
B. PI < 1.5, RI < 0.7, prominence of renal pyramids.
C. PI > 1.8, RI < 0.7, loss of cortico-medullary differentiation.
D. PI > 1.8, RI < 0.7, prominence of renal pyramids.
E. PI < 1.5, RI > 0.9, loss of cortico-medullary differentiation.
F. PI < 1.5, RI > 0.9, prominence of renal pyramids.
G. PI > 1.8, RI > 0.9, loss of cortico-medullary differentiation.
H. PI > 1.8, RI > 0.9, prominence of renal pyramids.

75. A 28-year-old para 0 + 0 female patient is referred from the gynaecology team for an MRI of pelvis, after presenting with pain in the RIF. On TVUS they have identified enlargement of the right ovary and have raised the possibility of a mass. On MRI, a 2-cm ovoid lesion is demonstrated within the right ovary. It is of high signal on T1WI and T1WI fat saturation sequences, and low signal on T2WI sequences. There is no evidence of a mural nodule or ascites and the uterus is not enlarged. What is the most likely diagnosis?

A. Fibrothecoma.
B. Endometriotic cyst.
C. Brenner tumour.
D. Simple follicular cyst.
E. Endometroid carcinoma.

chapter

4

GENITO-URINARY, ADRENAL, OBSTETRICS AND GYNAECOLOGY, AND BREAST

ANSWERS

1. A. Xanthogranulomatous pyelonephritis (XGP).

This is most commonly secondary to proteus infection. XGP is discussed elsewhere in this chapter.

2. D. Adenomyosis.

This appears as focal or diffuse thickening of the junctional zone of 12 mm or greater. Thickening of 8–12 mm is indeterminate, while thickening less than 8 mm usually allows exclusion of the disease. The bright foci on T2WI correspond to islands of ectopic endometrial tissue and cystic dilatation of glands, and have been reported to be present in up to 50% of cases of adenomyosis. Occasionally haemorrhage within these areas of ectopic endometrial tissue can result in areas of high signal within the junctional zone on T1WI.

Pseudothickening of the junctional zone can mimic adenomyosis. It occurs in the menstrual phase (especially the first 2 days) and thus scanning should not be performed at this time. Myometrial contractions can also mimic adenomyosis, but they result in focal, rather than diffuse, thickening of the junctional zone. The contractions are transient and thus will not persist on different sequences. They can therefore be more easily detected with multiphase–multisection imaging, rather than static fast SE. Neither pseudothickening nor myometrial contractions alone would result in high T2WI foci.

The appearances are not consistent with endometrial carcinoma or hyperplasia.

Tamai K, Togashi K, Ito T, Morisawa N, Fujiwara T, and Koyama T. MR imaging findings of adenomyosis: correlation with histopathologic features and diagnostic pitfalls. *RadioGraphics* 2005; 25: 21–40.

3. B. Transitional cell carcinoma (TCC).

The appearance of ureteral dilatation around and below an intraluminal filling defect is described as the 'goblet' sign. This sign indicates that the filling defect is caused by a chronic process, which allows dilatation of the ureter immediately below to accommodate the lesion. In addition to TCC, this appearance may rarely be seen with metastatic disease or endometriosis.

Chronic analgesic use is a risk factor for TCC.

Pyeloureteritis cystica appears as multiple small filling defects in the renal pelvis and ureter, typically seen in diabetics.

Browne RFJ, Meehan CP, Colville J, Power R, and Torreggiani WC. Transitional cell carcinoma of the upper urinary tract: spectrum of imaging findings. *RadioGraphics* 2005; 25: 1609–1627.

4. C. Gynaecomastia.

Most male breast lumps are benign, with breast cancer accounting for <1% of all breast lesions. Gynaecomastia is the most common benign condition of the male breast. The radiological description is in keeping with early nodular gynaecomastia. Lipomas are encapsulated fatty masses on mammography, which are mildly hyperechoic on ultrasound. Approximately 85% of male breast cancer is invasive ductal carcinoma. This is typically retroareolar and hyperdense on mammography with irregular margins. Secondary features such as nipple retraction and skin thickening are usually present. Ultrasound will show a non-parallel, hypoechoic mass. Posterior acoustic features and internal blood flow are not useful for distinguishing benign versus malignant lesions. Lymphoma will exhibit multiple hyperdense lymph nodes on mammography. Dermatofibrosarcoma is hyperechoic on ultrasound.

Chen L, Chantra PK, Larsen LH, Barton P, Rohitopakarn M, Zhu EQ et al. Imaging characteristics of malignant lesions of the male breast. *RadioGraphics* 2006; 26: 993–1006.

5. C. Fibrothecoma of the ovary.

Ovarian fibroma is the most common sex-cord stromal neoplasm and is almost always benign. Occasionally there will be histologic features of both fibroma and thecoma, giving rise to the term 'fibrothecoma'. These are typically solid lesions on ultrasound and have marked acoustic shadowing in 18–52% of cases. This shadowing is not secondary to calcification, but is related to marked attenuation of sound by the dense hypoechoic mass itself. This can be a useful sign for identifying fibrothecoma on ultrasound.

Classification of ovarian neoplasms is based on histologic features and typically includes the general categories of epithelial, germ cell, sex cord-stromal, and metastatic neoplasms. Cystadenomas/adenocarcinomas belong to the epithelial group of malignancies and make up over 90% of primary ovarian malignancies.

Sertoli–Leydig cell tumours, granulosa cell tumours, and fibrothecomas belong to the sex cord-stromal group of neoplasms. Sertoli–Leydig cell tumours may be subtle on ultrasound, as many are small and solid. They can secrete androgens and cause virilization. Granulosa cell tumours often have a sponge-like consistency and may produce oestrogen and cause endometrial disease.

Dysgerminomas and embryonal cell carcinomas are very rare germ cell neoplasms. The most common germ cell neoplasm is of course a mature cystic teratoma (dermoid cyst). A hyperechoic area (not usually as intensely echogenic as calcification) with acoustic shadowing is highly predictive of this lesion. Hyperechoic lines and dots, sometimes known as the dermoid mesh, are also highly predictive of a mature teratoma. Less common associated signs include a fluid–fluid level and floating globules. Calcification can be seen, but is not specific to dermoids, as other ovarian neoplasms can calcify.

Brown DL, Dudiak KM, and Laing FC. Adnexal masses: US characterisation and reporting. *Radiology* 2010; 254: 342–354.

6. C. Grade 3.

Whilst most commonly associated with congenital reflux in children, acquired reflux is also seen, most commonly due to bladder outlet obstruction or recurrent cystitis. Grade 1 reflux demonstrates reflux into the ureter, grade 2 has reflux into the pelvicalyceal system, grade 3 as described, and grade 4 is as grade 3 but with increased pelviureteric dilatation and calyceal blunting, and with persisting papillary impressions. Grade 5 demonstrates a markedly dilated pelvis and tortuous ureter with obliteration of the forniceal angles and papillary impressions.

Dahnert W. *Radiology Review Manual*, 5th edn, Lippincott Williams & Wilkins, 2007, p. 983.

7. C. recommend a repeat trans-abdominal ultrasound in 6 weeks' time.

At ultrasound, a functional ovarian cyst is typically anechoic with a thin, smooth wall and posterior acoustic enhancement. Regardless of size, these cysts are unlikely to be malignant. A unilocular cyst greater than 3 cm in a premenopausal or greater than 5 cm in a postmenopausal female patient should be rescanned in approximately 6 weeks (which will usually be at a different stage of the menstrual cycle in the case of premenopausal patients). Premenopausally this is the case, even if there are some internal echoes (but not other findings raising the possibility of malignancy), as these quite often represent haemorrhage within a cyst. In the premenopausal patient, the follow-up scan is to ensure there is reduction in size or resolution of what is usually a benign finding and commonly merely a dominant follicle; in the postmenopausal patient, it is to ensure there is no interim enlargement.

If the cyst is smaller than the above dimensions (i.e. <3 cm pre and <5 cm post menopausal) then, in the absence of other sinister findings or history, it can be assumed that the cysts are benign. Sonographic findings which increase the likelihood of malignancy include wall thickening, solid elements, septations, blood flow within solid elements, abnormal blood flow, and findings of metastatic disease. If a cyst displays any of the latter features or increases in size on interval scanning, then options A, B, and D may be valid steps in management.

Alty J, Hoey E, Wolstenhulme S, and Weston M. *Practical Ultrasound: An Illustrated Guide*, Royal Society of Medicine Press Ltd., 2006, p. 200.
Levine D. Gynaecologic ultrasound. *Clinical Radiology* 1998; 53: 1–9.

8. B. Renal imaging.

Mullerian duct anomalies are associated with renal tract anomalies in up to 30% of cases due to the close embryologic relationship between the Mullerian and mesonephric ducts. The most common renal tract abnormality is renal agenesis. Other associated anomalies include duplicated collecting system, renal duplication, horseshoe kidney, crossed renal ectopy. and cystic renal dysplasia. Renal imaging is therefore essential in all patients with Mullerian duct anomalies.

Surgical intervention is not required in patients with a unicornuate uterus and a non-functioning rudimentary horn.

Junqueira BLP, Allen LM, Spitzer RF, Lucco KL, Babyn PS, and Doria AS. Mullerian duct anomalies and mimics in children and adolescents: correlative intraoperative assessment with clinical imaging. *RadioGraphics* 2009; 29: 1085–1103.

9. D. Dot-dash.

Malignant calcifications vary in shape and size. Pleomorphic calcifications that are more linear or dot-dash in appearance are associated with intraductal carcinoma. DCIS is often detected as a result of such calcifications. Egg-shell calcification is seen in the walls of an oil cyst. Sedimented calcium appears as curvilinear on the lateral projection and as smudged on the cranio-caudal view. This is a feature of benign cysts. Arterial calcification presents as tubular, parallel calcification. Fibroadenomas typically exhibit large, coarse, and irregular calcification.

Brant WE and Helms CA. *Fundamentals of Diagnostic Radiology*, 3rd edn, Lippincott Williams & Wilkins, 2007, pp. 580–582.

10. B. The presence of aneurysmal blood vessels within the lesion.

Both well-differentiated retroperitoneal liposarcomas and exophytic renal angiomyolipomas can be very large in size and thus size is not a discriminating factor. Both contain large amounts of mature lipid, thus significant portions of the lesion will have negative Hounsfield attenuation values on CT imaging.

Aneurysmal blood vessels are commonly seen in large angiomyolipomas, whereas well-differentiated liposarcomas are generally rather hypovascular lesions. Both angiomyolipomas and retroperitoneal liposarcomas may contain areas of soft tissue density. Liposarcoma is probably more likely to have an irregular margin and may contain areas of fluid density.

Israel GM and Bosniak MA. Pitfalls in renal mass evaluation and how to avoid them. *RadioGraphics* 2008; 28: 1325–1338.

11. D. XGP.

Whilst the patient presents with the classical renal cell carcinoma (RCC) triad of loin pain, haematuria, and a mass, this triad is actually only present in 30% of patients with RCC. These features are also typically found in XGP. The key finding in this case is of areas of fatty attenuation within the mass, in association with a staghorn calculus. Calculi are found in 80–90% of cases of XGP. The long history of symptoms is also typical of XGP, which can be present for up to 6 months prior to diagnosis. Lymphoma, RCC, and renal oncocytoma would not typically have areas of fatty tissue within them. Angiomyolipomas, in the absence of tuberous sclerosis, are typically solitary. They are usually well defined, unlike in this case, and would rarely reach this size without having previously caused symptoms. XGP is typically found in diabetic patients and is due to proteus infection. Treatment is with nephrectomy.

Dahnert W. *Radiology Review Manual*, 5th edn, Lippincott Williams & Wilkins, 2007, p. 944.

12. D. Eagle Barrett syndrome.

Eagle Barrett syndrome or prune belly syndrome is classically defined as a triad of partial or complete absence of abdominal musculature (resulting in bulging flanks), cryptorchidism, and urinary abnormalities as described above. In addition a number of respiratory, GI, musculoskeletal, and cardiovascular anomalies are associated with this syndrome.

It occurs almost exclusively in males. The cause and embryogenesis remain controversial. Bladder outlet obstruction, mesodermal arrest, and dysgenesis of the yolk sac have been proposed as possible causes.

Berrocal T, Lopez-Pereira P, Arjonilla A, and Gutierrez J. Anomalies of the distal ureter, bladder, and urethra in children: embryologic, radiologic and pathologic features. *RadioGraphics* 2002; 22: 1139–1164.

13. B. Spiculated margin.

A recent study examining incidental breast lesions detected by CT found that spiculated breast lesions and axillary lymphadenopathy should raise concern for malignancy and be referred to the breast clinic. These features were significantly more likely to be present in malignant breast lesions. Genuine mass lesions and spiculation are more easily appreciated in non-dense breasts. The mammographic features of ill-definition and calcification do not appear to be suggestive of malignancy on CT, probably due to poorer resolution, as normal breast glandular tissue appears ill-defined on CT and malignant microcalcification is poorly demonstrated. Lesion size and location also do not differentiate between benign and malignant disease.

Porter G, Steel J, Paisley K, Watkins R, and Holgate C. Incidental breast masses detected by computed tomography: are any imaging features predictive of malignancy? *Clinical Radiology* 2009; 64: 529–533.

14. B. Renal oncocytoma.

This is a benign renal cell neoplasm responsible for about 5% of all adult primary renal epithelial neoplasms. It typically occurs in elderly men. They usually appear as solitary, well-demarcated, unencapsulated, fairly homogeneous renal cortical tumours. Bilateral, multicentric oncocytomas are seen in hereditary syndromes of renal oncocytosis and Birt–Hogg–Dubé syndrome. A central stellate scar is seen in approximately one-third. However, distinguishing them from RCC on imaging is not reliable. Leiomyoma of the kidney is a benign smooth muscle neoplasm. It appears as a well-circumscribed, homogeneous, exophytic solid mass that shows uniform enhancement on contrast-enhanced CT. It may occasionally be cystic.

Metanephric adenoma is a benign renal neoplasm that is more common in middle-aged to elderly females. It is associated with polycythaemia in 10%. It typically appears as a well-defined, unencapsulated, solitary mass that may be hyperattenuating on unenhanced CT. Calcification can be seen in up to 20%.

Hemangioma of the kidney occurs as an unencapsulated, solitary lesion that frequently arises from the renal pyramids or the pelvis. Contrast-enhanced CT or MRI may show early intense enhancement, with persistent enhancement on delayed images.

Juxtaglomerular cell (JGC) neoplasm or reninoma is an extremely rare, benign renal neoplasm of myoendocrine cell origin, which is associated with a clinical triad of hypertension, hypokalaemia, and high plasma renin activity. It typically appears as a unilateral, well-circumscribed, cortical tumour and often measures less than 3 cm, but otherwise is indistinguishable from other cortical neoplasms.

Prasad SR, Swabhi VR, Menias CO, Raut AA, and Chintapalli KN. Benign renal neoplasms: cross-sectional imaging findings. *American Journal of Roentgenology* 2008; 190: 158–164.

15. B. Emphysematous pyelitis.

The combination of these radiological findings in a septic diabetic patient indicates an infection with a gas-forming organism, usually *E. coli*. The gas is located entirely within the pelvicalyceal system, as opposed to the renal parenchyma, which would indicate a diagnosis of emphysematous pyelonephritis. The importance is in the urgency of treatment and prognosis. Emphysematous pyelonephritis carries a grave prognosis and often requires nephrectomy for life-saving treatment, whereas the prognosis with emphysematous pyelitis is not as grave and it often responds to antibiotics with possible urinary drainage procedures if necessary.

Dahnert W. *Radiology Review Manual*, 5th edn, Lippincott Williams & Wilkins, 2007, p. 944.
Narlawar R, Raut A, Nagar A, Hira P, Hanchate V, and Asrani A. Imaging features and guided drainage in emphysematous pyelonephritis: a study of 11 cases. *Clinical Radiology* 2004; 59: 192–197.

16. D. Referral for surgery.

The findings are consistent with a mature cystic teratoma or dermoid cyst. They are derived from all three germ cell layers and thus contain fat and may contain desquamated epithelium, skin, hair, and teeth. The classical finding is of high T1WI signal, which suppresses on fat saturation imaging. They can often have a fat–fluid level. The low signal on T2WI may represent tooth or calcification. Soft-tissue protuberances represent Rokintansky nodules or 'dermoid plugs' of sebaceous material.

It is the most common ovarian tumour, accounting for 20% of all ovarian neoplasms. Dermoids can be bilateral in 8–25% of cases. The chance of malignant transformation is low but surgical resection is indicated, not just for relief of symptoms, but because of the risk of torsion (in 4–16% of cases) or rupture (the latter is rare but can lead to chemical peritonitis). Adjuvant treatment need not be considered unless the case is complicated by malignant transformation.

Izumi I, Wada A, Kaji Y, Hayashi T, Hayashi M, and Matsuo M. Developing an MR imaging strategy for diagnosis of ovarian masses. *RadioGraphics* 2006; 26: 1431–1448.
Dahnert W. *Radiology Review Manual*, 5th edn, Lippincott Williams & Wilkins, 2003, pp. 1028–1029.

17. D. Utero-ovarian anastomosis is identified in less than 5% of cases.

Uterine arteries are the predominant source of blood supply to the fibroids in most cases. There is considerable variation in the pelvic arterial anatomy, a thorough knowledge of which is essential to carry out uterine artery embolization safely and effectively.

The internal iliac artery bifurcates into anterior and posterior divisions in 57–77% of the general population. The uterine artery arises as the first or second branch of the anterior division of internal iliac artery in 51% of cases. The internal iliac artery trifurcates into uterine artery, the anterior, and the posterior divisions in 15–40% of the general population. The uterine artery arises as the first branch of the internal iliac artery in 6% of cases.

The uterine artery may be replaced by small branches or may be absent. The ipsilateral ovarian artery often replaces an absent uterine artery. Ovarian arterial supply to fibroids is more common in those with previous history of pelvic surgery or tubo-ovarian disease and/or large fundal fibroids. The extent of ovarian supply should be assessed with flush pelvic aortography, preferably after uterine artery embolization.

The ovarian artery arises from the aorta just below the renal arteries in 80–90% of cases and has a characteristic corkscrew appearance. Normal ovarian arteries are not usually identified on angiography because of their small calibre.

Utero-ovarian anastomosis is seen in 10–30% of cases and left-to-right uterine anastomosis in 10% of cases.

Pelage J-P, Cazejust J, Plout E, le Dref O, Laurent A, Spies JB et al. Uterine fibroid vascularization and clinical relevance to uterine fibroid embolisation. *RadioGraphics* 2005; 25: S99–S117.

18. C. Multiple curvilinear lines of low T2WI signal within the implant.

Silicone gel implants are high signal on T2WI. Capsular contracture is caused by constriction of the fibrous capsule that invariably forms to some degree around the implant as a reaction to the foreign object. This is seen on MRI as increased thickening of the T2WI hypointense margin surrounding the implant. Rupture of the prosthesis is the most common complication with breast implants, occurring in up to 10–20%, although many are not noticed clinically. With intracapsular ruptures, the silicone gel is contained by the capsule. Curvilinear strands of low T2 signal within the capsule may be seen, representing the collapsed implant shell. This finding is known as the 'linguine' sign. T2WI hyperintense globules surrounding the implant are indicative of an extracapsular rupture. Inferior extension beyond the inframammary fold implies implant migration, which is a relatively uncommon occurrence. Marginal T2WI hypointense radial folds within the implant are a normal finding.

DeAngelis GA, de Lange EE, Miller LR, and Morgan RF. MR imaging of breast implants. *RadioGraphics* 1994; 14: 783–794.

19. A. Lymphoma.

Clinically testicular lymphoma is distinct from other testicular neoplasms in that it occurs in a much older age group. It is the most common testicular neoplasm over the age of 60 years. It is also the most common bilateral testicular neoplasm (up to 38% of cases). The epididymis and spermatic cord are commonly involved. The sonographic appearance is variable and indistinguishable from germ cell tumours. Typically they are discrete hypoechoic lesions that may completely infiltrate the testicle.

Primary leukaemia of the testis is rare, although it is a common site of leukaemia recurrence in children. The sonographic appearances are very variable, as the tumour may be unilateral or bilateral, focal or diffuse, hypoechoic or hyperechoic.

Testicular metastases, other than those from lymphoma or leukaemia, are very rare. Primary sites reported include prostate and lung. They are generally seen in the setting of widespread disease and are rarely the presenting complaint.

Seminoma is the most common germ cell tumour. The average age of presentation is approximately 40 years. It is typically uniformly hypoechoic on ultrasound and they are only rarely bilateral (2%).

Granulomatous orchitis may manifest as a testicular mass, but this would be very unusual. Typically this process tends to involve the epididymis first and to a much greater degree than the testis. Pathogens include TB, syphilis, fungi, and parasites.

Woodward PJ, Sohaey R, O'Donoghue MJ, and Green DE. From the archive of the AFIP – tumor and tumorlike conditions of the testis: radiologic-pathologic correlation. *RadioGraphics* 2002; 22: 189–216.

20. A. Malakoplakia.

This is an inflammatory response to chronic *E. coli* infection. It is more common in females and in diabetic/immunocompromised patients. It most commonly occurs in the bladder and distal ureter and is multifocal in 75% of cases.

Dahnert W. *Radiology Review Manual*, 5th edn, Lippincott Williams & Wilkins, 2007, p. 924.
Wasserman N. Inflammatory diseases of the ureter. *Radiological Clinics of North America* 1996; 34: 1131–1156.

21. A. Serum parathyroid hormone assay and ^{99m}Tc sestamibi scan.

Clinical findings, blood tests, and CT of the abdomen are diagnostic of pancreatitis. The most common causes for pancreatitis are alcohol and choledocholithiasis. Rarely, it may be caused by hyperparathyroidism. The associated findings on CT are suggestive of hyperparathyroidism, therefore further assessment with serum parathyroid hormone assay and ^{99m}Tc sestamibi scintigraphy is indicated. ^{99m}Tc sestamibi washes out more rapidly from the thyroid gland than from hyperfunctioning parathyroid glands and therefore it can be used on its own.

MIBG, a noradrenaline analogue, is used in the evaluation of neuroblastomas and paragangliomas.

^{99m}Tc pertechnetate is taken up by the thyroid gland only and is therefore not useful on its own in parathyroid imaging. However, it can be used in combination with ^{201}Tl, which is taken up by both thyroid and parathyroid. Subtracting the two scintigrams allows parathyroid localization.

Eslamy HK and Zeissman HA. Parathyroid scintigraphy in patients with primary hyperparathyroidism: ^{99m}Tc sestamibi SPECT and SPECT/CT. *RadioGraphics* 2008; 28: 1461–1476.

22. A. Irregular margin.

A woman over the age of 30 years who is a BRCA1 or BRCA2 carrier should be offered MRI annually for breast cancer surveillance. The description of the margin of the mass is the most predictive feature of the breast MR image interpretation. Irregular or spiculated margins have a positive predictive value of 84–91%. T2W signal hyperintensity is suggestive of benign pathology, but not in the setting of an irregular or spiculated mass. There is overlap in enhancement kinetics between benign and malignant disease, and thus reliance on kinetic assessment alone is not recommended. Progressive enhancement (type I) is associated with benign pathology, whereas plateau (type II) and washout (type III) curves are suggestive of malignant disease. Due to the importance of lesion morphology, the MRI technique should focus on optimizing high spatial and temporal resolution.

Macura KJ, Ouwerkerk R, Jacobs MA, and Bluemke DA. Patterns of enhancement on breast MR images: interpretation and imaging pitfalls. *RadioGraphics* 2006; 26: 1719–1734.

23. D. Tubular ectasia of the rete testis.

This is also known as cystic transformation of the rete testis and results from partial or complete obliteration of the efferent tubules, which causes ectasia and eventually cystic transformation. It is frequently bilateral, but may be asymmetric. The site is in or adjacent to the mediastinum testis and there are often associated epididymal cysts or spermatoceles. The key to the correct identification of this abnormality is the elongated shape that replaces the mediastinum.

Intratesticular varicoceles can occur, but they are very rare. It would be even rarer for it to be thrombosed.

Testicular abscess would not usually be multicystic, but would be more rounded with an irregular wall and low-level internal echoes.

Testicular infarction usually manifests as a hypoechoic mass that is largely avascular. It is not usually cystic.

Epidermoid cyst is a rare benign tumour of germ cell origin. It is usually rounded or oval in shape and classically has a target or 'onion skin' appearance of alternating layers of hyper- and hypo-echogenicity. The outer wall is typically hyperechoic and sometimes calcified.

Dogra VS, Gottlieb RH, Rubens DJ, and Liao L. Benign intratesticular cystic lesions: US features. *RadioGraphics* 2001; 21: S273–S281.

24. E. No intervention.

The factors described are all indicators of poor outcome following renal artery intervention. Reduced renal size bilaterally indicates advanced bilateral renal disease, unlikely to respond to intervention. The renal ultrasound Doppler patterns are also not suggestive of renal artery stenosis, which is indicated by a peak systolic velocity of greater than 180 cm/s. Resistive indices of greater than 0.7 indicate a likelihood of improvement after intervention.

Morgan R and Waltzer E. *Handbook of Angioplasty and Stenting Procedures*. Springer, 2010, p. 152.

25. D. Bartholin's gland cyst.

Bartholin's glands are located behind the labia minora and their ducts open onto the posterolateral vestibules on each side. The cysts are due to blockage of the ducts and retention of secretions. They are common in reproductive age and are usually cystic in appearance (high T2WI signal). Their T1WI signal is variable and can be high due to mucoid content. They are usually discovered as incidental findings on imaging for another cause, although they may be palpable or clinically visible. The radiologist should recognize them as a benign pathology.

Primary carcinoma of the vagina is rare, as 80–90% of tumours affecting the vagina are due to extension of primary bladder, cervical, vulval, or rectal tumours. Ninety per cent of primary carcinomas are squamous cell carcinoma. The majority occur in elderly women and the two most common presenting complaints are vaginal discharge and bleeding. Squamous cell carcinomas of the vagina are usually of low T1WI and intermediate T2WI signal. As for vulval and cervical squamous cell carcinoma, human papilloma virus (HPV) infection is a risk factor.

Urethral divertcula are best seen on T2WI sequences as hyperintense lesions adjacent to or surrounding the urethra: a connection to the urethra is not always seen. They are usually of low signal on T1WI sequences. They predispose to stones (low signal on T2WI sequences) and carcinoma (enhancing on T1W fat saturation post gadolinium).

Nabothian cysts are found at the external os of the cervix. They are benign retention cysts that develop secondary to obstruction of endocervical glands. They have high T2WI signal and may have high T1WI signal due to mucinous content. They are usually multiple and measure less than 2 cm. They become clinically relevant when they are mistakenly diagnosed as adenoma malignum, a subtype of mucinous adenocarcinoma of the cervix.

A vaginal septum is a low-signal T2WI band. If transverse, it may present in adolescence with primary amenorrhea and abdominal pain, and an abdominal mass if complete. A longitudinal septum is usually asymptomatic and is associated with duplication of the uterus, cervix, or vagina.

Lopez C, Balogun M, Ganesan R, and Olliff JF. MRI of vaginal conditions. *Clinical Radiology* 2005; 60: 648–662.

Siegelman E. *Body MRI*. Elsevier Saunders, 2004, p. 291.

26. A. Repeat fine needle aspiration.

The features suspicious for malignancy on ultrasound are calcification, irregularity, solid lesion, and irregular halo- and hypervascularity. A repeat biopsy should be considered if there is discordance between imaging findings and cytology.

Iyer NG and Shaha AR. Management of thyroid nodules and surgery for differentiated thyroid cancer. *Clinical Oncology* 2010; 22: 405–412.

27. E. Two lives are saved for every over-diagnosed case.

Over-diagnosis is defined as the diagnosis of cancer as a result of screening that would not have been diagnosed in the woman's lifetime had screening not taken place. Approximately 5.7–8.8 breast cancer deaths are prevented per 1000 women screened for 20 years starting at age 50 compared with 2.3–4.3 over-diagnosed cases per 1000 women screened for 20 years. The WHO International Agency for Research on Cancer determined that there is a 35% reduction in mortality from breast cancer among screened women aged 50–69.

The NHS Breast Screening Programme provides screening every 3 years for women between the ages of 50 and 70. After the age of 70, women are still screened, although they are not automatically called for. Expansion is planned to cover women from 47 to 73. A two-view (cranio-caudal and mediolateral oblique) mammogram is taken, performed with breast compression, which can be uncomfortable for the patient.

www.cancerscreening.nhs.uk/breastscreen
Duffy SW, Tabar L, Olsen AH, Vitak B, Allgood PC, Chen THH et al. Absolute numbers of lives saved and overdiagnosis in breast cancer screening, from a randomized trial and from the breast screening programme in England. *Journal of Medical Screening* 2010; 17: 25–30.

28. D. Succenturiate placenta.

This is an additional lobule separate from the main bulk of the placenta. The significance of this variant is the rupture of vessels connecting the two components or retention of the accessory lobe with resultant post-partum haemorrhage.

Circumvallate placenta has a chorionic plate smaller than the basal plate, with associated rolled placental edges. There is known to be an increased risk of placental abruption and haemorrhage with this type of placenta.

A bilobed placenta is a placenta with two evenly sized lobes connected by a thin bridge of placental tissue. This has no known increased risk of morbidity.

Placenta membranacea is a thin membranous structure circumferentially occupying the entire periphery of the chorion. There is an increased risk of placenta praevia, as a portion of the placenta completely covers the internal os.

Placenta acreta is not a variant of placental morphology. It occurs when there is superficial invasion of the chorionic villi of the placenta into the basalis layer of the uterine wall. Deeper invasion of the myometrium is termed 'placenta increta'. Even deeper invasion involving the serosa or adjacent pelvic organs is termed 'placenta percreta'. The risk of this is catastrophic intrapartum haemorrhage at the time of placental delivery.

Elsayes KM, Trout AT, Friedkin AM, Liu PS, Bude RO, Platt JF, and Menias CO. Imaging of the placenta: a multimodality pictorial review. *RadioGraphics* 2009; 29: 1371–1391.

29. B. Patients C and D.

A 70% stenosis is taken as the cut-off for significant stenosis. Patient B is atypical in their age. They also have imaging characteristics typical of fibromuscular dysplasia. Patients C and D have classical imaging features of renal artery stenosis (RAS). With regard to ultrasound diagnosis using Doppler, this is made by either showing flow acceleration immediately distal to the site of stenosis or showing dampened flow in the segmental arteries. In the renal artery, a peak systolic velocity of over 180 cm/s combined with a renal/aortic velocity ratio of over 3 is reported as being the most sensitive method of detecting RAS.

House M, Dowling R, King P, and Gibson R. Using Doppler sonography to reveal renal artery stenosis: an evaluation of optimal imaging parameters. *American Journal of Roentgenology* 1999; 173: 761–765.
Morgan R and Waltzer E. *Handbook of Angioplasty and Stenting Procedures*, Springer, 2010, pp. 151–156.

30. B. Adrenal cortical carcinoma.

The clinical picture is one of undiagnosed Cushing's syndrome with obesity and hypertension. In this case it is adrenocorticotropic hormone (ACTH) independent Cushing's, as the negative feedback from the cortisol producing adrenal carcinoma causes reduction in ACTH levels and atrophy of the contra-lateral, normal adrenal gland.

Adrenal adenoma can cause Cushing's syndrome, but the features described point to adrenal carcinoma. They have a bimodal distribution (first and fourth decades). On average 55% are functional, manifesting with Cushing' syndrome, feminization, virilisation, or a mixture of these. Hypertension is common in all syndrome types. The majority of masses measure more than 6 cm. They are inhomogenous on unenhanced CT, owing to necrosis. They enhance heterogeneously, often peripherally, with a thin rim of enhancing capsule in some cases. In 19–33% of cases calcification or microcalcifications have been identified. The liver is the most common metastatic site, followed by the lung and lymph nodes. Direct extension and tumour thrombus can also occur. Compression of the IVC can lead to presentation with abdominal pain, lower extremity oedema or pulmonary embolism.

Neuroblastoma is a disease of childhood. Myelolipoma is a relatively uncommon benign adrenal mass containing fat and haemopoeitic tissue.

Phaeochromocytoma is classically brightly enhancing, but can have a variety of CT appearances. It would explain hypertension, but not atrophy of the contra-lateral adrenal gland. Phaeochromocytoma rarely invades the IVC.

Johnson PT, Horton KM, and Fishman EK. Adrenal mass imaging with multidetector CT: pathologic conditions, pearls, and pitfalls. *RadioGraphics* 2009; 29: 1333–1351.
Rockall AG, Babar SA, Sohaib SA, Isidori AM, Diaz-Cano S, Monson JP et al. CT and MR imaging of the adrenal glands in ACTH-independent Cushing syndrome. *RadioGraphics* 2004; 24: 435–452.

31. B. Calcitonin.

Medullary thyroid carcinoma arises from the parafollicular C cells of the thyroid that secrete calcitonin, therefore calcitonin is a useful tumour marker for medullary thyroid carcinoma. CEA is another tumour marker produced by neoplastic C cells.

Thyroglobulin is produced by follicular cells and is therefore not useful in medullary carcinomas.

Pacini F, Castagna MG, Cipri C, and Schlumberger M. Medullary thyroid carcinoma. *Clinical Oncology* 2010; 22: 475–485.

32. A. Reassurance and discharge with advice.

The clinical and radiological findings in this case are typical for fibroadenoma. Standard practice for investigating breast lumps involves triple assessment with clinical examination, imaging with ultrasound, and tissue diagnosis (with either cytology or histology). However, in women under the age of 25 who present with a clinically and radiologically benign lump, biopsy is not needed unless there is overriding clinical concern. To be assessed as definitely benign on ultrasound, there should be no malignant features (spiculation, angular margins, acoustic shadowing, calcification, and marked hypoechogenicity) and the lesion should follow tissue planes (wider than it is tall). The ultrasound should also be performed by an experienced operator. The patient should be advised to seek further assessment if there is any increase in size or change to the mass.

Smith GEC and Burrows P. Ultrasound diagnosis of fibroadenoma – is biopsy always necessary? *Clinical Radiology* 2008; 63: 511–515 (commentary by Dall BJG, *Clinical Radiology*, 2008; 63: 516–517).

33. B. Cortico-medullary phase.

Imaging in the cortico-medullary phase is helpful for showing the normal cortico-medullary pattern in pseudotumours such as prominent columns of Bertin or focal renal hypertrophy. It is also useful for suspected abnormalities such as vascular malformations and pseudoaneurysms of the kidney. The nephrographic phase is best to characterize renal masses. Small parenchymal renal lesions may be hidden in the renal medulla on the cortico-medullary phase and excretory phases. Excretory phases are best to assess for collecting system lesions and the unenhanced scan is best for detection of renal calculi and for using as a baseline in assessing the enhancement characteristics of parenchymal renal lesions.

Israel GM and Bosniak MA. Pitfalls in renal mass evaluation and how to avoid them. *RadioGraphics* 2008; 28: 1325–1338.

34. D. Arterial phase CT abdomen.

The IVU has surprisingly been helpful in showing a delayed increasing nephrogram, a classical, although uncommon, appearance of renal vein thrombosis. This is also indicated by the history of glomerulonephritis, which can manifest as nephrotic syndrome, the most common cause for renal vein thrombosis. Ultrasound is often successful at identifying a thrombosed right renal vein, but is not useful in assessing the longer left renal vein. Gradient and SE sequences are both helpful in assessing the renal venous system, with GE giving low-signal thrombus and SE giving high-signal thrombus. Arterial phase CT would be too early to show a venous filling defect and thus may not contribute, although it may show a rim nephrogram. Portal venous phase CT is reasonably sensitive at detecting the lack of enhancement within the renal vein and abnormal enhancement pattern within the affected kidney.

Adam A and Dixon A. *Grainger and Allison's Diagnostic Radiology. A textbook of medical imaging, Vol 1*, 5th edn, Churchill Livingstone, 2008, Ch 39.

35. D. In- and out-of-phase T1WI.

This is a T1WI technique and will reveal the presence of intracellular lipid via a dropout of signal on the out-of-phase imaging when compared to the in-phase imaging. Thus a benign adrenal adenoma will show such signal dropout (20% or greater in quantity is diagnostic; 10–20% is highly suggestive), whilst adrenal metastases will not. However, approximately 15% of benign adenomas do not accumulate intracellular lipid and may retain signal on the out-of-phase imaging; in such cases, dynamic gadolinium-enhanced images can increase specificity to over 90–95% (by showing washout characteristics as seen on CT). If there is still doubt, PET-CT is useful. Adrenal hyperplasia may also show loss of signal on the out-of-phase imaging. Of note an adrenal cortical carcinoma can show dropout of signal in portions on the out-of-phase sequence, but there is not the uniform loss of signal as seen with adenomas.

The T1WI with fat saturation will show signal dropout in areas of extracellular lipid, e.g. macroscopic fat in lipomas, dermoid cysts, or the subcutaneous tissues. T2WI is not of much benefit in distinguishing benign from malignant adrenal masses unless the tumour is a phaeochromocytoma, which can show very high T2WI signal.

Martin D, Brown M, and Semelka, R. *Primer on MR Imaging of the Abdomen and Pelvis*, Wiley, 2005, 223–256.

36. C. Medullary sponge kidney.

Hyperparathyroidism, renal tubular acidosis, and medullary sponge kidney are the three most common causes of medullary nephrocalcinosis. The former two conditions are associated with hypercalciuria that results in uniform medullary nephrocalcinosis. Sarcoidosis and multiple myeloma are associated with hypercalcemia resulting in bilateral nephrocalcinosis. Medullary sponge kidney can affect the kidney segmentally, unilaterally, or bilaterally, therefore unilateral nephocalcinosisis is suggestive of medullary sponge kidney.

Medullary sponge kidney is characterized by cystic dilatation of collecting tubules. Urine stasis within the dilated tubules predisposes to infection and calculus formation within the dilated tubules or urinary tracts. On excretory urogram, contrast within the dilated tubules produces a striated 'paintbrush' appearance of the renal pyramids.

Joffe SA, Servaes S, Okon S, and Horowitz M. Multi-detector row CT urography in the evaluation of hematuria. *RadioGraphics* 2003; 23: 1441–1455.
Dyer RB, Chen MY, and Zagoria RJ. Abnormal calcifications in the urinary tract. *RadioGraphics* 1998; 18: 1405–1424.

37. D. Phyllodes tumour.

This most commonly manifests as a rapidly growing mass, which is lobulated on mammography. Calcifications are rarely seen. A solid mass containing cystic spaces on ultrasound and demonstrating posterior acoustic enhancement is strongly suggestive of phyllodes tumour. Phyllodes tumour can be benign or malignant, but both have a tendency to recur if not widely excised. Adenoid cystic carcinoma is a slow-growing mass that is well defined on mammography. Fibromatosis presents as an indistinct mass on mammography, which is hypoechoic with posterior acoustic shadowing on ultrasound, simulating malignancy. Granular cell tumours are thought to arise from Schwann cells and have a very variable appearance. Metastatic disease to the breast is much more likely to be multiple or bilateral. Diffuse skin thickening is also a feature.

Feder JM, Shaw de Paredes E, Hogge JP, and Wilken JJ. Unusual breast lesions: radiologic-pathologic correlation. *RadioGraphics* 1999; 19: 511–526.

38. D. Close application of the soft tissue to the adjacent vertebrae.

Unfortunately attempts to consistently distinguish benign retroperitoneal fibrosis (RPF) from malignancy are fraught with danger, but there are certain CT findings which are more commonly seen in one or other of these conditions.

Malignancy tends to be larger and bulkier, displaying mass effect and displacing the aorta and IVC anteriorly from the spine and the ureters laterally. The purely fibrotic process of benign RPF tends to tether these structures to the adjacent vertebrae.

Malignancy is more likely to extend cephalad to the renal hila, with benign RPF remaining caudal to the hila. Neoplasia also more typically has a nodular outline, whereas benign RPF usually manifests as a plaque-like density. There are, of course, exceptions to both these features.

Contrast enhancement is not a reliable feature for distinguishing benign RPF from malignancy, as both malignancy and active RPF can enhance with contrast. Similarly, the degree of hydronephrosis caused is not a good distinguisher.

Cronin CG, Lohan DG, Blake MA, Roche C, McCarthy P, and Murphy JM. Retroperitoneal fibrosis: a review of clinical features and imaging findings. *American Journal of Roentgenology* 2008; 191: 423–431.

39. A. Repeat scan in 4 weeks.

There are a number of important points in this question. Firstly, the date from biopsy must be known to avoid misinterpreting haemorrhage as disease on MRI. Fortunately the urologists have provided you with the salient information necessary to estimate disease stage from the Partin's tables. Whilst these are clinical features, they are essential to know when interpreting MRI. The features described indicate a <1% risk of this patient having extracapsular disease. In combination with the unknown date of the biopsy, it would be prudent to exclude the possibility that this low signal in the seminal vesicles is not haemorrhage by repeating the scan. If this does represent disease invasion of the seminal vesicles, then it would indicate T3b disease.

Partin A, Kattan M, Subong E, Walsh P, Wojno K, Oesterling J et al. Combination of prostate-specific antigen, clinical stage, and Gleason score to predict pathological stage of localised prostate cancer. A multi-institutional update. *Journal of the American Medical Association* 1997; 277: 1445–1451.

40. A. Krukenberg tumours.

The history points towards a GI source, namely gastric carcinoma. Approximately 5–15% of ovarian tumours are metastatic lesions. They are bilateral in 75% of cases. They are often asymptomatic and may present before the primary tumour. They should be considered, along with serous epithelial tumours of the ovary, when bilateral complex ovarian masses are demonstrated. Krukenberg tumours represent ovarian metastases that contain mucin-secreting 'signet-ring' cells from colonic or gastric neoplasms. Other primary neoplasms that less commonly metastasize to the ovary are breast, lung, and the contra-lateral ovary (not strictly Krukenberg tumours due to the cell types). Imaging findings in metastatic lesions are non-specific, consisting of predominately solid components or a mixture of cystic and solid areas. In Krukenberg tumours, there are distinctive findings, including solid components secondary to stromal reaction that are low T2WI and high T1W signal.

A Sertoli–Leydig tumour is a sex cord-stromal tumour that occurs in young women (less than 30 years old). It manifests as a well-defined, enhancing solid mass with intra-tumoral cysts. They constitute 0.5% of ovarian tumours. They are rarely bilateral.

Dysgerminomas are rare ovarian tumours that occur predominantly in young women. Serum β-HCG is increased in 5%. Calcification may be present in a speckled pattern. Characteristic imaging findings include multilobulated solid masses with prominent fibrovascular septa. They are rarely if ever bilateral.

Fibromas are benign solid tumours of the ovary, which are of low signal on T1W and very low signal on T2W sequences. They can be associated with ascites and pleural effusions (Meigs syndrome), and dense calcifications are often seen. Together with fibrothecomas they form a spectrum of benign tumours.

Endodermal sinus tumour, also known as yolk sac tumour, is a rare malignant ovarian tumour that usually occurs in the second decade of life. These tumours manifest as a large, complex pelvic mass that extends into the abdomen and contains both solid and cystic components. They are rarely bilateral. They grow rapidly and have a poor prognosis. Affected patients have an elevated serum alpha feta protein.

Hamm B and Forstner R (eds). *MRI and CT of the Female Pelvis*, Springer, 2007, p. 259.
Jung SE, Lee JM, Rha SE, Byun JY, Jung JI, and Hahn ST. CT and MR imaging of ovarian tumors with emphasis on differential diagnosis. *RadioGraphics* 2002; 22: 1305–1325.

41. C. A relative percentage washout (RPW) of 60%.

Findings consistent with an adrenal adenoma are: a pre-contrast attenuation of 10 HU or less, an absolute percentage washout (APW) of 60% or greater, or an RPW of 40% or greater.

The percentage washout is calculated by comparing the attenuation value at 15 minutes post contrast (delayed H), to the value in the portal venous phase (enhanced H), and in the case of APW, the pre-contrast value.

RPW = 100 × (enhanced H – delayed H)/enhanced H

APW = 100 × (enhanced H – delayed H)/(enhanced H – pre-contrast H)

In practice, an unenhanced scan is not usually performed and thus only the RPW is calculated.

Adrenal cortical carcinomas usually have an RPW of less than 40% although exceptions have been reported. Their large size (usually greater than 6 cm), heterogeneity pre-contrast (necrosis), and heterogeneous enhancement are more reliable indicators of the diagnosis. Phaeochromocytomas and hypervascular metastases may mimic adenomas, but most metastases show RPW < 40% and APW < 60%.

Johnson PT, Horton KM, and Fishman EK. Adrenal mass imaging with multidetector CT: pathologic conditions, pearls, and pitfalls. *RadioGraphics* 2009; 29: 1333–1351.

42. A. Coagulation necrosis.

HIFU is a non-invasive method to treat solid tumours or haemorrhage. As HIFU is essentially ultrasound, it requires an acoustic window to transmit ultrasound energy and is subject to similar artefact.

The principle effect of HIFU is heat generation from absorption of acoustic energy. This causes coagulation necrosis within seconds. Hyperthermia also induces apoptosis, which can be an important delayed effect in tissue exposed to lower energy HIFU. This mechanism is also a potential limitation of HIFU as adjacent tissue may be at risk.

Mechanical effects such as cavitation and microstreaming are also seen with the use of higher ultrasound intensity.

Dubinsky TJ, Cuevas C, Dighe MK, Kolokythas O, and Hwang JH. High-intensity focused ultrasound: current potential and oncologic applications. *American Journal of Roentgenology* 2008; 190: 191–199.

43. B. Architectural distortion.

ILC is the second most common form of invasive breast cancer, after ductal carcinoma. It exhibits the same mammographic features as invasive ductal carcinoma, although architectural distortion is the most common mammographic finding. Due to the pattern of small cells growing around ducts ('Indian files'), mammographic findings are subtle and thus ILC is the most frequently missed breast cancer. Prognosis is generally poor due to late diagnosis.

Dahnert W. *Radiology Review Manual*, 6th edn, Lippincott Williams & Wilkins, 2007, p. 558.

44. D. Double decidual sac sign.

All the other answers are findings in the uterus that may be associated with ectopic pregnancy. In normal pregnancies, TVUS can demonstrate an intradecidual sign approximately 4.5 weeks after the last menstrual period. The intradecidual sign is a small collection of fluid that is eccentrically located within the endometrium and is surrounded by a hyperechoic ring. At approximately 5 weeks, the double decidual sac sign can be visualized. This consists of two concentric hyperechoic rings that surround an anechoic gestational sac in a normal intrauterine pregnancy. The secondary yolk sac may be identified at TVUS at approximately 5.5 weeks. Embryonic cardiac activity should also be visualized at TVUS at approximately 5–6 weeks, when the gestational sac measures at least 18 mm or when the embryonic pole measures at least 5 mm.

A pseudogestational sac is a thick decidual reaction surrounding intrauterine fluid and is seen in approximately 10% of ectopic pregnancies. A trilaminar endometrium is formed during the late proliferative phase of the menstrual cycle. When an abnormal pregnancy is suspected on the basis of laboratory results, the absence of a true gestational sac in the presence of a trilaminar endometrium is highly suggestive of ectopic pregnancy. Thin-walled decidual cysts are seen at the junction of endometrium and myometrium, and may be seen in both normal and abnormal pregnancies. The thin wall differentiates it from a true gestational sac.

Lin EP, Bhatt S, and Dogra V. Diagnostic clues to ectopic pregnancy. *RadioGraphics* 2008; 28: 1661–1671.

45. E. All of them.

MRI is not a primary investigation in the diagnosis of prostate cancer but it is used in staging known disease. Occasionally, in a patient with a high risk of prostate carcinoma, as in this case, when the urologists have repeatedly failed biopsies, MRI can be used to help guide biopsy. In this setting MRS can also be used to increase confidence in the diagnosis. As with all prostate imaging for cancer, the results are more reliable in the peripheral zone due to the variability of appearances in the transitional zone. Choline is elevated in prostate cancer, and is thought to reflect increased cell membrane turnover. Creatine, also detected on MRS, is unchanged. Polyamine is reduced. Citrate, which is stored in normal prostatic cells, is reduced, presumably because of reduced normal function within cancerous cells. The (creatine + choline)/citrate ratio has been used to help discriminate prostate cancer from normal prostate. The role of MRS in the transitional zone is unclear.

Fuchsjager M, Shukla-Dave A, Akin O, Barentsz J, and Hricak H. Prostate cancer imaging. *Acta Radiologica* 2008; 49(1): 107–120.

46. A. Hypovolaemic shock.

Marked adrenal enhancement may be the only sign of significant hypovolaemic shock. This is thought to be due to hyperperfusion of the adrenal glands because of their crucial role in this clinical situation. Other signs that may accompany this sign, the 'hypoperfusion complex' described in shock due to trauma, are collapsed IVC, small hypodense spleen, small aorta and mesenteric arteries, shock nephogram (lack of renal contrast excretion), intense pancreatic enhancement, dilatation of fluid-filled intestine with thickening of folds, and increased enhancement of the wall. However, in cases of hypovolaemic shock due to sepsis, where there has been rapid fluid replacement, the IVC and aorta may be of normal calibre and persisting marked adrenal enhancement has been described as the only abnormality.

Phaeochromocytomas are bilateral in only approximately 10% and this would be even less likely in the presence of another neoplasm. Hypervascular metastases are uncommon in colonic carcinoma. Adrenal hyperplasia may occur as a response to stress but the adrenals would enhance normally. In tuberculous adrenalitis, the adrenal glands show areas of necrosis and sometimes calcification, with possible rim enhancement. In all four of these alternative options the adrenal glands would be enlarged.

Cheung SCW, Lee R, Tung HKS, and Chan FL. Persistent adrenal enhancement may be the earliest CT sign of significant hypovolaemic shock. *Clinical Radiology* 2003; 58: 315–318.
Dahnert W. *Radiology Review Manual*, 5th edn, Lippincott Williams & Wilkins, 2003, p. 872.
Wang YX, Chen CR, He GX, and Tang AR. CT findings of adrenal glands in patients with tuberculous Addison's disease. *Journal Belge de Radiologie* 1998; 81: 226–228.

47. D. Ovarian dysfunction.

Ovarian dysfunction is a known complication of fibroid embolization. The exact mechanism is not known, but inadvertent embolization of the ovaries via a uterine–ovarian anastomosis has been suggested. There is a higher prevalence of uterine–ovarian anastomosis in women over 45 years of age and that puts them at increased risk.

Kitamura Y, Ascher S, Cooper C, Allison SJ, Jha RC, Flick PA et al. Imaging manifestations of complications associated with uterine artery embolization. *RadioGraphics* 2005; 25: S119–S132.

48. B. Ultrasound guided needle aspiration.

Breast abscess is a potential complication of mastitis that may occur during breast-feeding, particularly in primiparous women. *Staphylococcus aureus* is the most common causative organism. Treatment of mastitis usually consists of breast-emptying procedures and antibiotics. Abscesses are difficult to detect clinically and so the patient should be investigated via ultrasound if mastitis does not promptly respond to appropriate therapy. Ultrasound-guided needle aspiration is a suitable method of treatment for abscesses less than 3 cm in maximum diameter. Continuing breast-feeding is not felt to be problematic.

Ulitzsch D, Nyman MKG, and Carlson RA. Breast abscess in lactating women: US-guided treatment. *Radiology* 2004; 232: 904–909.

49. E. 60 pre-contrast attenuation, 70 post-contrast attenuation.

The attenuation of the normal renal parenchyma typically ranges from 30 to 40 HU. That of hyperattenuating renal masses usually is at least 40 HU but no higher than 90 HU on CT without intravenous contrast. Benign cysts are overwhelmingly the most common type of hyperattenuating renal mass and are also known as hyperdense renal cysts. They are usually cysts containing haemorrhage or proteinaceous material. Hyperattenuating cysts should not enhance and therefore cannot be diagnosed with confidence by using unenhanced CT alone. A proper CT examination includes scanning both before and after the administration of intravenous contrast material. Masses that increase in attenuation by 10 HU or less are considered non-enhancing. Masses that increase in attenuation by more than 10 HU are considered enhancing. However, because the standard deviation of attenuation measurements may be more than 10 HU, an attenuation difference of 20 HU or more is a more specific criterion of enhancement.

Silverman SG, Mortele KJ, Tuncali K, Jinzaki M, and Cibas ES. Hyperattenuating renal masses: etiologies, pathogenesis, and imaging evaluation. *RadioGraphics* 2007; 27: 1131–1143.

50. C. Perinephric and periureteric stranding.

Whilst this observation is sensitive and specific for detecting calculi, it does not have a bearing on stone outcome or urgency of treatment. The site is of value because if the stone impacts, it dictates the therapeutic approach. The size of the calculus can be used to assess the likelihood of spontaneous passage, with calculi over 5 mm more likely to cause obstruction. The density of the calculus has been found to predict the success of extracorporeal shock wave lithotripsy (ESWL). The presence of anatomical variations is also of interest to the urologists in treatment planning, if this becomes necessary.

Sandhu C, Anson K, and Patel U. Urinary tract stone – Part 1: Role of radiological imaging in diagnosis and treatment planning. *Clinical Radiology* 2003; 58: 415–421.

51. C. Uterine leiomyomas.

Also known as uterine fibroids, these are very common. They are usually of low signal on T2WI and intermediate signal on T1WI. Benign metastasizing leiomyoma is an unusual variant, with tumours in the lungs, lymph nodes, or peritoneal nodules, not uncommonly from a benign uterine fibroid, which has been removed many years earlier. Malignant transformation to leiomyosarcoma is very rare and it is thought the latter may arise de novo even in the presence of leiomyomas.

Endometrial sarcoma might produce peritoneal metastases, but would be expected to show a large heterogenous mass with indistinct or irregular borders arising from the endometrial canal.

Endometriosis and adenomyosis are diseases of the reproductive years. Metastases to the uterus are rare and if present represent advanced malignancy. There is usually diffuse enlargement of the myometrium, which can be of low or high signal.

Martin D, Brown M, and Semelka R. *Primer on MR Imaging of the Abdomen and Pelvis*, Wiley, 2005, 437–439.
Szklaruk J, Tamm EP, Choi H, and Varavithya V. MR imaging of common and uncommon large pelvic masses. *RadioGraphics* 2003; 23: 403–424.

52. C. Vesico-ureteric reflux.

The abnormality described on ultrasound is multicystic dysplastic kidney (MCDK). It is the most common form of cystic disease in infants and the second most common cause of an abdominal mass in a neonate (after hydronephrosis). Obstruction/atresia of the ureter during the developmental stage is thought to be the etiology.

Bilateral MCDK is uncommon, but associated anomalies of the contra-lateral kidney are seen in up to 50% of cases. Vesico-ureteric reflux (30–40%) is the most common associated anomaly, followed by pelvi-ureteric junction obstruction (10–20%).

Mercado-Deane M-G, Beeson JE, and John SD. US of renal insufficiency in neonates. *RadioGraphics* 2002; 22: 1429–1438.
Dahnert W. Multicystic dysplastic kidney, in *Radiology Review Manual*, 6th edn, Lippincott Williams & Wilkins, 2007, pp. 937–938.

53. C. Deep laceration to the collecting system.

Renal injuries are classified into five grades of severity by the American Association for the Surgery of Trauma (AAST), with approximately 80% classified as grade 1 (Table 4.1). Most significant injuries manifest as haematuria and no significant urinary tract injury occurs in the absence of gross haematuria and shock. In addition, most significant renal trauma is associated with additional visceral injury.

Table 4.1 AAST grading of renal trauma

Grade	Injury
1	Parenchymal contusion Isolated subcapsular haematoma
2	Superficial cortical laceration <1 cm Non-expanding perirenal haematoma
3	Laceration >1 cm without extension to collecting system
4	Deep laceration to collecting system Segmental infarctions without associated lacerations Injury to main renal artery without devascularization
5	Shattered kidney Ureteropelvic junction avulsion Devascularization to renal pedicle

Alonso RC, Nacenta SB, Martinez PD, Guerrero AS, and Fuentes CG. Kidney in danger: CT findings of blunt and penetrating renal trauma. *RadioGraphics* 2009; 29: 2033–2053.

54. C. Repeat CT in 3–6 months.

Solid masses smaller than 1 cm are challenging. Firstly, there is a reasonable chance that a very small solid mass is benign. Secondly, it is often difficult to characterize a mass smaller than 1 cm as solid and enhancing, despite a meticulous technique using state-of-the-art CT and MR imaging. Thirdly, these masses are often too small to biopsy, therefore when encountering a mass that is believed to be solid and is less than 1 cm in size, it is reasonable to observe them with an initial examination with CT or MR at 3–6 months followed by yearly examinations. A full work-up could ensue when the mass reaches 1 cm in size.

Silverman SG, Israel GM, Herts BR, and Richie JP. Management of the incidental renal mass. *Radiology* 2008; 249: 16–31.

55. B. Bladder calcification.

Whilst this can be seen in TB, it is more typically associated with schistosomiasis. TB usually causes scarring and a reduced capacity bladder. Renal calcification is typical. The areas of increased attenuation within the calyceal system represent areas of coalescing caseating granulomas, and may have associated calcification. Scarring can also cause stenosis of calyces, causing focal obstruction. Occasionally a small calcified kidney is found, evidence of autonephrectomy. Passage of the infection via the urine into the ureters causes focal stenoses, which can coalesce to cause a long stricture, or give a beaded or corkscrew appearance to the ureter. Whilst renal TB results from spread from a primary pulmonary infection, the CXR is only abnormal in 25–50% of cases and is therefore not helpful.

Gibson M, Puckett M, and Shelly M. Renal tuberculosis. *RadioGraphics* 2004; 24: 251–256.

56. B. Multiple small peripheral rounded high T2WI signal areas with hypointense central stroma in both ovaries.

The clinical features suggest polycystic ovarian syndrome (PCOS). The diagnosis is based on hormonal imbalance and patients often show an abnormality in the ratio of luteinizing hormone to follicle stimulating hormone. The MRI findings are those described, with multiple small peripheral cysts with low signal central stroma. MRI is not specific or sensitive, and 25% of patients with PCOS can have normal appearing ovaries. Multiple small, T2WI hyperintense cysts have been seen in patients with anovulation, medication-stimulated ovulation, or vaginal agenesis.

The other descriptions are associated with infertility, but not particularly hirsutism or obesity. Option A describes bilateral hydrosalpinx. Option D describes a unicornuate uterus, which is associated with the poorest foetal survival among all uterine anomalies. Option E describes adenomyosis and using a junctional zone thickness of 12 mm or above optimizes the accuracy of MRI for this diagnosis.

Imaoka I, Wada A, Matsuo M, Yoshida M, Kitagaki H, and Sugimura K. MR imaging of disorders associated with female infertility: use in diagnosis, treatment, and management. *RadioGraphics* 2003; 23: 1401–1421.

57. B. Wilms tumour.

Sporadic aniridia is associated with nephroblastomatosis (multiple nephrogenic rests) and an increased risk of Wilms tumour. At CT, the nephrogenic rests appear as homogenous, hypodense nodules/peripheral rind, with little or no enhancement compared to the compressed normal cortical tissue.

Any new, enlarging, or heterogenous mass in the setting of nephroblastomatosis indicates the development of a Wilms tumour.

Sethi AT, Das Narla L, Fitch SJ, and Frable WJ. Wilms tumor in the setting of bilateral nephroblastomatosis. *RadioGraphics* 2010; 30: 1421–1425.

58. E. Urine leak.

Lacerations generally contain clotted blood and therefore do not enhance on scans obtained with intravenous contrast. Contrast enhancement during the pyelographic phase of the CT examination indicates the presence of a urine leak. A delayed scan of 10–15 minutes may show the extent of the urinary extravasation. Intense enhancement within a laceration during the early phase indicates active haemorrhage. Focal areas of infarction do not enhance (unlike contusions). The cortical rim nephrogram is a sign of a devascularized kidney, which occurs due to laceration of the main renal artery.

Harris AC, Zwirewich CV, Lyburn, ID, Torreggiani WC, and Marchinkow LO. CT Findings in blunt renal trauma. *RadioGraphics* 2001; 21: S201–S214.

59. C. Multiple thin non-enhancing septa.

The criteria for a Bosniak IIF cyst are multiple hairline-thin septa with or without perceived (not measurable) enhancement, minimal smooth thickening of wall or septa that may show perceived (not measurable) enhancement, calcification may be thick and nodular but no measurable enhancement present, no enhancing soft-tissue components, and intrarenal non-enhancing high-attenuation renal mass (> 3cm). The follow-up is CT or MRI at 6 months, 1 year, and then yearly up to 5 years.

The criteria for a Bosniak II cyst that does not require follow-up include few hairline-thin septa with or without perceived (not measurable) enhancement, fine calcification or a short segment of slightly thickened calcification in the wall or septa, homogeneously high-attenuating masses (<3 cm) that are sharply marginated and do not enhance.

Thickened irregular or smooth walls or septa, with measurable enhancement, are features of a Bosniak III cyst and these are surgical lesions unless there are co-morbidities or limited life expectancy, when they may be observed.

Silverman SG, Israel GM, Herts BR, and Richie JP. Management of the incidental renal mass. *Radiology* 2008; 249: 16–31.

60. B. HIV-positive patient on antiretroviral therapy.

Whilst CT KUB has 95–99% sensitivity for renal calculi, occasionally calculi due to antiretroviral therapy can be undetectable even to CT. Proteus is associated with formation of staghorn calculi and chronic dehydration with calcium oxalate calculi, both of which are radio-opaque. Xanthine calculi and urate calculi are classically not detectable on plain film KUB, but are usually visible on CT KUB.

Sandhu C, Anson K, and Patel U. Urinary tract stone – Part 1: Role of radiological imaging in diagnosis and treatment planning. *Clinical Radiology* 2003; 58: 415–421.

61. B. Tamoxifen therapy.

The normal endometrial stripe is of high T2WI signal and measures 3–6 mm in diameter in the follicular phase and 5–13 mm in the secretory phase. The description of the endometrium in this case is consistent with endometrial hyperplasia, but there is in addition myometrial enlargement. An enlarged uterus is frequently encountered in the presence of endogenous or exogenous hormonal abnormalities. In these cases the uterus usually has normal zonal anatomy, although the signal intensity of the endometrium and myometrium is abnormally increased. However, with tamoxifen, the uterus can display marked zonal anatomy distortion. It is a weak oestrogen agonist and can result in endometrial hyperplasia, polyps, and carcinoma. The findings of multiple cysts or lattice-like enhancement of the endometrium post contrast are encountered frequently in relation to tamoxifen therapy and favour a benign diagnosis.

IUCDs are widely used for contraception. A study has found that the IUCD-bearing uterus is enlarged. IUCD placement most likely results in myometrial hypertrophy. The associated findings are symmetrical globular enlargement of the uterine corpus, cervical elongation and enlargement, and diffuse or localized myometrial thickening. The IUCD will usually be seen as a band of low signal intensity within the endometrium.

The uterus is rarely the primary site for lymphoma, but when it does occur, the most common manifestation is diffuse symmetrical uterine enlargement with relatively high signal on T2WI and epithelial preservation: the endometrium is usually normal. The myometrium will also lack its standard zonal appearance. There will almost always be associated lymphadenopathy.

Endometrial stromal sarcoma invariably exhibits myometrial involvement. Imaging will typically show a large mass that replaces the endometrial cavity and infiltrates the myometrium: at the very least the endometrial-myometrial border will be obscured. Myometrial involvement is commonly so extensive that a myometrial component predominates. Bands of low signal may be present within the area of myometrial invasion and these correspond to preserved bundles of myometrium at histologic examination. Extension along the vessels, fallopian tubes, or ligaments is another characteristic of the tumour.

Pelvic congestion syndrome involves symptoms, including chronic pelvic pain, that are associated with dilated ovarian veins and pelvic varices resulting from left renal vein reflux. This results in a thickened myometrium containing multiple large signal voids, the latter corresponding to engorged arcuate vessels. Additional findings include varicose veins around the uterus and ovaries with retrograde filling of ovarian veins.

Kido A, Togashi K, Koyama T, Toshihide Y, Fujiwara T, and Fujii S. Diffusely enlarged uterus: evaluation with MR imaging. *RadioGraphics* 2003; 23: 1423–1439.

62. C. Ablation zone unchanged in size over time.

Following ablation the treatment zone is larger than the original lesion, as a margin of normal tissue is intentionally ablated to prevent recurrence. This should reduce in size/involute over time. If the ablation zone remains the same or increases in size, recurrence should be suspected.

Lack of enhancement is a reliable indicator of successful treatment. It is not uncommon to find peripheral enhancement in the immediate post-treatment period due to reactive hyperaemia. Any nodular or central enhancement indicates incomplete treatment or recurrence.

Allen BC and Remer EM. Percutaneous cryoablation of renal tumors: patient selection, technique, and postprocedural imaging. *RadioGraphics* 2010; 30: 887–900.

63. A. Anterior urethral injury.

Urethral injuries are rarely life-threatening but have significant long-term morbidity. Complications include stricture, incontinence, and impotence. The male urethra extends from the bladder base to the external meatus and is divided into the posterior (prostatic and membranous) and anterior (bulbous and penile) urethra. The anterior and posterior urethra are separated by the urogenital diaphragm. The Goldman classification of urethral injury emphasizes anatomic location (Table 4.2).

Table 4.2 The Goldman classification of urethral injury

Type	Injury description	Urethrographic appearance
I	Stretching of an intact posterior urethra	Intact but stretched urethra
II	Urethral disruption above the urogenital diaphragm, membranous segment intact	Contrast extravasation above the urogenital diaphragm only
III	Disruption of membranous urethra extending to anterior urethra	Contrast extravasation below the urogenital diaphragm possibly extending to the perineum
IV	Bladder neck injury extending into the proximal urethra	Extraperitoneal contrast extravasation, bladder neck disruption
IVa	Bladder base injury simulating type IV	Bladder base disruption, periurethral contrast extravasation
V	Isolated anterior urethral injury	Contrast extravasation below the urogenital diaphragm

Data from Goldman SM, Sandler CM, Corriere JN, and McGuire EJ. Blunt urethral trauma: anatomical mechanical classification. *Journal of Urology* 1997; 157: 85–89.

Ingram MD, Watson SG, Skippage PL, and Patel U. Urethral injuries after pelvic trauma: evaluation with urethrography. *RadioGraphics* 2008; 28: 1631–1643.

64. D. Maintenance of reniform shape.

Advanced TCC of the collecting system in the kidney can cause distortion of the renal architecture, but typically the reniform shape of the kidney is maintained. As RCC arises in the renal cortex, large tumours of this nature typically distort the normal renal outline.

Calcification can rarely occur in both RCCs and TCCs, although perhaps more commonly in RCC. TCC demonstrates calcification in less than 3%, when it is usually diffuse and punctate.

Necrosis can occur in both large RCCs and large TCCs, giving a heterogenous enhancement pattern on CT. Renal vein invasion is a more typical manifestation of RCC and both these tumours may be hypovascular compared to normal renal parenchyma on a nephrographic phase of the CT examination.

Browne RFJ, Meehan CP, Colville J, Power R, and Torregiani WC. Transitional cell carcinoma of the upper urinary tract: spectrum of imaging findings. *RadioGraphics* 2005; 25: 1609–1627.
Anderson EM, Murphy R, Rennie ATM, and Cowan NC. Multidetector computed tomography urography (MDCTU) for diagnosing urothelial malignancy. *Clinical Radiology* 2007; 62: 324–332.

65. C. Chronic non-steroidal anti-inflammatory drug (NSAID) analgesic overuse.

The appearances described are those of renal papillary necrosis. This can be due to a number of causes, most commonly analgesic abuse, but also severe renal infection in diabetics, sickle cell disease, haemophilia, and renal vein thrombosis. The causes of chronic renal disease can be subdivided by the effects noted on the renal parenchyma and the papillary/pelvicalyceal system, and whether these are uni- or bilateral. In bilateral cases such as this, no radiological abnormality suggests possible glomerulonephritis, acute tubular necrosis (ATN), acute cortical necrosis, or pyelonephritis. Generalized infiltration of the renal parenchyma suggests amyloid or malignant infiltration (e.g. lymphoma or leukaemia). Papillary/pelvicalyceal abnormalities, in the presence of normal parenchyma, indicate papillary necrosis, medullary sponge kidney, or renal TB. Papillary calyceal abnormality with focal parenchymal loss indicates reflux nephropathy, TB, or calculus. Both parenchymal loss and papillary calyceal abnormalities indicate obstructive nephropathy or severe reflux nephropathy.

Adam A and Dixon A. *Grainger and Allison's Diagnostic Radiology. A textbook of medical imaging, Vol 1*, 5th edn, Churchill Livingstone, 2008, Ch 39.

66. D. Minimal deviation adenocarcinoma of the cervix.

This is also known as adenoma malignum and, as in this scenario, is often associated with Peutz–Jeghers syndrome (characterized by mucocutaneous pigmentation, multiple hamartomatous polyps of the GI tract, and mucinous tumours of the ovary). Adenoma malignum makes up about 3% of adenocarcinoma of the cervix. Its MRI appearances are as described in the question, but the differential diagnosis includes deep nabothian cysts, florid endocervical hyperplasia, and even well-differentiated adenocarcinoma. It disseminates into the peritoneal cavity even in the early stage of the disease and its response to radiation or chemotherapy is poor.

Cervical squamous carcinoma makes up to 90% of cervical carcinoma. The tumour is of high signal compared to the hypointense cervical stroma, but not cystic as in our vignette. It advances predominantly by direct extension and local spread; haematogenous dissemination is only occasionally seen in the form of hepatic metastases.

Carcinoid tumour of the cervix is a subgroup of small cell carcinoma of the cervix. It cannot be differentiated from squamous cell carcinoma of the cervix on MRI findings.

Malignant melanoma of the female genital tract accounts for 1–5% of all melanomas. It usually occurs in the vaginal mucosa and occasionally involves the cervix. Malignant melanoma arising in the cervix is very rare (only about 30 reported cases). There is usually high signal intensity on T1WI.

The incidence of cervical pregnancy has been increasing, possibly due to the increased number of induced abortions. Reported risk factors include multiparity, prior cervical surgical manipulation, cervical or uterine leiomyomas, atrophic endometrium, and septate uterus. The major symptom is painless vaginal bleeding. At MR it is characterized by a mass with heterogenous signal intensity and a partial or complete dark ring on T2WI sequences. As it contains haematoma, it often consists of some high signal on T1WI.

Okamoto Y, Tanaka YO, Nishida M, Tsunoda H, Yoshikawa H, and Itai Y. MR imaging of the uterine cervix: imaging-pathologic correlation. *RadioGraphics* 2003; 23: 425–445.

67. A. Cervical carcinoma.

This patient has developed lymphangitis carcinomatosis. In 50% of cases the septal thickening is focal or unilateral and this is useful in distinguishing lymphangitis from other causes of septal thickening, such as pulmonary oedema or sarcoidosis. Hilar adenopathy is present in 50% and pleural effusion in 30–50%. The interlobular septal thickening can be smooth (as in pulmonary oedema and alveolar proteinosis) or nodular (also found in sarcoidosis and silicosis).

Lymphangitis carcinomatosis usually occurs secondary to the spread of (adeno-) carcinoma, most commonly bronchogenic, breast, and stomach. The mnemonic **C**ertain **C**ancers **S**pread **B**y **P**lugging **T**he **L**ymphatics (**C**ervix **C**olon **S**tomach **B**reast **P**ancreas **T**hyroid **L**arynx) is useful. Lymphangitis carcinomatosis is occasionally associated with cervical carcinoma and certainly more so than with the other options presented.

Dahnert W. *Radiology Review Manual*, 5th edn, Lippincott Williams & Wilkins, 2003, p. 502.

68. C. Adenomyosis.

This is a condition in which the endometrium extends into the myometrium in either a diffuse or a focal distribution. It generally manifests as pelvic pain or abnormal bleeding. It is more commonly detected on MR imaging as thickening of the junctional zone or on ultrasound as diffuse or focal heterogenous myometrium. On HSG, adenomyosis appears as small diverticula extending from the endometrial cavity into the myometrium.

Salpingitis isthmica nodosa appears as small outpouchings from the isthmic portion of the fallopian tube.

Multiple uterine synechiae (linear filling defects in the uterine cavity) associated with infertility is known as Asherman syndrome.

Polyps would appear as filling defects on HSG.

Simpson Jr WL, Beitia LG, and Mester J. Hysterosalpingography: a reemerging study. *RadioGraphics* 2006; 26: 419–431.

69. A. Uterus didelphys.

This is caused by complete failure of fusion of the paramesonephric ducts, resulting in a completely duplicated system (two uterine cavities and two cervices) with no communication between the two cavities. It is associated with complete or partial vaginal septum in 75% of cases, which can result in obstruction and haematometrocolpos. Ipsilateral renal agenesis is associated with a vaginal septum.

Bicornuate uterus is caused by partial fusion of the paramesonephric ducts. Bicornuate bicollis uterus demonstrates a septum extending from the fundus to the external os, but some degree of communication remains between the two horns.

Septate uterus is the most common mullerian/paramesonephric duct anomaly. It is also the most common anomaly associated with infertility and recurrent miscarriage. A complete or partial septum divides the uterine cavity, but there is no fundal cleft.

Arcuate uterus is associated with a small indentation in the fundal endometrial canal but the external contour is normal. It has no pathological consequence and is considered by some to be a normal variant.

Junqueira BLP, Allen LM, Spitzer RF, Lucco KL, Babyn PS, and Doria AS. Mullerian duct anomalies and mimics in children and adolescents: correlative intraoperative assessment with clinical imaging. *RadioGraphics* 2009; 29: 1085–1103.

70. C. Extraperitoneal rupture.

Over 70% of patients with traumatic bladder injury have a coexisting pelvic fracture. CT cystography is considered to be as accurate as conventional cystography. Extraperitoneal rupture accounts for 80% of all cases of traumatic bladder injury. It occurs as a result of shearing forces or penetrating injury from bony fragments at the base of the bladder. Contrast can also track down into the scrotum or thigh. Intraperitoneal rupture (15% of cases) follows a direct blow to a distended bladder, with the tear involving the bladder dome. Contrast will be seen to outline small bowel loops. Combined injuries occur in 5%. Interstitial injuries are rare and are detected by contrast dissecting into the bladder wall. Imaging is frequently normal in the setting of bladder contusion.

Bent C, Lyngkaran T, Power N, Matson M, Hajdinjak T, Buchholz N et al. Urological injuries following trauma. *Clinical Radiology* 2008; 63: 1361–1371.

71. E. Focus of increased radionuclide activity within the lower pole of the right lobe of thyroid on delayed images only.

Solitary parathyroid adenoma accounts for 85% of cases of primary hyperparathyroidism, with parathyroid hyperplasia (10%), multiple adenomas (4%), and carcinoma (1%) making up the remainder. When ^{99m}Tc MIBI is used for parathyroid imaging, immediate and delayed images of the neck and mediastinum are performed. Parathyroid adenomas may or may not be visualized on initial imaging, but they retain radiopharmaceutical on delayed (1–2 hours) images, whereas the normal thyroid washes out.

Brant WE and Helms CA. *Fundamentals of Diagnostic Radiology*, 3rd edn, Lippincott Williams & Wilkins, 2007, pp. 1412–1414.

72. A. Localized cystic renal disease.

This is an uncommon, non-familial, and non-progressive disorder of the kidney characterized by the replacement of all or localized areas of a kidney by multiple variably sized cysts. These cysts form clusters that are separated by thin areas of normal renal parenchyma. The aggregated cysts in localized cystic disease can frequently appear like a multi-septate mass, but they do not form a distinct encapsulated mass and do not show mural irregularities, which are characteristics of cystic neoplasms.

Multilocular cystic nephroma in adults is much more common in females (female:male 9:1) and manifests as a multi-loculated cystic lesion with hair-like septa and minimal mural enhancement. It is distinguished from localized cystic disease by the presence of a capsule. Typically extension into the central renal sinus is found and multilocular cystic nephroma is often classified on imaging as Bosniak III lesions.

Lymphangioma of the kidney is a rare benign cystic tumour that most often arises from the peripelvic region or renal sinus. It may more rarely arise from the lymphatics of the capsule or cortex. In the diffuse form of lymphangiomatosis, the cystic changes occur diffusely in the renal sinus or perinephric region, with a relatively normal appearing renal parenchyma. Clear cell RCC presents as a solid or a cystic lesion, the cystic variant accounting for 4–15% of all RCCs. These lesions typically have nodular or septal enhancement, distinguishing them from benign cystic renal lesions.

Multicystic dysplastic kidney is a congenital maldevelopment in which the kidney is completely replaced by cysts with no normal renal parenchyma remaining.

Feire M and Remer EM. Clinical and radiological features of cystic renal masses. *American Journal of Roentgenology* 2009; 192: 1367–1372.

73. D. Refer for immediate venous intervention.

There are a number of complications to be aware of in the immediate post-transplant period. The most efficient and cost-effective method of surveillance for these is ultrasound. Acute rejection and acute tubular necrosis (ATN) both occur early in the post-transplant phase and can be difficult to differentiate. Both can cause elevation of pulsatility index (PI) (normal <1.5) and resistive index (RI) (normal <0.7), although these tend to be higher with rejection. ATN is more common with cadaveric transplants. It usually resolves within a matter of days or weeks, but ultimately biopsy can be necessary to reliably differentiate these processes. This patient probably had a degree of ATN initially. Arterial occlusion is uncommon and is evident by reduced/absent arterial flow in the main artery as well as in the interlobar arteries, which can demonstrate loss of flow with any cause of severe oedema (e.g. renal vein thrombosis or acute rejection). Renal vein thrombosis causes pain and anuria. It is associated with early treatment with cyclosporine and steroids. It also causes a rise in the RI and PI. The key feature to notice is the persistent flow in the main renal artery, reducing the likelihood of renal arterial thrombosis. There is also a tubular structure noted in the hilum, which is what a thrombosed renal vein looks like, and reversal of diastolic flow on arterial traces.

Baxter G. Ultrasound of renal transplantation. *Clinical Radiology* 2001; 56(10): 802–818.
Sandhu C and Patel U. Renal transplantation dysfunction: the role of interventional radiology. *Clinical Radiology* 2002; 57(9): 772–783.

74. B. PI < 1.5, RI < 0.7, prominence of renal pyramids.

PI < 1.5 or RI < 0.7 can be regarded as normal, whilst a PI > 1.8 or RI = 0.9 should be regarded as abnormal. Although both ATN and acute rejection cause the PI and RI to rise, the likelihood of acute rejection is greater with higher values. Complete absence of diastolic flow, or flow reversal, is due to acute rejection in the majority of cases.

Morphologically, the transplant kidney is very similar to the native and many of the subtle differences are attributed to the improved resolution of the former. There is a well-defined renal parenchyma peripherally, with a highly reflective echogenic sinus centrally. In distinction to the native kidney, the renal pyramids are more commonly visualized within the transplant, being hypoechoic, relative to the parenchyma itself.

Loss of cortico-medullary differentiation is pathological and is a B mode finding that can be associated with acute rejection.

Baxter GM. Pictorial review: ultrasound of renal transplantation. *Clinical Radiology* 2001; 56: 802–818.

75. B. Endometriotic cyst.

Also known as a chocolate cyst, the methaemoglobin within the lesion causes T1 shortening, resulting in increased signal on the T1WI sequence. This high signal remains and becomes more conspicuous on the T1WI with fat saturation sequence.

Endometriosis is characterized by the presence of tissue resembling endometrium outside the uterus. The ovaries are the most commonly involved site, and endometriotic cysts usually have a thick fibrotic wall with chocolate-coloured hemorrhagic material. An endometriotic cyst may be high or low signal on T2WI sequences. Chronic cyclical haemorrhage and increased viscosity of the cyst material will produce T2 shortening, leading to the low signal, or 'T2 shading'. The patient usually presents with cyclical pain. The cysts have a propensity for multicentric growth and are often associated with fibrous adhesions. These latter features increase the MR sensitivity. Small peritoneal implants of endometriosis may be identified elsewhere and their conspicuity is increased by the use of fat saturation techniques.

Endometroid and clear cell carcinoma of the ovary are malignancies associated with endometriosis and these represent 17.5 and 7.4% of ovarian carcinomas, respectively. Chocolate cysts with multiple locules, mural foci, or nodules within the cyst are suspicious for malignancy and contrast should be administered if this appearance is seen.

The findings in this question are not consistent with a follicular cyst, which would show low T1WI and high T2WI signal.

Brenner tumours show low T2WI signal due to their abundant fibrous content and calcification, but also low T1WI signal. Fibrothecomas show intermediate T1WI signal and usually low (although sometimes it can be mixed high and low) T2WI signal. They sometimes show associated uterine enlargement, as they may be oestrogenic.

Izumi I, Wada A, Kaji Y, Hayashi T, Hayashi M, Matsuo M et al. Developing an MR imaging strategy for diagnosis of ovarian masses. *RadioGraphics* 2006; 26: 1431–1448.

chapter 5 PAEDIATRICS

QUESTIONS

1. An HRCT chest is carried out on a 3-year-old girl. This child has a history of mild wheeze and tachypnoea, which has developed in the last few months. Standard treatment with bronchodilators and inhaled steroid for presumed asthma has been unsuccessful. The CXR is abnormal, showing mild increased airspace density. The HRCT shows a bilateral pattern of ground-glass change. The interlobular septa are markedly thickened, giving a 'crazy paving' pattern. What is the most likely diagnosis?

A. *Pneumocystis jirovecii* pneumonia.
B. Lymphocytic interstitial pneumonitis.
C. Alveolar proteinosis.
D. Childhood idiopathic pulmonary haemosiderosis.
E. Childhood sarcoidosis.

2. A baby boy is born prematurely at 30 weeks gestation. Cranial ultrasound demonstrates bilateral multiseptate cystic lesions within the frontal lobe white matter with associated ex vacuo dilatation of the ventricles. Which of the following is the most likely diagnosis?

A. Periventricular leucomalacia.
B. Porencephaly.
C. Supratentorial arachnoid cysts.
D. Vein of Galen malformation.
E. Subependymal cysts.

3. A 10-year-old girl presents with pain in the left hip which she first noticed when playing sports at school. Apart from pain on movement and several prominent café-au-lait spots, there is nothing else to find on examination. The patient is apyrexic and her WCC and CRP are normal. A plain film of the pelvis reveals a lucent lesion in the proximal femoral metaphysis. The margins of the lesion are well defined and the metaphysis is expanded with adjacent cortical thinning. The lesion extends as far as, but does not involve, the physis. There is GGO in the centre of the lesion. There is no periosteal reaction. What is the most likely diagnosis?

A. Osteomyelitis.
B. Chondroblastoma.
C. Aneurysmal bone cyst.
D. GCT.
E. Fibrous dysplasia.

4. **A 2-day-old term neonate with an antenatal history of enlarged kidneys undergoes ultrasound of the renal tracts, which reveals bilateral enlarged and diffusely echogenic kidneys, with loss of cortico-medullary differentiation. Further assessment with a high-resolution linear probe reveals multiple small radially oriented cysts. Which of the following statements regarding this condition is false?**
   - A. It is associated with congenital hepatic fibrosis.
   - B. The severities of renal and hepatic involvement are inversely proportional to each other.
   - C. Severe renal compromise is the immediate cause of death in the perinatal group.
   - D. Potter facies may be found in severely affected neonates.
   - E. It is associated with clubfoot deformity.

5. **A 4-month-old infant presents with shortness of breath. A CXR is performed and this shows evidence of cardiac failure. The liver is noted to be enlarged and slightly irregular on examination. Ultrasound demonstrates multiple mixed echogenicity masses. A subsequent dynamic contrast-enhanced CT shows multiple lesions that show progressive centripetal enhancement. What is the most likely diagnosis?**
   - A. Hepatoblastoma.
   - B. Multifocal hepatoma.
   - C. Mesenchymal hamartoma.
   - D. Metastases.
   - E. Infantile haemangioendothelioma.

6. **You are attending a paediatric cardiac MRI list. The next patient is a 4-year-old girl who has undergone previous surgical correction of tetralogy of Fallot. Which of the following is the part of the report of most interest to the referring clinical team?**
   - A. Pulmonary valve function.
   - B. Left ventricular function.
   - C. Presence of thrombus in the graft between IVC and pulmonary artery.
   - D. Situs position.
   - E. Ventricular septum.

7. **A 2-year-old girl is investigated for slow motor development via MRI. Which of the following radiological features would suggest a diagnosis of Dandy–Walker malformation, as opposed to Dandy–Walker variant?**
   - A. Cerebellar dysgenesis.
   - B. Enlargement of the posterior fossa.
   - C. Agenesis of the corpus callosum.
   - D. Holoprosencephaly.
   - E. Cystic dilatation of the fourth ventricle.

8. A 10-year-old boy presents with pain in his left leg following a minor fall whilst playing football. A plain film shows a mixed lytic/sclerotic lesion in the distal femoral metaphysis extending across the physis to involve the epiphysis. The lesion appears centred in the medulla and is causing cortical destruction. There is periosteal reaction and a Codman's triangle. No significant soft tissue component is visible. What advice do you give as a radiologist?

A. Arrange urgent skeletal survey and CT brain.
B. Advise treatment with antibiotics and arrange outpatient MRI.
C. Arrange CT guided bone biopsy and MIBG scan.
D. Arrange MRI, CT chest, and isotope bone scan.
E. Perform CT chest, abdomen, and pelvis to look for a primary neoplasm elsewhere.

9. A 7-year-old girl presents with a history of continuous dribbling incontinence. On imaging she is found to have bilateral duplex kidney, complete ureteral duplication, and ectopic ureter. Which of the following statements regarding ectopic ureters and ureteral duplication is true?

A. Ectopic insertion is more commonly associated with solitary ureter than complete ureteral duplication.
B. Urinary incontinence with ectopic ureter is more common in boys.
C. In complete ureteral duplication, the ureter of the upper pole moiety inserts into the bladder superior to the ureter of lower pole moiety.
D. The upper moiety ureter is associated with ureterocele whereas the lower moiety ureter is associated with vesicoureteric reflux.
E. The obstructed lower moiety may not be visualized on IVU.

10. A 14-year-old girl has an episode of pancreatitis. An MRCP examination is subsequently performed to assess for any biliary disease or pancreatic duct anomaly. You notice failure of fusion of the ventral and dorsal ducts, and suspect pancreas divisum. What other appropriate finding do you notice on the scan?

A. Longer dorsal duct draining via major papilla/shorter ventral duct draining via minor papilla.
B. Longer dorsal duct draining via minor papilla/shorter ventral duct draining via major papilla.
C. Longer dorsal duct and shorter ventral duct both draining via the major papilla.
D. Shorter dorsal duct draining via major papilla/longer ventral duct draining via minor papilla.
E. Shorter dorsal duct draining via minor papilla/longer ventral duct draining via major papilla.
F. Shorter dorsal duct and longer ventral duct both draining via the minor papilla.

11. A 4-month-old boy is having a barium swallow done in your department for suspected reflux. There is no relevant past medical history. On the AP view you notice a filling defect in the mid oesophagus. Your consultant recommends doing a lateral swallow to further assess this. This reveals a focal area of compression of the oesophagus anteriorly in the mid oesophagus. On the screening images you also notice a posterior impression on the trachea at this level. What is the most likely cause for this finding?

A. Duplication cyst.
B. Double aortic arch.
C. Lymphadenopathy.
D. Aberrant right subclavian artery.
E. Aberrant left pulmonary artery.

12. A 5-year-old boy is admitted for investigation of headache and vomiting. Unenhanced CT demonstrates a hyperdense mass centred on the cerebellar vermis and effacing the fourth ventricle. Homogenous enhancement is demonstrated on contrast administration. What is the most likely diagnosis?

A. Ependymoma.
B. Pilocytic astrocytoma.
C. Haemangioblastoma.
D. Brainstem glioma.
E. Medulloblastoma.

13. A 2-month-old boy is brought to A&E by his mother with a swollen, tender ankle which she had noticed that afternoon. She does not recall any injury and the child is otherwise well. You are in A&E out of hours for an unrelated matter when the A&E doctor shows you the plain film, which reveals a metaphyseal fracture of the distal tibia. What is the next appropriate radiological step?

A. To arrange a follow-up film 2 weeks after treatment.
B. To arrange an urgent 'babygram' (single plain film of the child).
C. To arrange a CT brain that night, followed by a skeletal survey the following morning.
D. To arrange an urgent out-of-hours skeletal survey.
E. To arrange an urgent isotope bone scan.

14. A 15-year-old female undergoes a pelvic MRI on which incidental note is made of a 1.5-cm lesion antero-lateral to the vagina and above the level of the inferior margin of the pubic symphysis. The lesion is hypointense on T1WI and hyperintense on T2WI. There is no displacement of or communication with the urethra. What is the likely diagnosis?

A. Urethral diverticulum.
B. Gartner duct cyst.
C. Bartholin gland cyst.
D. Skene duct cyst.
E. Urethral caruncle.

15. A 6-week-old neonate presents with several episodes of bilious vomiting. You suspect the child may have a malrotation. Which of the following findings on imaging is the most specific for midgut volvulus having occurred?

A. Reversal of the normal orientation of the superior mesenteric artery and vein on ultrasound.
B. High medial position of the caecum on a contrast enema.
C. Positioning of the duodenal-jejunal flexure to the right of midline on an upper GI contrast study.
D. Duodenal-jejunal corkscrew appearance on an upper GI contrast study.
E. Duodenal obstruction on an upper GI contrast study.

16. You are reviewing the daily radiograph on a 4-week-old neonate in the neonatal ICU. This patient was born at 32 weeks and was diagnosed with uncorrected transposition of the great arteries with an intact ventricular septum for which he underwent an emergency balloon atrial septostomy for palliation, whilst awaiting an arterial switch operation (ASO). As part of your routine practice, you review the position of the lines. The ET tube is located 9 mm from the carina. The right internal jugular vein central line is sited in the mediastinum, 8 mm inferior to the carina. The umbilical venous catheter (UVC) passes superiorly from the umbilicus, with its tip at the inferior aspect of the right atrium. The umbilical arterial line (UAC) passes inferiorly before passing superiorly, with its tip located at the level of T9. The nasogastric tube tip is below the diaphragm. Which of these pieces of apparatus may be incorrectly sited?

A. ET tube.
B. Nasogastric tube.
C. UAC.
D. Central line.
E. UVC.

17. A 14-month-old girl is brought to A&E with a head injury following a fall at home. Clinical examination reveals that the child is unkempt and has multiple bruising. Which of the following potential findings on CT raises the greatest suspicion for non-accidental injury (NAI)?

A. Parietal skull fracture.
B. Temporal lobe extradural haematoma.
C. Inter-hemispheric subdural haematoma.
D. Bilateral frontal enlargement of the subarachnoid space.
E. Soft-tissue swelling overlying the occiput.

18. A child is diagnosed with neuroblastoma. He is referred for staging and you are asked to advise on the standard radiological investigation of bony metastases. What do you advise?

A. Whole body MRI.
B. Whole body 18-FDG PET-CT.
C. ^{123}I-metaiodobenzylguanidine (MIBG) scan.
D. ^{99m}Tc methylene-diphosphonate (MDP) isotope bone scan.
E. MIBG and isotope bone scan.

19. A 15-year-old boy is homozygous for the delta F508 mutation for CF. He has poor weight gain and is diagnosed as having pancreatic insufficiency. What is the most likely imaging finding in his pancreas?

A. Diffuse pancreatic swelling.
B. Diffuse fatty infiltration and fibrosis.
C. Diffuse scattered microcysts (less than a few millimetres in size) within the pancreas.
D. Complete replacement of the pancreas with macrocysts.
E. Diffuse pancreatic calcification.

20. A cardiac MRI is being carried out on an infant for a conotruncal rotational abnormality. It is clear that this infant has 150 clockwise rotation of the great vessels. What conotruncal rotation abnormality does this infant have?

A. Normal rotation.
B. Situs inversus.
C. L-transposition.
D. D-transposition.
E. Double-outlet right ventricle.

21. A 12-year-old boy is investigated via MRI brain for headache, nystagmus, and ataxia. Which of the following radiological findings would suggest a diagnosis of Chiari I malformation as opposed to Chiari II?

A. Lacunar skull.
B. Myelomeningocoele.
C. Elongation of the fourth ventricle.
D. Caudal displacement of the cerebellar tonsils.
E. Cervicomedullary kinking.

22. A 12–year-old who is a keen athlete presents with left groin pain. A plain film of the pelvis reveals avulsion of the apophysis of the left ischial tuberosity. Which muscle attachment has he injured?

A. Sartorius.
B. Hamstrings.
C. Adductors.
D. Rectus femoris.
E. Iliopsoas.

23. An infant with ambiguous genitalia is referred for ultrasound of pelvis. This shows a normal uterus and ovaries, suggesting female pseudohermaphroditism. There is elevated 17-hydroxy-progesterone. What further investigation is recommended?

A. Ultrasound of adrenal glands.
B. MRI of pelvis.
C. Fluoroscopic genitography.
D. Laparoscopy.
E. Ultrasound of inguinal region.

24. A 6-day-old neonate presents with persistent vomiting. A plain x-ray of abdomen shows a dilated stomach and proximal duodenum, suggesting a high-grade duodenal obstruction. A subsequent upper GI contrast study confirms obstruction in the second part of the duodenum with a 'windsock' type deformity evident. What is the most likely diagnosis?

A. Duodenal atresia.
B. Midgut volvulus.
C. Annular pancreas.
D. Preduodenal portal vein.
E. Duodenal web.

25. A male neonate born at 38 weeks gestation develops acute respiratory distress within 36 hours of delivery. Clinical examination reveals coarse breath sounds. Serial CXRs carried out in the Special Care Baby Unit (SCBU) reveal reduced lung volumes and widespread granular opacities. There is reduced transradiancy in the right hemithorax and an ultrasound reveals that this is secondary to a mild-moderate pleural effusion. What is the most likely diagnosis?

A. Surfactant deficiency.
B. Meconium aspiration.
C. Bronchopulmonary dysplasia (BPD).
D. Beta haemolytic streptococcal pneumonia.
E. Pulmonary interstitial emphysema (PIE).

26. A 4-year-old boy is investigated via MRI brain for developmental delay and intractable seizures. Which of the following findings is in keeping with a diagnosis of schizencephaly?

A. Intracerebral cleft lined by gray matter connecting the lateral ventricle to the subarachnoid space.
B. Smooth cortical surface with absence of convolutions.
C. Multiple small, irregular cortical convolutions without intervening sulci.
D. Column of grey matter extending from the subependymal to the pial surface.
E. Circumferential, symmetric band of heterotopic grey matter deep to the cortical surface.

27. A 6-year-old child attends A&E with neck pain and tenderness after landing badly whilst trampolining in a neighbour's back garden. Which of the following findings is most concerning?

A. C2/3 subluxation.
B. Overhang of the lateral masses of C1 on C2 of 6 mm.
C. An atlanto-dens interval (ADI) of 6 mm.
D. Prevertebral soft tissue of 6 mm at C3.
E. Anterior wedging of C3.

28. A 6-week-old infant presents with a history of failure to thrive. Plain abdominal radiograph demonstrates punctate calcification in the region of the adrenal glands. Which of the following findings on CT of abdomen is most specific for Wolman disease?

A. Hepatosplenomegaly.
B. Enlarged retroperitoneal lymph nodes.
C. Diffuse fatty infiltration of the liver.
D. Enlarged calcified adrenals that maintain their normal triangular configuration.
E. Thickening of small bowel.

29. A 4-week-old neonate presents with persistent jaundice. The hyperbilirubinaemia is conjugated. An ultrasound scan of liver and gallbladder does not reveal a significant abnormality. A subsequent Hepatobiliary Iminodiacetic Acid (HIDA) scan shows decreased parenchymal extraction and clearance of radioisotope from the bloodstream, but tracer does eventually reach the gut. What is the jaundice is most likely to be due to?

A. Biliary atresia.
B. Caroli's disease.
C. Neonatal hepatitis.
D. Physiological jaundice of the newborn.
E. Hypothyroidism.

30. A male neonate born at 26 weeks gestation is currently being treated in your neonatal ICU. The patient's mother received corticosteroids prior to delivery and prophylactic surfactant administration as per your department's standard practice. The CXR was clear for the first 7 days. Despite this the child developed streaky perihilar granular opacities and respiratory difficulties. Further surfactant administration has been carried out, but the CXR carried out today (day 28 postpartum) shows small streaky linear densities along with cystic bubbly lucencies, which have been becoming increasingly prominent over the last 7 days and are distributed in an irregular pattern bilaterally. What is the most likely explanation for this appearance?

A. Surfactant deficiency.
B. Meconium aspiration.
C. BPD.
D. Beta haemolytic streptococcal pneumonia.
E. PIE.

31. A 14-year-old boy is having a follow-up MRI brain for a known seizure disorder. Axial T2WI demonstrates gyriform low signal in the left occipital and temporal lobes with corresponding volume loss. Leptomeningeal enhancement is present on the axial T1WI post contrast. A right-sided developmental venous anomaly (DVA) is also present. What is the most likely diagnosis?

A. Neurofibromatosis type 1.
B. Neurofibromatosis type 2.
C. Sturge Weber syndrome.
D. Tuberous sclerosis.
E. Von Hippel–Lindau disease.

32. A child presents after trauma to the elbow. Which configuration of the following ossification centres is most suspicious for significant injury?

A. Capitellum present before radial head.
B. Radial head present before trochlea.
C. Trochlea present before internal epicondyle.
D. Internal epicondyle present before olecranon.
E. Olecranon present before external epidondyle.

33. A 5-year-old girl with a history of precocious puberty and increased serum inhibin levels is referred for ultrasound of the pelvis. On ultrasound, there is a complex solid/cystic mass in the adnexa. MRI of the pelvis confirms a solid/cystic ovarian mass with a 'sponge-like appearance' on T2WI. What is the likely diagnosis?

A. Sertoli–Leydi cell tumour.
B. Juvenile granulosa cell tumour.
C. Mature cystic teratoma.
D. Fibroma.
E. Mucinous cystadenocarcinoma.

34. A 4-month-old child presents with abdominal distension and signs of obstruction. A plain film of abdomen shows mild small bowel distension with some displacement of loops in the lower abdomen and pelvis by a homogenous density. A subsequent ultrasound of the abdomen and pelvis shows a 7-cm cystic lesion in the lower abdomen. It is anechoic, but has a definable wall that has an inner echogenic line and an outer hypoechoic layer. What is the most likely diagnosis?

A. Mesenteric cyst.
B. Omental cyst.
C. Ovarian cyst.
D. Lymphangioma.
E. Duplication cyst.

35. A 3-month-old child presents to the paediatric outpatient clinic with a history of recurrent respiratory distress. The child had an uneventful delivery, but has had recurrent problems since birth. The child had a CXR taken prior to discharge home, aged 2 days, which showed a density in the left upper lobe, felt by the paediatrician to represent the thymus. Whilst the infant has never required admission, the mother is concerned due to recurrent coughing and dyspnoea. A CXR obtained at the clinic shows a large hyperlucent area in the left upper lobe. What is the most likely diagnosis?

A. Congenital lobar emphysema.
B. Congenital cystic adenomatoid malformation.
C. Pulmonary sequestration.
D. Persistent PIE.
E. Congenital diaphragmatic hernia.

36. A 12-year-old boy presents with a painless neck mass which recently increased in size after an upper respiratory tract infection. Which of the following radiological findings are in keeping with a second branchial cleft cyst?

A. Anechoic cystic mass posterior to sternocleidomastoid in the posterior triangle.
B. Lateral echogenic mass with hypoechoic vascular channels.
C. Anechoic cystic mass anterior to sternocleidomastoid near the angle of the mandible.
D. Anechoic cystic mass in an infrahyoid midline location.
E. Anechoic cystic mass inferior and posterior to the tragus.

37. A 12-year-old boy injures his ankle whilst playing football. The plain film reveals a lucent line through the distal metaphysis of the tibia and touching, but not crossing, the physis into the epiphysis. This represents a:

A. Salter–Harris type 1 injury.
B. Salter–Harris type 2 injury.
C. Salter–Harris type 3 injury.
D. Salter–Harris type 4 injury.
E. Normal variant.

38. An antenatal ultrasound of foetus at 20 weeks gestation reveals an occipital encephalocele. Foetal MRI demonstrates bilateral enlarged kidneys with cystic dysplasia and polydactyly. What is the diagnosis?

A. Autosomal recessive polycystic kidney disease.
B. Bardet–Biedl syndrome.
C. Meckel Gruber syndrome.
D. Tuberous sclerosis.
E. Zellweger syndrome.

39. A 7–day-old neonate presents with delayed passage of meconium and abdominal distension. There is no vomiting. An AXR shows non-specific gas-filled loops of bowel extending distally with air/fluid levels. A water-soluble contrast enema is performed and this shows a large filling defect in the proximal descending colon. There is a calibre change at this site between a small distal colon and mildly distended proximal colon. The colon wall is otherwise smooth, with no abnormal contractions or wall irregularity. What is the most likely diagnosis?

A. Hirschsprung's disease.
B. Meconium plug syndrome.
C. Meconium ileus syndrome.
D. Small left colon syndrome.
E. Colonic atresia.

40. One of the obstetricians in your hospital refers a pregnant patient, who is at 34 weeks gestation, to your department for assessment, as an antenatal ultrasound has shown a mass in the chest of the foetus. A repeat ultrasound does confirm a hyperechoic mass confined to the inferior aspect of the left hemithorax. This mass is vascular. Incidental note is also made of a ventricular septal defect. An MRI confirms the presence of a high-signal intrathoracic mass in the left lower thorax, which derives its blood supply from the abdominal aorta. The lung surrounding this area appears unremarkable. What is the most likely diagnosis?

A. Congenital diaphragmatic hernia.
B. Intralobar sequestration.
C. Congenital cystic adenomatoid malformation.
D. Foregut duplication cyst.
E. Extralobar sequestration.

41. An 18-month-old girl presents with increasing incoordination and developmental regression. T2WI demonstrates confluent high signal within the periventricular white matter and centrum semiovale, with radiating linear low signal intensity, giving a 'tigroid' pattern. Sparing of subcortical U fibres is also noted. What is the most likely diagnosis?

A. Krabbe disease.
B. Metachromatic leucodystrophy.
C. X-linked adrenoleucodystrophy.
D. Alexander disease.
E. Canavan disease.

42. A 10-year-old boy presents with left hip pain. Which of the following radiographic features makes the diagnosis of Perthes' disease more likely than slipped upper femoral epiphysis (SUFE)?

A. Failure of intersection of the superior femoral epiphysis by the line of Klein.
B. Widening of the physis.
C. Irregularity of the physis.
D. Sclerosis in the regional femoral neck.
E. Widening of the joint space.

43. A 10-year-old girl presents with right hip pain. Which of the following radiographic features makes the diagnosis of SUFE more likely than Perthes' disease?

A. Reduction in size of the proximal femoral epiphysis.
B. Loss of overlap between the medial femoral metaphysis and acetabulum.
C. Regional femoral demineralization.
D. A crescent of subcortical lucency in the femoral head.
E. Fragmentation of the femoral head.

44. A full-term infant with unilateral cryptorchidism is referred for ultrasound assessment. Which is the most common location of a cryptorchid testis?

A. Inguinal canal.
B. Superficial inguinal ring.
C. Deep inguinal ring.
D. Femoral triangle.
E. Abdomen.

45. An 8-month-old child presents with gradually increasing abdominal swelling. An ultrasound scan of abdomen is performed and this shows a large liver mass, which is well-defined and slightly hyperechoic to surrounding hepatic parenchyma. A subsequent biphasic CT scan confirms a solitary heterogeneous, but predominantly hypodense, liver mass on both phases with some calcification. The serum alphafetoprotein is elevated. What is the most likely diagnosis?

A. Hepatic angiosarcoma.
B. Mesenchymal hamartoma.
C. Undifferentiated embryonal sarcoma.
D. Hepatoblastoma.
E. Hepatocellular carcinoma.

46. A 6-year-old presents to A&E with a history of a productive cough associated with green sputum and mild wheeze. This child had a similar event 2 years earlier. Clinical examination reveals mild tachypnoea and coarse breath sounds. A CXR is requested. Your consultant points out the salient findings on the CXR as being the presence of hyperinflation, possible areas of air trapping, peribronchial wall oedema bilaterally, subsegmental atalectasis in the right midzone, and slight perihilar haziness. Your consultant asks you what you would do with this child given the findings. What do you say?

A. Send them home and reassure the parents.
B. Repeat CXR in 4 weeks to look for resolution.
C. Start antibiotics and reassess in 2 weeks.
D. Do expiratory films to rule out inhaled foreign body.
E. Respiratory consult and HRCT chest due to air-trapping.

47. A premature baby girl is noted to have a skull deformity consistent with scaphocephaly. Fusion of which vault suture or sutures gives rise to this craniosynostosis?

A. Coronal suture.
B. Sagittal suture.
C. Lambdoid suture.
D. Metopic suture.
E. Sagittal, coronal, and lambdoid sutures.

48. A 12-year-old male presents with a history of sudden onset of severe pain in the right testis. On examination, the right testis is tender and higher in position compared to the left side. An ultrasound of testes is requested. Which of the following statements regarding testicular torsion is true?

A. Torsion results in arterial obstruction first followed by venous obstruction.
B. The testis is usually salvageable if corrected within 24 hours.
C. Bell clapper deformity predisposes to testicular torsion.
D. Enlargement and heterogenous echogenicity of the testis is specific for torsion.
E. Clinical differentiation between testicular torsion and epididymo-orchitis is straightforward.

49. A 6-week-old male child presents with non-bilious vomiting after feeds, which has more recently become projectile in nature. You clinically suspect hypertrophic pyloric stenosis. Which of the following ultrasound findings would be inconsistent with this diagnosis?

A. A pyloric muscle thickness of 4 mm.
B. The presence of retrograde gastric contractions.
C. A pyloric thickness (serosa to serosa) of 10 mm.
D. The presence of hyperperistaltic gastric contractions.
E. A pyloric channel length of 12 mm.

50. A CT chest has been requested for a neonate in the neonatal ICU. This infant was born at 27 weeks gestation and developed right-sided PIE during the first week of life. The neonatologists practiced selective left bronchial intubation and no further air leak sequelae occurred. Also present on the CXR is a hyperlucent lesion in the right lower lobe. This is not clearly seen on the initial radiographs due to the generalized haziness present due to the surfactant deficiency. This lesion is not increasing in size and is not causing any significant respiratory embarrassment, but requires further assessment to define treatment. On CT a focal lesion is present confined to the right lower lobe, which consists of multiple cystic structures with central linear densities. This area demonstrates mild expansion. What is the diagnosis?

A. Congenital cystic adenomatoid malformation.
B. Persistent PIE.
C. Congenital diaphragmatic hernia.
D. Congenital lobar emphysema.
E. Bronchogenic cyst.

51. A 10-year-old boy of Japanese origin presents with episodes of right transient hemiparesis and declining intellect. MRI brain is performed. Which of the following are the most likely radiological findings?

A. Multiple flow voids within the basal ganglia bilaterally.
B. Irregular beading of the left extracranial internal carotid artery.
C. Hypoplasia of the left internal carotid artery.
D. Distal left middle cerebral artery aneurysm.
E. Normal study.

52. A 13-year-old boy presents with activity-related knee pain and locking. A plain film is unremarkable. An MRI reveals a defect in the lateral aspect of the medial femoral condyle. There is increased signal in the adjacent bone marrow on T2WI. What is the most likely diagnosis?

A. Distal femoral cortical irregularity.
B. Osteochondritis dissecans.
C. Sinding–Larsen–Johanssen disease.
D. Osgood–Schlatter disease.
E. Avulsion of the anterior tibial spine.

53. A 5-year-old girl presents with a pelvic mass with extension into the gluteal region through the sciatic foramen. Which of the following statements regarding sciatic foraminal anatomy is correct?

A. Piriformis muscle forms the boundary between the greater and lesser sciatic foramen.
B. The sacrotuberous ligament divides the greater sciatic foramen into superior and inferior compartments.
C. The pudendal nerve and internal pudendal vessels pass through the lesser sciatic foramen.
D. The sciatic nerve passes through the superior part of greater sciatic foramen.
E. The superior gluteal vessels and nerve pass through the inferior part of the greater sciatic foramen.

54. A pregnant mother is having an antenatal foetal anomaly scan and the ultrasonographer asks for your opinion on a large hernia arising from the anterior abdominal wall of the foetus, to try and determine between an omphalocele and a gastroschisis. Which of the following findings makes an omphalocele more likely than a gastroschisis?

A. The lack of a peritoneal covering.
B. The presence of the stomach in the herniated defect.
C. The umbilical cord inserting at the apex of the hernia.
D. The site of the hernia slightly lateral to the midline.
E. The lack of any other associated congenital anomalies.

55. A 4-day-old cyanosed infant is admitted as an emergency to SCBU following a home birth. The history is of episodes of severe cyanosis developing when the infant is distressed. A CXR is carried out and shows a normal mediastinal contour with slightly decreased pulmonary vascularity. What do you think the most likely cause of this infant's cyanosis is based on these findings?

A. Truncus arteriosus.
B. Pulmonary valve atresia with an intact ventricular septum.
C. Pulmonary valve hypoplasia with a VSD and overriding aorta.
D. D-transposition of the great arteries.
E. Coarctation of the aorta.

56. An 18-month-old boy is referred for CT after presenting with a right-sided white eye reflex (leucocoria). Which radiological feature is most in keeping with a diagnosis of retinoblastoma, as opposed to non-neoplastic causes of leucocoria (pseudoretinoblastoma)?

A. Contrast enhancement.
B. Calcification.
C. Microophthalmia.
D. Mass extension into the vitreous.
E. Secondary retinal detachment.

57. An 11-year-old boy falls and injures his elbow. Which of the following combination of injuries is most likely?

A. Posterior dislocation and capitellum fracture.
B. Anterior dislocation and lateral epicondyle fracture.
C. Posterior dislocation and medial epicondyle fracture.
D. Anterior dislocation and trochlea fracture.
E. Posterior dislocation and radial head fracture.

58. A 6-year-old boy undergoes an ultrasound examination of the renal tracts that shows dilated, polygonal, multifaceted calcyces in the right kidney. The infundibula, renal pelvis, and ureter are normal in calibre. IVU confirms the ultrasound findings and there is normal contrast excretion. What is the diagnosis?

A. Congenital megacalcyces.
B. Obstructive hydronephrosis.
C. Multicystic dysplastic kidney.
D. Congenital megacystis-microcolon syndrome.
E. Vesico-ureteric reflux.

59. A 10-year-old boy presents with a 1-day history of severe epigastric pain radiating to the back. Serum amylase is elevated. The patient has an ultrasound scan of abdomen performed which does not show evidence of gallbladder or biliary disease. Pancreatitis is suspected. What is the most useful sign with regard to the pancreas on ultrasound that would support this diagnosis?

A. Increased pancreatic echogenicity.
B. Decreased pancreatic echogenicity.
C. Pancreatic duct dilatation.
D. Pancreatic atrophy.
E. Pancreatic calcification.

60. A male neonate is born at 40 weeks gestation. There is a history of polyhydramnios during pregnancy. During baby checks, the baby is noted to have a sacral dimple. At this time the mother reports that the baby has been unable to feed properly during the initial 24 hours, during which it dribbles and spits out milk. She also reports the baby has had recurrent coughing episodes. The paediatrician is unable to pass an nasogastric tube and suspects a tracheoesophageal fistula. A contrast swallow is requested. This demonstrates termination of the proximal oesophagus, with a fistulous connection between the proximal oesophagus and the trachea. Contrast does not pass into the distal oesophagus. What class of tracheoesophageal fistula is this likely to be?

A. Type A.
B. Type B.
C. Type C.
D. Type D.
E. Type E.

61. An 8-year-old boy presents with a painful scalp swelling over the right frontal region for the last 6 weeks. An initial skull radiograph demonstrates a punched out oval osteolytic lesion with an apparent double contour or bevelled edge. The lesion does not have a sclerotic margin and no periosteal reaction is seen. Which of the following is the most likely diagnosis?

A. Epidermoid cyst.
B. Neuroblastoma metastasis.
C. Langerhans cell histiocytosis (LCH).
D. Haemangioma.
E. Osteoma.

62. A 12-year-old boy undergoes a plain film of his left knee after minor trauma playing rugby. The film reveals a lucent, cortically based lesion with a sclerotic rim in the metadiaphysis of the proximal tibia. There is no periosteal reaction or soft-tissue component and the boy denies pain prior to the injury. As the reporting radiologist you advise:

A. plain films of the extremities to look for similar lesions
B. MRI of the left lower leg and CT chest
C. Isotope bone scan
D. CT of left lower leg
E. none of the above.

63. A 15-year-old male undergoes a pelvic MRI on which an incidental note is made of absent bilateral seminal vesicles. Which of the following is commonly associated with bilateral seminal vesicle agenesis?

A. Renal agenesis.
B. CF.
C. Calcified vas deferens.
D. Ectopic ureter.
E. Rotation anomaly of one kidney.

64. A neonate is born at 34 weeks gestation. During the first week of life it presents with bloody diarrhoea and abdominal distension. You wonder about the possibility of necrotising enterocolitis. Which one of the following radiological investigations is unlikely to be helpful in the acute setting?

A. Supine AXR.
B. Left lateral decubitus AXR.
C. Water-soluble contrast enema.
D. Ultrasound of abdomen.
E. Supine cross-table lateral AXR.

65. A 7-year-old boy is being investigated for a history of mild exertional dyspnoea. A CXR has been carried out that shows normal lungs but does demonstrate a linear density passing inferiorly from the right lower hemithorax to the level of the diaphragm. A cardiac MRI has been requested, which shows normal pulmonary venous drainage on the left side. On the right side, the lower pulmonary vein drains into the right atrium, the superior pulmonary vein drains into the left atrium, and the arterial supply for the entire right lung arises from the pulmonary artery. No cardiac abnormality is identified. What form of abnormality does this child have?

A. Total anomalous pulmonary venous return.
B. Partial anomalous pulmonary venous return (PAPVR).
C. Extralobar sequestration.
D. Cor triatriatum.
E. Scimitar syndrome.

66. A 14-year-old boy presents with a slow-growing painless mass at the angle of the mandible on the left. Ultrasound demonstrates a hypoechoic left parotid mass containing echogenic calcific foci. On follow-up contrast-enhanced MRI, the mass demonstrates mild increased enhancement. Which of the following is the most likely diagnosis?

A. Warthin tumour.
B. Primary lymphoma.
C. Parotitis.
D. Pleomorphic adenoma.
E. Haemangioma.

67. A 5-year-old boy with bilateral wrist pain undergoes a plain film which reveals several peduncuated bony outgrowths from the metaphyses of both radii, which point away from the adjacent joints. What is the most likely diagnosis?

A. Ollier disease.
B. Maffucci syndrome.
C. Morquio syndrome.
D. Diaphyseal aclasia.
E. Hunter syndrome.

68. A 15-year-old female undergoes an ultrasound of pelvis that demonstrates uterine abnormality with a differential diagnosis of bicornuate or septate uterus. An MRI of the pelvis is requested for further assessment. Which of the following findings on MRI is suggestive of a bicornuate uterus?

A. Two uterine cavities.
B. Fundal concavity of less than 1 cm.
C. Intercornual distance of more than 4 cm.
D. Convex external fundal contour.
E. Thin fibrous low-intensity septum separating the uterine cavities.

69. A 2-year-old boy presents with abdominal pain and clinical signs of GI bleeding. The clinical team wish to exclude a Meckel's diverticulum and request a radionuclide 'Meckel's scan'. What ectopic tissue is required in the Meckel's diverticulum for the scan to be successful?

A. Colonic tissue.
B. Gastric mucosa.
C. Exocrine pancreatic tissue.
D. Pancreatic islet cells.
E. Thyroid tissue.

70. A 6-year-old girl is brought to your local paediatric outpatients with a history of night sweats, tiredness, and new onset wheeze not responding to bronchodilators. A CXR is done which shows increased mediastinal soft tissue noted superiorly. The paravertebral lines are maintained. The aortic knuckle is not visible. A lateral CXR has been carried out at the request of the paediatrician, which shows increased soft tissue displacing the trachea posteriorly, causing mild narrowing. What is the most likely diagnosis?

A. Tuberculosis.
B. Lymphangioma.
C. Bronchogenic cyst.
D. Thymic/nodal malignant infiltration.
E. Teratoma.

71. Follow-up MRI is performed on a foetus of 26 weeks gestational age after ultrasound raised the suspicion of agenesis of the corpus callosum (ACC). This subsequently confirms that the callosum is absent. What is the most likely additional radiological finding?

A. None, isolated abnormality.
B. Parenchymal T2WI signal hypointensity.
C. Periventricular nodular heterotopia.
D. Dysplastic brainstem.
E. Delayed sulcation.

72. An infant is of short stature and undergoes a skeletal survey. This reveals markedly shortened femora and humeri, although the other long bones are also greatly affected. The vertebral bodies are moderately flattened and there is a reduction in the interpedicular distance in a caudal direction in the spine. What is the diagnosis?

A. Thanatophoric dysplasia.
B. Achondroplasia.
C. Chondrodysplasia punctata.
D. Jeune syndrome.
E. Cleidocranial dysplasia.

73. A 14-year-old girl presents with sudden onset of severe right-sided lower abdominal pain, nausea, and vomiting. An ultrasound of the pelvis is requested with a suspected diagnosis of ovarian torsion. Which of the following is the most constant ultrasound finding in ovarian torsion?

A. Enlarged ovary.
B. Absent ovarian blood flow.
C. Pelvic free fluid.
D. Twisted ovarian pedicle.
E. 'String of pearls' sign.

74. A 15-year-old boy presents with severe abdominal pain. He has a known history of a 'polyposis' syndrome. A plain AXR shows small bowel obstruction. A subsequent CT scan of abdomen indicates that this is due to a small bowel intussusception. Which 'polyposis' syndrome does he most probably have?

A. Cronkhite–Canada syndrome.
B. Familial adenomatous polyposis syndrome.
C. Cowden disease.
D. Gardner's syndrome.
E. Peutz–Jehger's syndrome.

75. With appropriate clinical suspicion, which of the following radiologically depicted injuries would most raise suspicion of NAI?

A. Posterior rib fracture.
B. Vertebral compression fracture.
C. Duodenal haematoma.
D. Spiral fracture of long bone.
E. Jejunal laceration.

chapter

5

PAEDIATRICS

ANSWERS

1. C. Alveolar proteinosis.

Intersitial lung disease in children is uncommon, but it is important to be aware of as 50% of children present with a history of wheeze. Chronic idiopathic pulmonary haemosiderosis does not cause a 'crazy paving' pattern. It is a rare disorder (although common in exams) and when present in children usually presents before 3 years of age. Whilst a 'crazy paving' pattern was originally described as being typical of alveolar proteinosis, it has since been described in numerous conditions and as such a knowledge of these processes is necessary to differentiate them. *Pneumocystis jirovecii* pneumonia would not normally be considered in the absence of a history of immunocompromise. Whilst NSIP can cause this appearance, in children it more typically has an upper zone and peripheral predominance with associated ground-glass changes and a degree of honeycombing. The imaging characteristics of NSIP, LIP and DIP overlap in children and often require lung biopsy to differentiate them. LIP is also usually associated with immunodeficiency disorders, as in adults. Sarcoidosis in children is very rare and usually presents in older children, around 13–15 years of age.

Koh D and Hansell D. Computed tomography of diffuse interstitial lung disease in children. *Clinical Radiology* 2000; 55(9): 659–667.

2. A. Periventricular leucomalacia.

This refers to white matter necrosis, typically involving the centrum semiovale, and is seen in premature infants. This results from hypoxic-ischaemic injury at the watershed areas, which in premature infants are present in a periventricular location. Porencephaly refers to an area of encephalomalacia, which may or may not communicate with the ventricular system and develops postnatally or in the third trimester. This is the end result of a destructive process, such as an intraparenchymal haemorrhage. Sylvian fissure cysts are the most common site for supratentorial arachnoid cysts. Vein of Galen malformations occur in the midline and exhibit Doppler flow. Subependymal cysts are detected in the caudothalamic groove.

Epelman M, Daneman A, Blaser SI, Ortiz-Neira C, Konen O, Jarrin J et al. Differential diagnosis of intracranial cystic lesions at head US: correlation with CT and MR imaging. *RadioGraphics* 2006; 26: 173–196.

3. E. Fibrous dysplasia.

The clue here is the café-au-lait spots, which are seen in McCune–Albright syndrome (unilateral polyostotic fibrous dysplasia, precocious puberty, and café-au-lait spots).

Osteomyelitis is unlikely because of the normal inflammatory markers, lack of systemic symptoms, and lack of periosteal reaction. Aneurysmal bone cyst and GCTs are possibilities (the former may even complicate fibrous dysplasia). Chondroblastoma is an epiphyseal lesion.

Manaster BJ, May DA, and Disler DG. *Musculoskeletal Imaging: The Requisites.* 3rd edn, Mosby, 2007, pp. 460–465.

4. C. Severe renal compromise is the immediate cause of death in the perinatal group.

The incidence of autosomal recessive polycystic kidney disease (ARPKD) is approximately 1:20,000 births. It is a disease of tubular ectasia and fibrosis that results in bilateral enlarged kidneys, with loss of cortico-medullary differentiation and multiple small radially arranged cysts. ARPKD is associated with congenital hepatic fibrosis, the severity of which is inversely proportional to the renal abnormality.

Four distinct groups of ARPKD are recognized based on age at presentation: perinatal, neonatal, infantile, and juvenile. The most severe renal involvement is seen in the perinatal group. In this group, severe renal impairment results in reduced urine output, oligohydramnios, and pulmonary hypoplasia. Severe respiratory compromise is the immediate cause of death in these patients. Oligohydramnios is also associated with Potter facies (low set and flattened ears, short and snubbed nose, deep eye creases, and micrognathia) and clubfoot deformity.

Lonergan GJ, Rice RR, and Suarez ES. Autosomal recessive polycystic kidney disease: radiologic-pathologic correlation. *RadioGraphics* 2000; 20: 837–855.

5. E. Infantile haemangioendothelioma.

Also known as infantile hepatic haemangioma, infantile haemangioendothelioma is a vascular neoplasm and the most common benign hepatic tumor of infancy. It may be a solitary mass or multifocal, and most are diagnosed before the age of 1 year. The lesion itself runs a benign course, but life-threatening clinical complications may occur. These include high-output cardiac failure secondary to large arterio-venous shunts and Kasabach–Merritt syndrome of coagulopathy secondary to intratumoral platelet sequestration. On ultrasound the lesions are well-demarcated and are generally hypoechoic or of mixed echogenicity. On CT and MRI the enhancement pattern of the lesion is similar to adult haemangioma. There is intense early peripheral nodular enhancement, with centripetal progression on the later images.

Hepatoblastoma rarely occurs in the newborn but can be seen in young infants. This tumour is distinguished by a heterogeneous rather than intense centripetal enhancement pattern and markedly elevated levels of alphafetoprotein (AFP) in 90% of patients. AFP level is rarely elevated in infantile haemangioendothelioma.

Mesenchymal hamartoma of the liver, like infantile haemangioendothelioma, may also be found in the perinatal period. This benign tumour differs in imaging appearance from infantile haemangioendothelioma in that it usually appears as a multicystic, multilocular mass with enhancement of only the septa and solid portions. Less commonly, mesenchymal hamartoma may be predominantly solid, but it differs from infantile haemangioendothelioma in that it is hypovascular at dynamic contrast-enhanced imaging.

Whilst metastases could occur in an infant (e.g. neuroblastoma), they would tend to be hypodense to normal liver on contrast-enhanced CT. Hepatoma is exceedingly rare in an infant and the imaging characteristics described would not be typical.

Chung EM, Cube R, Lewis RB, and Conran RM. Pediatric liver masses: radiologic-pathologic correlation Part 1. Benign tumors. *RadioGraphics* 2010; 30: 801–826.

6. A. Pulmonary valve function.

As a general rule, pre-operative imaging of paediatric cardiac malformations focuses on the morphology, to allow accurate characterization of the abnormality pre-operatively. Post-operative imaging focuses more on function, to assess the success of the treatment given and need for further intervention. With regard to a corrected tetralogy of Fallot, the situs will be known and the ventricular septum assessed and usually repaired at surgery. A graft between the systemic venous system and pulmonary artery is a feature of a Fontan/Glenn procedure and these are most commonly carried out for tricuspid atresia, not tetralogy of Fallot. Assessment of the pulmonary valve, along with right ventricular function, is essential in this post-operative patient, as re-stenosis of the pulmonary valve or progressive right ventricular impairment are associated with increased morbidity.

Krisnamurthy R. Pediatric cardiac MRI: anatomy and function. *Pediatric Radiology* 2008; 38 (Suppl 2): S192–S199.

7. B. Enlargement of the posterior fossa.

Dandy–Walker variant is more common, accounting for a third of all posterior fossa malformations, but less severe than the malformation. Enlargement of the posterior fossa is not a feature. Cystic dilatation of the fourth ventricle with vermian dysgenesis is characteristic of both. Associated CNS anomalies, usually of the midline, are also seen, as is ventriculomegaly, although both are more common with Dandy–Walker malformation.

Dahnert W. Radiology Review Manual, 6th edn, Lippincott Williams & Wilkins, 2007, pp. 280–281.

8. D. Arrange MRI, CT chest, and IBS.

The lesion described is probably an osteosarcoma. Ewing's sarcoma is high on the differential diagnosis, but is less often found in the metaphysis and usually has a soft-tissue component. Osteosarcomas commonly arise from the metaphysis (only 2–11% arise from the diaphysis). They are most common in the distal femur followed by the proximal tibia. If osteoid matrix is present on plain film, osteosarcoma is the diagnosis until proven otherwise. The appropriate action would be to refer to a regional orthopaedic centre for discussion at a multidisciplinary meeting with imaging followed by biopsy or surgery as thought appropriate. An MRI is used to evaluate local extent, the CT chest and IBS to search for pulmonary and bony metastases, respectively. Surgery is often performed after repeat imaging following the administration of neoadjuvant chemotherapy, when the oedema surrounding the tumour is less pronounced.

The findings are not particularly suspicious for NAI (option A). It is not safe to assume the appearances are caused by osteomyelitis and in any case more urgent investigation would be required to confirm such a diagnosis. A CT of the area might be useful but involves ionizing radiation, which MRI avoids; the MIBG scan would be appropriate for neuroblastoma, which is unlikely in this age group (90% occur before the age of 5) (option C). A metastasis is very unlikely in this age group.

Kan J. and Kleinman P. *Pediatric and Adolescent Musculoskeletal MRI*, Springer, 2007, 116–126.

9. D. The upper moiety ureter is associated with ureterocele whereas the lower moiety ureter is associated with vesicoureteric reflux.

Ectopic ureter results when the ureteral bud fails to separate from the Wolffian duct and as a consequence is carried more caudally than normal. In females, the ectopic ureter can insert distal to the external sphincter, resulting in incontinence. Approximately 70% of ectopic insertion is associated with complete ureteral duplication.

According to the Weigert–Meyer rule of complete ureteral duplication, the ureteric orifice of the upper moiety inserts into the bladder medial and inferior to the lower moiety. The ureter draining the Upper moiety is associated with Ureterocele and Obstruction (note the vowels), whereas the lower pole moiety is associated with vesico-ureteric reflux. The obstructed upper moiety may not be visualized on IVU. The absence of upper pole calyx and displaced ('drooping lily') lower moiety calyces help in making the diagnosis.

Berrocal T, Lopez-Pereira P, Arjonilla A, and Gutierrez J. Anomalies of the distal ureter, bladder, and urethra in children: embryologic, radiologic and pathologic features. *RadioGraphics* 2002; 22: 1139–1164.

10. B. Longer dorsal duct draining via the minor papilla/shorter ventral duct draining via the major papilla.

Pancreas divisum is the most common congenital anomaly of the pancreatic duct and has a prevalence of 4–10% of the general population. Although it is usually asymptomatic and an incidental finding, it can lead to recurrent episodes of pancreatitis in children and adults. By definition, the dorsal and ventral ducts fail to fuse during embryological development, which results in the following features seen at MRCP: (a) a prominent dorsal pancreatic duct, which drains directly into the minor papilla, and (b) a ventral duct, which does not communicate with the dorsal duct, but joins with the distal bile duct to enter the major papilla (ampulla of Vater). Typically, the ventral duct is short and narrow, while the dorsal duct normally has a larger caliber.

Anupindi SA. Pancreatic and biliary anomalies: imaging in 2008. *Pediatric Radiology* 2008; 38(2): S267–S271.
Patel HT, Shah AJ, Khandelwal SR, Patel HF, and Patel MD. MR cholangiopancreatography at 3.0 T. *RadioGraphics* 2009; 29: 1689–1706.

11. E. Aberrant left pulmonary artery.

Double aortic arch compresses the trachea anteriorly and the oesophagus posteriorly. Aberrant right subclavian (with a left-sided aortic arch) causes posterior indentation of the oesophagus, but no indentation of the trachea. An identical appearance is seen on the lateral view with a right-sided aortic arch and an aberrant left subclavian.

Aberrant left pulmonary artery commonly presents any time up to early childhood, with stridor, wheezing, recurrent infections, and feeding problems being amongst the most common symptoms. It can be associated with a PDA or ASD.

Donnelly L. *Fundamentals of Pediatric Radiology*, 1st edn, Saunders, 2001, p. 14.
Dahnert W. *Radiology Review Manual*, 6th edn, Lippincott Williams & Wilkins, 2007, p. 603.

12. E. Medulloblastoma.

This is the most common malignant posterior fossa tumour in children, generally occurring before 10 years of age. The vast majority (85%) arise in the cerebellar vermis. They are hyperdense due to their high cellular content. Calcification is uncommon, occurring in up to 20% of cases. Pilocytic astrocytoma typically present as a cystic mass with an enhancing nodule. The most common location is the cerebellum, but they usually occur in other sites when associated with neurofibromatosis type 1. Haemangioblastomas are rare in children and even in the setting of von Hippel–Lindau syndrome typically manifest in early adulthood. Ependymomas are usually more heterogenous owing to calcification, cystic change, and haemorrhage. The tumour arises from ependymal cells that line the ventricular system and central canal of the spinal cord. Brainstem gliomas are hypodense on CT and may show exophytic growth into the adjacent cisternal spaces.

Brant WE and Helms CA. *Fundamentals of Diagnostic Radiology*, 3rd edn, Lippincott Williams & Wilkins, 2007, pp. 136–140.

13. C. To arrange a CT brain that night, followed by a skeletal survey the following morning.

A metaphyseal fracture in a non-ambulant child is due to NAI until proven otherwise. Of all the injuries described in NAI, none is more specific than the metaphyseal fracture. Royal College guidelines state that skeletal surveys should be performed by two radiographers and the films reviewed by a consultant radiologist before the child leaves the x-ray department in cases of suspected NAI. Thus, it is more appropriate that such a skeletal survey should be performed within normal hours, although usually within 24 hours of admission. Also, the guidelines state that any child under the age of 1 year who has evidence of physical abuse should undergo neuroimaging (as well as any child with evidence of physical abuse and encephalopathic features/focal neurology/haemorrhagic retinopathy). Thus a CT brain is indicated. The guidelines infer this CT brain should be performed as soon as the child is stabilized following admission. IBSs and follow-up imaging may be relevant depending on the circumstances. A 'babygram' (a film which includes the whole of the infant) is not appropriate.

At radiology trainee level it is important to remember that, due to the severe consequences for child and family of correctly/incorrectly making or missing the diagnosis of NAI, consultant involvement is necessary, both of the clinical and radiological teams.

Standards for Radiological Investigations of Suspected Non-accidental Injury, Intercollegiate report from the Royal College of Radiologists and Royal College of Paediatrics and Child Health, March 2008. Available at: http://www.rcpch.ac.uk/doc.aspx?id_Resource=3521.

14. B. Gartner duct cyst.

Anatomical location is useful in the differential diagnosis of periurethral cysts. A Gartner duct cyst is a retention cyst arising from Wolffian (mesonephric duct remnant). It is typically located in the antero-lateral aspect of the vagina above the level of the pubic symphysis. It is usually solitary and less than 2 cm in size. At MRI, the lesion may appear hypo- or hyperintense on T1WI depending on whether the contents are simple fluid or haemorrhagic/proteinaceous. They do not displace or deform the urethra.

A Bartholin cyst is located in the posterolateral aspect of the lower vagina, at or below the level of the pubic symphysis. Skene cysts are located lateral to the external urethral meatus, below the level of pubic symphysis. It may be difficult to differentiate Bartholin and Skene cysts. Urethral diverticula communicate with the urethra whereas periurethral cysts do not. A urethral caruncle manifests as T2 hyperintense soft tissue surrounding the external urethral meatus.

Chaudhari VV, Patel MK, Douek M, and Raman SS. MR imaging and US of female urethral and periurethral disease. *RadioGraphics* 2010; 30: 1857–1874.

15. D. Duodenal-jejunal corkscrew appearance on an upper GI contrast study.

In individuals with malrotation, the mesenteric attachment of the midgut, particularly the portion from the duodenal-jejunal junction to the caecum, is abnormally short. The gut is therefore prone to twist counterclockwise around the superior mesenteric artery and vein—midgut volvulus. Options A to C are all imaging findings in malrotation, but not specifically that midgut volvulus has occurred. With regard to option E duodenal obstruction can, of course, be seen with midgut volvulus, but obstruction may also occur due to obstructive bands and there is also an increased risk of congenital duodenal anomalies in malrotation, such as duodenal atresia, stenosis, and webs.

It is the finding of an abnormally located duodenal-jejunal flexure and a corkscrew appearance to the duodenum and proximal jejunum that is the most specific for malrotation complicated by midgut volvulus.

Applegate KE, Anderson JM, and Klatte EC. Intestinal malrotation in children: a problem-solving approach to the upper gastrointestinal series. *RadioGraphics* 2006; 26: 1485–1500.

16. D. Central line.

The tip of the central line is ideally situated superior to the level of the carina to ensure that it is not within the right atrium. Whilst placement inferior to this may be satisfactory, it can result in placement within the right atrium or coronary sinus, which are associated with an increased risk of complications. When assessing the ET tube in neonates, the tip should lie between the carina and the thoracic inlet, as more accurate placement is difficult given the size of the patient. UACs are divided into high and low lines. High lines should have their tip between T8 and T10. Low lines should be sited below L3. Lines should not be sited between T10 and L3 as they can cause thrombosis of the mesenteric or renal vessels. UVCs pass superiorly into the portal vein, along the ductus venosus into the IVC.

Teele S, Emani S, Thiagarajan R, and Teele R. Catheters, wires, tubes and drains on postoperative radiographs of pediatric cardiac patients: the whys and wherefores. *Pediatric Radiology* 2008; 38: 1041–1053.
Donnelly L. *Fundamentals of Pediatric Radiology*, 1st edn, Saunders, 2001, pp. 27–29.

17. C. Inter-hemispheric subdural haematoma.

NAI is a difficult and controversial subject with no absolute pathognomonic features. It is, however, the leading cause of morbidity and mortality in abused children. Inter-hemispheric subdural haematoma has the highest specificity of abuse for any intracranial injury. Subarachnoid haemorrhage is also a much more common injury in NAI. Skull fractures are relatively common in both accidental and non-accidental injury. In addition, there are no fracture patterns that are specific for abuse, although fractures that cross sutures and bilateral fractures are more common in the setting of NAI. Skull radiography is preferred over CT for fracture assessment. Extradural haematoma is much more often accidental than inflicted and may result from relatively short-distance falls. Bilateral frontal enlargement of the subarachnoid space is a feature of benign external hydrocephalus.

Lonergan GJ, Baker AM, Morey MK, and Boos SC. Child abuse: radiologic-pathologic correlation. *RadioGraphics*, 2003; 23: 811–845.

18. C. ^{123}I-metaiodobenzylguanidine (MIBG) scan.

Owing to the high specificity and sensitivity in neuroblastoma, MIBG imaging has superseded the use of ^{99m}Tc bone scans for the detection of skeletal metastases in the majority of children with neuroblastoma, which take up the tracer in >90% of cases, and has been recommended by the last international consensus conference as a standard element of staging and response evaluation. False-negative scans may be observed in approximately 10% of neuroblastomas that do not concentrate MIBG. In addition, very small amounts of bone marrow tumour will often not be detected and therefore the MIBG scan must be supplemented with bilateral bone marrow biopsy. For those patients whose tumours are negative for MIBG uptake at diagnosis, the ^{99m}Tc MDP bone scan is the standard test recommended to evaluate skeletal metastases. However, the low specificity of this test and the difficulty in interpreting uptake in young children with actively growing bones make investigation of alternative methods preferable. Whole-body MRI is also a sensitive test for neuroblastoma tumours, including bone and bone marrow metastases, although the specificity is much lower than for MIBG.

MRI and CT are appropriate in the staging of neuroblastoma, but for the assessment of local invasion rather than bony involvement in particular. There currently is no consensus about the optimal imaging modality for assessing local disease. Both MRI and CT are routinely used, depending on local availability and the radiologist's preference. 18-FDG PET-CT imaging is not as sensitive as MIBG imaging for bony metastases, although it may be more sensitive for small soft tissue tumours and nodal metastases. The use of PET-CT is not at present well defined and delivers a high radiation dose.

Matthay KK, Shulkin B, Ladenstein R, Michon J, Giammarile F, Lewington V et al. Criteria for evaluation of disease extent by (123)I-metaiodobenzylguanidine scans in neuroblastoma: a report for the International Neuroblastoma Risk Group (INRG) Task Force. *British Journal of Cancer* 2010; 102(9): 1319–1326.
Brisse HJ, McCarville MB, Granata C, Krug KB, Wootton-Gorges SL, Kanegawa K et al. Guidelines for Imaging and Staging of Neuroblastic Tumors: Consensus Report from the International Neuroblastoma Risk Group Project. *Radiology* 2011 (May 17), doi: 10.1148/radiol.11101352 (epub ahead of print).

19. B. Diffuse fatty infiltration and fibrosis.

Pancreatic insufficiency is almost invariable in patients who have the delta F508 mutation for CF. The most commonly described imaging abnormality in patients with CF is diffuse fatty infiltration and fibrosis. While pancreatic cysts are described, their size does not usually exceed a few millimetres. Larger pancreatic cysts have only been described in a few patients and complete replacement of the pancreas by macrocysts is very unusual.

Ryan S and Finn S. Pancreatic replacement by cysts in cystic fibrosis. *Pediatric Radiology* 2008; 38: 1141.

20. B. Situs inversus.

The primitive truncus is a midline structure that persists to a degree in truncus arteriosus abnormality. During normal development the truncus divides into the aortic and pulmonary trunks, which then undergo 150° anticlockwise rotation. In situs inversus there is 150° clockwise rotation. Transposition of the great arteries (TGA) is characterized by 30° rotation, anticlockwise in D-TGA and clockwise in L-TGA. Double-outlet right ventricle displays 90° anticlockwise rotation.

Donnelly L. *Fundamentals of Pediatric Radiology*, Saunders, 2001, pp. 87–92.
Dahnert W. *Radiology Review Manual*, 6th edn, Lippincott Williams & Wilkins, 2007, p. 603.

21. D. Caudal displacement of the cerebellar tonsils.

Chiari II is seen in all patients with open spinal dysraphisms, such myelomeningocoele. Lacunar skull (luckenshadel) is also associated with Chiari II. Cervicomedullary kinking is common to both, although more so with Chiari II. Caudal displacement of the cerebellar tonsils is a feature of Chiari I, whereas in Chiari II the vermis herniates into the foramen magnum and the tonsils are lateral to the medulla.

Tortori-Donati P and Rossi A. *Pediatric Neuroradiology*, Springer, 2005, pp. 172–184.

22. B. Hamstrings.

Avulsion fractures in the pelvis are generally uncommon injuries and are seen almost exclusively in adolescent athletes. They occur at the apophyses, which while growing are more prone to injury than the adjacent tendons. The hamstrings attach at the ischial tuberosity. Sartorius attaches at the anterior superior iliac spine, rectus femoris at the anterior inferior iliac spine, the adductors at the symphysis pubis, and iliopsoas at the lesser trochanter. Care should be taken not to mistake an old avulsion, which can produce irregularity, marked periostitis, and adjacent soft-tissue mineralization, for a more sinister lesion.

Donnelly LF. *Fundamentals of Pediatric Radiology*, Saunders, 2001, pp. 177–178.

23. A. Ultrasound of adrenal glands.

Congenital adrenal hyperplasia (CAH) is the most common cause of ambiguous genitalia. It causes virilization in females and precocious puberty in males. Most cases are caused by 21-hydroxylase deficiency resulting in elevated 17-hydroxy-progesterone level.

Enlarged adrenal glands, limbs over 20 mm in length and 4 mm width, with nodular contour and normal cortico-medullary differentiation are suggestive of CAH. Stippled echogenicity producing 'cerebriform' appearance is considered specific for CAH. Normal adrenal glands do not, however, exclude the diagnosis.

Chavhan GB, Parra DA, Oudjhane K, Miller SF, Babyn PS, and Pippi Salle FL. Imaging of ambiguous genitalia: classification and diagnostic approach. *RadioGraphics* 2008, 28, 1891–1904.

24. E. Duodenal web.

A duodenal web is classically associated with the 'windsock sign' seen on an upper GI contrast study. Over time, the web or diaphragm passively elongates as a result of continual peristalsis, to form the windsock configuration of an intraluminal duodenal diverticulum.

Duodenal atresia is commonly associated with the 'double bubble' appearance on AXR. The atresia is most commonly just distal to the ampulla of Vater. Associated anomalies are common, such as congenital heart disease, Down's syndrome, and malrotation.

Midgut volvulus is usually a complication of malrotation. The AXR may be normal, gasless, or show signs of duodenal/high small bowel obstruction. The upper GI contrast study shows an abnormal position of the duodenal-jejunal flexure (to the right of midline) or duodenal obstruction in severe cases. More often the volvulus is intermittent, when the 'corkscrew' appearance is classical, due to clockwise twisting of the jejunum around the superior mesenteric artery.

Annular pancreas and preduodenal portal vein are exceedingly rare. In preduodenal portal vein (persistent left vitelline vein), the portal vein lies in an abnormal position anterior to the duodenum and may cause compression. However, in this entity, the primary obstruction is more usually due to an associated obstructing duodenal lesion, such as an intraluminal membrane or web, and not to the abnormal position of the vein.

Materne R. The duodenal windsock sign. *Radiology* 2001, 218, pp. 749–750.
Rao P. Neonatal gastrointestinal imaging. *European Journal of Radiology* 2006, 60, 171–186.

25. D. Beta-haemolytic streptococcal pneumonia.

This is the most common neonatal pneumonia and differs from other common patterns of pneumonia as it causes this pattern on CXR, whereas other neonatal pneumonias commonly cause high lung volumes and streaky perihilar densities. Transient tachypnoea of the newborn (TTN) and meconium aspiration syndrome also classically cause increased lung volumes and streaky perihilar density, although the radiographic appearance of meconium aspiration can also often be difficult to differentiate from beta-haemolytic streptococcal pneumonia. A useful differentiation is that pleural effusions are uncommon in meconium aspiration, but are commonly seen in beta-haemolytic streptococcal pneumonia. TTN is also characterized by rapid clearance and would not be expected to persist on serial radiographs. The other common cause for low lung volumes and granular densities described is surfactant deficiency. This would be very unlikely in an infant born at 38 weeks gestation.

Donnelly L. *Fundamentals of Pediatric Radiology*, Saunders, 2001, pp. 23–26.

26. A. Intracerebral cleft lined by gray matter connecting the lateral ventricle to the subarachnoid space.

Schizencephaly can be defined as open or closed lip, depending on the presence of separation of the cleft walls. The remaining options describe lissencephaly, polymicrogyria, transmantle heterotopia, and subcortical band heterotopia, respectively. Transmantle heterotopia can potentially be confused with closed lip schizencephaly.

Tortori-Donati P and Rossi A. *Pediatric Neuroradiology*, Springer, 2005, pp. 100–138.

27. C. An atlanto-dens interval (ADI) of 6 mm.

There are appearances that are normal for a paediatric cervical spine, which would be considered pathological in an adult and of which it is important to be aware. Pseudo-subluxation at C2/3 and C3/4 is common (it was observed in 46% of patients less than 8 years old at C2/3 in one study and has been seen up to 14 years). The anterior aspects of the spinous processes of C1, C2, and C3 should line up within 1 mm of each other on flexion and extension (assessed by drawing the posterior cervical line, a line from the anterior aspect of the spinous process of C1 to the equivalent point at C3). The anterior aspect of the spinous process of C2 is allowed to pass through, touch, or lie up to 1 mm behind the posterior cervical line in physiological subluxation.

The normal ADI (the distance between the anterior aspect of the dens and the posterior aspect of the ring of the atlas) in adults is 3 mm, but is normal up to 5 mm in children. 'Pseudo-Jefferson' fractures (pseudospread of the lateral masses of C1 on C2) can be seen on the peg view, and up to 6 mm of displacement is common up to 4 years old and may be seen in patients up to 7 years old. Anterior wedging of up to 3 mm of the vertebral bodies should not be confused with compression fracture. This finding can be profound at C3. Prevertebral swelling of 6 mm or less is considered normal at C3. Widening of prevertebral soft tissues in children can be due to expiration, and if suspected, a repeat lateral film in inspiration and mild extension should be performed.

Lustrin ES, Karakas SP, Ortiz AO, Cinnamon J, Castillo M, Vaheeson K et al. Pediatric cervical spine: normal anatomy, variants and trauma. *RadioGraphics* 2003, 23, 539–560.

28. D. Enlarged, calcified adrenals that maintain their normal triangular configuration.

Wolman disease is a rare, autosomal recessive, primary familial xanthomatosis with involvement and calcification of the adrenal glands. Deficiency of acid esterase or acid lipase results in lipid deposition in multiple organs, including the liver, spleen, lymph nodes, adrenal cortex, and small bowel. It has a poor prognosis. Most patients die within 6 months of life due to malabsorption.

All the above-mentioned features are noted in Wolman disease but the most specific finding is enlarged, calcified adrenal glands that maintain their normal configuration.

Fulcher A, Lakshmana Das Narla, and Hingsbergen EA. Pediatric case of the day – Wolman disease (primary familial xanthomatosis with involvement and calcification of the adrenal glands). *RadioGraphics* 1998; 18: 533–535.

29. C. Neonatal hepatitis.

Physiological jaundice of the newborn usually resolves within 2 weeks and thus is unlikely to be the cause in this case. It is also unconjugated, as is jaundice secondary to hypothyroidism. Caroli's disease (type V of the Todani choledochal cyst classification) would typically have an abnormal ultrasound, demonstrating cystic dilatation of the intrahepatic bile ducts.

The key distinction in this question is between biliary atresia and neonatal hepatitis. The question stated that the ultrasound was normal and visualization of a normal-sized gallbladder has been said to favour neonatal hepatitis. However, 20% of patients with biliary atresia may have a normal sized gallbladder, which also empties after a feed. Despite this, in the presence of a suggestive clinical picture, an absent or small gallbladder in the fasting state, a gallbladder with irregular and echogenic walls, or a large gallbladder that does not empty post feed are highly suggestive of biliary atresia. Distinction can be clarified with a HIDA scan. In early biliary atresia prior to cirrhosis, there is rapid extraction of radionuclide from the bloodstream, which persists and accumulates in the hepatic parenchyma with failure of excretion into the gut. Thus, visualization of isotope activity within the gut excludes the diagnosis of biliary atresia. In severe or late biliary atresia, hepatocyte function eventually deteriorates, resulting in sluggish tracer uptake by the hepatocytes. Patients with neonatal hepatitis often have decreased parenchymal extraction and clearance of radioisotope from the bloodstream but tracer does reach the intestines.

Rao P. Neonatal gastrointestinal imaging. *European Journal of Radiology* 2006, 60, 171–186.

30. C. BPD.

Whilst surfactant deficiency is undoubtedly a feature of this case, the evolution of the clinical scenario indicates that a further condition is evolving to explain the findings and clinical condition. In this case the two likeliest conditions are BPD and PIE, both most commonly associated with immature lungs and both of which give bubbly lucencies on radiography. PIE is a feature of air leak phenomena which occur in stiff lungs and is due to either high airway pressure or alveolar overdistention causing passage of gas into the interstitial spaces. It is associated with other airleak phenomena such as pneumopericardium. BPD was originally described to occur in four stages, but the advent of refined ventilation, surfactant, and prophylactic administration of corticosteroids, have changed the typical progression. A complete discussion of these diseases is found in the article referenced below. BPD tends to develop more gradually than PIE (as described in the clinical vignette) and tends to occur later than PIE.

Agrons G, Courtney S, Stocker J, and Markowitz R. Lung disease in premature neonates: radiologic-pathologic correlation. *RadioGraphics* 2005; 25: 1047–1073.

31. C. Sturge Weber syndrome.

The gyriform low T2WI signal corresponds to cortical calcification, which in association with unilateral atrophy and leptomeningeal enhancement is characteristic of Sturge Weber syndrome, one of the neurocutaneous phakomatoses. Other findings include calvarial thickening and choroid plexus angiomas. Associated facial port wine stain in the distribution of the trigeminal nerve is classic.

Pope TL. *Aunt Minnie's Atlas and Imaging-Specific Diagnosis*, 3rd edn, Lippincott Williams & Wilkins, 2009, pp. 263–264.

32. C. Trochlea present before internal epicondyle.

The appearance of the ossification centres can be remembered by using the mnemonic CRITOE (Capitellum, Radial head, Internal epicondyle, Trochlea, Olecranon, and External epicondyle). These appear at years 1, 5, 5, 7, 10, and 11, respectively. This sequence is very important in the recognition of elbow fractures in children. The apparent appearance of the trochlea or olecranon before the internal (also called medial) epicondyle infers avulsion of the internal epicondyle into the joint space to pose as the not yet formed trochlea or olecranon.

Donnelly LF. *Fundamentals of Pediatric Radiology*, 1st edn, Saunders, 2001, pp. 175–176.

33. B. Juvenile granulosa cell tumour.

This is a sex cord stromal tumour arising from the granulose-thecal cells. They typically affect prepubescent girls and are unilateral. They are usually hormonally active (secrete oestrogen), resulting in precocious puberty. Granulosa cell tumours have a varied appearance on imaging. They may be completely solid with or without haemorrhagic or fibrotic changes, multilocular solid/cystic, or a completely cystic neoplasm. On T2WI they have a characteristic sponge-like appearance with innumerable cystic areas in a solid lesion of intermediate signal. Inhibin is the tumour marker used to monitor these lesions.

Sertoli–Leydig cell tumour is also hormonally active, but it results in virilization and hirsutism.

Malignant epithelial neoplasms of the ovaries are extremely rare in prepubertal girls. Mature cystic teratoma is the most common type of ovarian neoplasm in the paediatric age group, containing derivatives of at least two of the three germ cell layers: ectoderm, mesoderm, or endoderm. Fibroma is rare in children.

Epelman M, Chikwava KR, Chauvin N, and Servaes S. Imaging of pediatric ovarian neoplasms. *Pediatric Radiology* 2011; 41(9): 1085–1099.

34. E. Duplication cyst.

The most common location for duplication cysts is in the terminal ileum. This is followed by oesophagus, duodenum, and stomach. Duplication cysts contain both mucosal and muscle layers. On ultrasound, the mucosa is represented by an inner echogenic line and the muscle as an outer hypoechoic layer. The cyst is usually anechoic, unless complicated by haemorrhage or infection.

Lymphangiomas, mesenteric, and omental cysts are rare. On ultrasound, they are usually anechoic, unless complicated by debris, haemorrhage, or infection. The wall is usually thin and does not have the double layer associated with duplication cysts.

Ovarian cysts arise from the pelvis and will not have the layered wall appearance of a duplication cyst.

Rao P. Neonatal gastrointestinal imaging. *European Journal of Radiology* 2006; 60: 171–186.

35. A. Congenital lobar emphysema.

This has a lobar predilection with around 40% being found in the left upper lobe. Congenital lobar emphysema initially presents as an area of soft tissue density due to retained foetal pulmonary fluid. This resolves and is replaced by hyperlucency. Most present in the neonatal period with respiratory distress, but they can present later. Congenital cystic adenomatoid malformations (CCAM) do not show a lobar predilection, but can be found anywhere. They can be either air or fluid filled and consist of multiple cysts. CCAM are graded on the size of the cysts with type 1 lesions containing one or more large cysts, type 2 have numerous small cysts, and type 3 contain microscopic cysts, but appear solid at imaging. Congenital diaphragmatic hernias are also initially solid on plain radiography and only contain air if there is bowel present within the hernia and this contains air. This would obviously have continuity with the diaphragm and not be contained entirely within the upper lobe. Persistent PIE occurs when PIE fails to resolve after 1 week. As PIE is almost always seen in infants with surfactant deficiency being ventilated, it would not be in the differential in this case. Sequestrations are usually solid masses on plain film radiography, unless there has been a history of infection within the sequestration.

Donnelly L. *Fundamentals of Pediatric Radiology*, Saunders, 2001, pp. 35–44.

36. C. Anechoic cystic mass anterior to sternocleidomastoid near the angle of the mandible.

The other options are typical locations for cystic hygroma, infantile haemangioma, thyroglossal cyst, and first branchial cleft cyst, respectively. The majority (75%) of branchial cleft cysts are remnants of the second branchial cleft. Cystic hygromas are lymphatic malformations (lymphangiomas) that result from blockage of lymphatic channels. Most present before 2 years of age. Most are slow growing, but can suddenly enlarge following infection or haemorrhage into the lesion. Infantile haemangiomas usually grow rapidly until 9–10 months of age, followed by spontaneous resolution, which can take up to 10 years. Thyroglossal cysts are remnants of the thyroglossal duct, which extends from the foramen caecum at the base of the tongue to the pyramidal lobe of the thyroid. The majority (65%) are infrahyoid.

Turkington JRA, Paterson A, Sweeney LE, and Thornbury GD. Neck masses in children. *British Journal of Radiology* 2005; 78, 75–85.

37. B. Salter–Harris type 2 injury.

The Salter–Harris classification is used to describe fractures involving the physis when it is not yet fused. Involvement of the growth plate may cause arrest in growth, with the higher Salter–Harris numbers having a greater rate of complications. Type 2 is the most common (75% of physeal injuries). A useful mnemonic is SALTR:

Type 1 Slip: only the physis
Type 2 Above: a metaphyseal fracture extending to the physis, but not involving the epiphysis

Type 3 Low: a fracture involving the epiphysis and physis but not the metaphysis
Type 4 Through: a fracture extending from the metaphysis, through the physis to involve the epiphysis
Type 5 Rammed: CRUSH injury to all or part of the physis

Dähnert W. *Radiology Review Manual*, 5th edn, Lippincott Williams & Wilkins, 2003, pp. 81–83.

38. C. Meckel Gruber syndrome.

All of the mentioned conditions are associated with multiple renal cysts, but the triad of bilateral enlarged cystic kidneys, occipital encephalocele, and polydactyly is diagnostic of Meckel Gruber syndrome. Bardet–Biedl syndrome is associated with enlarged cystic dysplasia of the kidneys with polydactyly.

Gupta P and Jain S. MRI in a fetus with Meckel–Gruber syndrome. *Pediatric Radiology* 2008; 38: 122.
Avni FE and Hall M. Renal cystic diseases in children: new concepts. *Pediatric Radiology* 2010; 40: 939–946.

39. B. Meconium plug syndrome.

This is a transient disorder of the neonatal colon characterized by delayed passage of meconium and proximal dilatation of the bowel. The obstruction is due to a colonic dysmotility and associated with a large meconium plug in the left colon. The colon may appear normal or distended proximal to the plug and small caliber distally. A water-soluble contrast enema is both diagnostic and therapeutic. If there is persistence of abdominal distension and/or failure to evacuate, then rectal biopsy may be needed to exclude Hirschsprung's disease.

Hirschsprung's disease is a disorder of the bowel resulting from absence of normal ganglionic cells in the Auerbach's and Meissner's plexuses. Aganglionosis always affects the rectum and extends proximally for a variable distance. Short segment disease occurs in the vast majority of cases, with the transition zone (the junction between the normal-sized distal aganglionic segment and the proximal dilated bowel) occurring in the region of the rectosigmoid. Contrast enema is used to delineate the level of the transition zone and care must be taken not to overfill the recto-sigmoid and thus mask the transition zone. Irregular, uncoordinated contractions in the aganglionic segment would more commonly be seen in the distal colon in Hirschsprung's disease than in a meconium plug syndrome.

Meconium ileus syndrome is a distal small bowel obstruction secondary to thick inspissated meconium in the ileum, usually associated with CF. Water-soluble contrast enema may be both diagnostic and therapeutic.

A small left colon syndrome is a subtype of meconium plug syndrome. Contrast enema shows an apparent transition zone at the splenic flexure. There is a normal-sized sigmoid colon, but a small descending colon, mimicking a microcolon, which becomes normal sized again around the splenic flexure. The caliber abnormality is therefore limited to the descending colon, which was not described in this case.

Colonic atresia is secondary to a vascular insult in utero and is extremely uncommon. A microcolon exists distal to the atretic segment.

Rao P. Neonatal gastrointestinal imaging. *European Journal of Radiology* 2006; 60: 171–186.

40. E. Extralobar sequestration.

Sequestrations are defined as lung tissue masses with no normal connection to the bronchial tree or pulmonary arteries. This diagnosis can often be difficult to make as extralobar sequestrations are associated with CCAM and congenital diaphragmatic hernia (CDH). The fact that the lesion is contained entirely within the thorax, with no abdominal connection described, means CDH is less likely. CCAM usually derive their blood supply from the pulmonary arteries.

Foregut duplication cysts would be expected to be hypoechoic on ultrasound and non-vascular. The differentiation between intralobar and extralobar sequestrations is more difficult. Previously the venous drainage has been used, with intralobar described as draining to the pulmonary veins and extralobar to systemic veins (IVC or azygous commonly). In actuality, the drainage is variable and the pleural covering the only constant difference, with intralobar having a separate visceral pleural covering, but extralobar having completely separate pleura. Extralobar sequestrations are more common in males and are usually in the left hemithorax (90%). They are also more commonly associated with other congenital abnormalities, such as cardiac malformations.

Berrocal T, Madrid C, Novo S, Gutierrez J, Arjonilla A, and Gomez-Leon N. Congenital anomalies of the tracheobronchial tree, lung and mediastinum: embryology, radiology and pathology. *RadioGraphics* 2003; 24(1): e17.

41. B. Metachromatic leucodystrophy.

Leucodystrophies are dysmyelinating inherited white matter diseases, which are secondary to lysosomal, peroxisomal, or mitochondrial dysfunction. Metachromatic leucodystrophy is caused by deficiency of the lysosomal enzyme ayrlsulfatase A. The 'tigroid' pattern relates to sparing of perivascular white matter.

Table 5.1 outlines characteristic radiological findings of the major leucodystrophies.

Table 5.1 Characteristic radiological findings of the major leucodystrophies

Organelle dysfunction	**Disease**	**Radiological findings**
Lysosome	Metachromatic leucodystrophy	U fibre sparing Perivascular sparing (tigroid pattern)
	Krabbe disease	Thalamic and caudate nuclei high attenuation on CT U fibre sparing
	Mucopolysaccharidosis	Well-defined high T2 signal foci in corpus callosum and basal ganglia
Peroxisome	X-linked adrenoleucodystrophy	Symmetrical peritrigonal and splenium high T2 signal Peripheral contrast enhancement
Mitochondria	MELAS	Multiple cortical and subcortical infarct-like lesions
Unclassified	Canavan disease	U fibres preferentially affected
	Alexander disease	Frontal lobe predilection Subcortical white matter affected early

Data from Cheon J-E, Kim I-O, Hwang YS, Kim KJ, Wang K-C, Cho B-K et al. Leukodystrophy in children: a pictorial review of MR imaging features. *RadioGraphics* 2002; 22: 461–476.

Cheon J-E, Kim I-O, Hwang YS, Kim KJ, Wang K-C, Cho B-K et al. Leukodystrophy in children: a pictorial review of MR imaging features. *RadioGraphics* 2002; 22: 461–476.

42. E. Widening of the joint space.

Explanation given with the answer to question 43.

43. B. Loss of overlap between the medial femoral metaphysis and acetabulum.

Perthes' disease and SUFE, along with transient synovitis and septic arthritis, are important paediatric causes of hip pain. The diagnosis of Perthes' disease and SUFE is usually made initially on plain film and it is important to be able to both pick up the abnormalities and to correctly attribute them to the correct disease process (Table 5.2).

The answer to question 42 is widening of the joint space. This occurs early in Perthes' disease. There is widening of the physis initially in SUFE (in advanced slip the physis can appear narrowed), but loss of joint space rather than widening may occur late in the disease, secondary to chondrolysis. In question 42, answers A, C, and D are also features of SUFE. The line of Klein is the line along the lateral aspect of the proximal femoral metaphysis, which should normally intersect the proximal femoral epiphysis, but does not in SUFE.

The answer to question 43 is loss of overlap between the medial femoral metaphysis and acetabulum. This has been termed the 'metaphyseal extrusion' sign and is a subtle early finding in SUFE. Answers A, D, and E are signs of Perthes' disease, although apparent reduction in size of the femoral epiphysis can occur later in SUFE as the epiphysis slips more posteriorly. Demineralization is not a good discriminating factor. It is more associated with Perthes' disease; it can occur in SUFE, but sclerosis of the proximal metaphysis occurs later (metaphyseal blanch sign).

Table 5.2 Diagnostic features of Perthes' disease and SUFE

	Perthes' disease	SUFE
Demographics	2–12 years, M:F 5:1, previous trauma in 30%	10–14 years, M > F, often overweight
Bilateral?	5–10%	25%
Radiographic features (early to late)	Small, sclerotic femoral epiphysis Widening of joint space Demineralization Subchondral radiolucent crescent Subcortical fracture on frog leg lateral view Fragmentation of femoral head Femoral head cysts Coxa plana, coxa magna	Initial widening and irregularity of physis Demineralization can occur early but sclerosis occurs later Metaphyseal extrusion sign (see above) Line of Klein abnormal Frank slip (easier seen with frog leg lateral) which can produce narrowing of physis on AP film

Data from: Hubbard AM. Imaging of pediatric hip disorders. *Radiologic Clinics of North America* 2001; 39: 721–732. Data from Dähnert W. *Radiology Review Manual*, 5th edn, Lippincott Williams & Wilkins, 2003, pp. 49, 71–72.

Hubbard AM. Imaging of pediatric hip disorders. *Radiologic Clinics of North America* 2001; 39: 721–732.
Dähnert W. *Radiology Review Manual*, 5th edn, Lippincott Williams & Wilkins, 2003, pp. 49, 71–72.

44. A. Inguinal canal.

The testes form in the retroperitoneum and descend through the inguinal canal into the scrotum. Failure to descend is known as cryptorchidism. A cryptorchid testis may be located at any point along the descent route. The most common location is the inguinal canal (70% of cases) followed by the prescrotal region, just beyond the superficial inguinal ring. On ultrasound, it is usually smaller and hypo or isoechoic compared to the normally located testis. Cryptorchidism is associated with an increased risk of malignancy even after correction.

Aso C, Enriquez G, Fite M, Toran N, Piro C, Piqueras J et al. Gray-scale and color Doppler sonography of scrotal disorders in children: an update. *RadioGraphics* 2005; 25: 1197–1214.

45. D. Hepatoblastoma.

This is the most common primary malignant hepatic tumour in children (approximately 80%). Most cases occur below the age of 3 years. Serum alphafetoprotein is elevated in 70–90%. The imaging features are as described. Calcification is seen in approximately 50%.

HCC is the next most common malignant liver tumour and has two peaks in childhood, at 2–4 years and 12–14 years. Serum alphafetoprotein is also elevated in approximately 80%. Imaging features are similar to those seen in an adult population, i.e. larger tumours are of heterogeneous echogenicity on ultrasound and on biphasic CT they show arterial enhancement with rapid washout on the portal venous phase.

Undifferentiated embryonal sarcoma (UES) is the third most common liver malignancy and is most common between the ages of 6 and 10 years. Serum alphafetoprotein levels are normal. The imaging hallmark of this tumour is the discrepancy between its appearance on ultrasound and that on CT. Ultrasound is used to confirm the solid nature of this tumour, which typically is isoechoic or hyperechoic. On CT, UES is seen as a well-circumscribed, multiseptate, fluid-attenuating lesion. Enhancement of solid-appearing septa and a pseudocapsule may be seen.

Mesenchymal hamartoma is the second most common benign hepatic lesion (to haemangioendothelioma). It is usually seen under the age of 2 years. Serum alphafetoprotein is not elevated. The typical ultrasound appearance is a multiseptate, cystic mass. Less commonly, the solid component of the lesion can be more predominant, with multiple smaller cysts giving the lesion a Swiss-cheese appearance. The usual CT finding is of a multilocular cystic mass with enhancing septa of varying thickness.

Angiosarcoma is not usually seen in children, but is a rare, highly vascular and highly malignant, hepatic tumour of adults.

Das CJ, Dhingra S, Gupta AK, Lyer V, and Agarwala S. Imaging of paediatric liver tumours with pathological correlation. *Clinical Radiology* 2009; 64: 1015–1025.

46. A. Send them home and reassure the parents.

This radiograph has all the classic hallmarks of a viral pneumonia in a child. Air-trapping is common due to the small airways, which become occluded secondary to peribronchial wall oedema. There is no focal consolidation or pleural effusion seen, features that would indicate a bacterial pneumonia requiring antibiotics. In children it is not necessary to repeat imaging to ensure appearances resolve as long as the symptoms settle. Bilateral inhaled foreign bodies, causing the bilateral air-trapping, would be very unusual, especially in a well child. Respiratory consult would only be indicated if the symptoms failed to settle or there was a significant associated history, e.g. CF.

Donnelly L. *Fundamentals of Pediatric Radiology*, Saunders, 2001, pp. 44–52.

47. B. Sagittal suture.

Craniosynostosis refers to premature closing of sutures and is often present at birth. It may be primary or secondary to bone dysplasias or haemoglobinopathy, or as part of a generalized syndrome. Scaphocephaly is the most common craniosynostosis and results in a long skull. Brachycephaly arises from bilateral closure of the coronal suture, resulting in a short, tall skull. Unilateral fusion of the lambdoid suture is seen in plagiocephaly, giving a lopsided skull. Trigonocephaly is a forward-pointing skull from premature closure of the metopic suture. Intrauterine closure of coronal, sagittal and lambdoid sutures gives rise to the cloverleaf skull, which may be associated with thanatophoric dysplasia.

Dahnert W. *Radiology Review Manual*, 6th edn, Lippincott Williams & Wilkins, 2007, p. 178.

48. C. Bell clapper deformity predisposes to testicular torsion.

Testicular torsion is an emergency. If it is not corrected within 6 hours, testicular salvage is less likely. Torsion results initially in venous obstruction followed by arterial obstruction. The severity of testicular ischemia depends on the duration and the degree of torsion (180–720°). Clinical differentiation between testicular torsion and epididymo-orchitis can be challenging.

Two types are described: intravaginal and extravaginal. 'Bell clapper' deformity is the term used to describe high attachment of the tunica vaginalis to the spermatic cord that leaves the testis free to rotate.

On ultrasound, the affected testis may have normal echogenicity in the early phase. In the later phase, the testis enlarges and demonstrates increased or heterogenous echogenicity. An enlarged and torted spermatic cord may be visualized. Absence of blood flow in the affected testis, with normal flow on the asymptomatic side, is most specific for torsion. Some arterial flow may persist in incomplete torsion (less than 360°). Decreased or reversed diastolic flow on pulsed-wave Doppler assessment assists in the diagnosis in such cases.

Aso C, Enriquez G, Fite M, Toran N, Piro C, Piqueras J et al. Gray-scale and color Doppler sonography of scrotal disorders in children: an update. *RadioGraphics* 2005; 25: 1197–1214.

49. E. A pyloric channel length of 12 mm.

Ultrasound is the primary imaging modality used for the diagnosis of hypertrophic pyloric stenosis, although the criteria are generally applied to infants of 6 weeks and older. These include muscle thickness >3 mm, pyloric channel length >14 mm, pyloric thickness (serosa to serosa) >10 mm, failure of the pylorus to open with pyloric elongation and displacement, as well as retrograde or hyperperistaltic gastric contractions. A pyloric ratio, which is the ratio of the wall thickness to the pyloric diameter, above 0.27 is stated to be 96% sensitive for the diagnosis. The standard measurements above are not always applicable to neonates and real-time assessment to look for passage of fluid from the stomach into the duodenum becomes more important.

Rao P. Neonatal gastrointestinal imaging. *European Journal of Radiology* 2006; 60: 171–186.

50. B. Persistent PIE.

Although alluded to in the clinical scenario, this should not be assumed to be the most likely diagnosis in the absence of the CT findings, as this is an extremely uncommon condition. The CT findings provide the diagnosis due to the linear densities within the cystic cavities representing the bronchopulmonary bundle surrounded by air within the interstitial space. This appearance is seen in over 80% of cases. The abnormality is often confined to a single lobe, but can be more widespread. Current optimal management is debated. Lesions increasing in size are thought to be best treated with surgical resection, with stable lesions often resolving over time with conservative management.

Donnelly L, Lacaya J, Ozelame V, Frush D, Strouse P, Sumner T, and Paltiel H. CT findings and temporal course of persistent pulmonary interstitial emphysema in neonates: a multi-institutional study. *American Journal of Roentgenology* 2003; 180(4): 1129–1133.

51. A. Multiple flow voids within the basal ganglia bilaterally.

The history and ethnic origin of the patient suggest moyamoya syndrome. This is an idiopathic progressive arteriopathy of childhood resulting in narrowing of the distal internal carotid arteries and lenticulostriate collateralization. This collateralization causes the multiple basal ganglia flow voids, likened to a 'puff of smoke' (moyamoya in Japanese) on angiography. Secondary causes of moyamoya collateralization include neurofibromatosis type 1, post-radiation therapy and sickle cell anaemia. Irregular beading of the extracranial internal carotid arteries is seen in fibromuscular dysplasia.

Osborn AG, Blaser SI, Salzman KL, Katzman GL, Provenzale J, Castillo M et al. *Diagnostic Imaging: Brain*, Amirsys, 2004, I-4: 42–45.

52. B. Osteochondritis dissecans.

This disease is thought to represent a fracture secondary to avascular necrosis of an area of subchondral bone and cartilage, and peak incidence is at 12–13 years of age. Repetitive trauma, ischaemia, and familial tendency are common predisposing factors. In the knee, 75% of cases involve the postero-Lateral Aspect of the MEdial femoral condyle, hence the mnemonic LAME. The disease is bilateral in one-third of patients. A purely cartilaginous fragment will go unrecognized on plain film; a bony fragment and its donor site will not. Instability on MRI is suggested by fragments >1 cm, cysts larger than 5 mm within the donor site, high T2WI signal between the donor site and fragment (even if the cartilage is intact), and loose bodies within the joint.

Distal femoral cortical irregularity (also referred to as cortical desmoid) is seen as a defect in the posterior aspect of the medial cortex of the distal femoral metaphysis, 1–2 cm proximal to the physis (at the attachment of adductor magnus). It appears low signal on T1WI and high signal on T2WI sequences. Plain film may show an ill-defined or scalloped appearance and may occasionally mimic an aggressive lesion (it is benign).

Sinding–Larsen–Johanssen disease represents osteochondrosis at the site of attachment of the patellar tendon to the patella (inferior pole). Osgood–Schlatter disease represents apophysitis at the site of attachment of the patellar tendon to the tibia, namely the anterior tibial tubercle. Both are causes of knee pain and are associated with activity and repetitive traction microtrauma.

An avulsion of the anterior tibial spine is the paediatric equivalent of an ACL tear (the chondro-osseous tibial spine is the weakest part of the ACL complex prior to physeal closure). MRI reveals a low signal T1WI line through the anterior tibial spine.

Sanchez R and Strouse PJ. The knee: MR imaging of uniquely pediatric disorders. *Radiologic Clinics of North America* 2009; 47: 1009–1025.

53. C. The pudendal nerve and internal pudendal vessels pass through the lesser sciatic foramen.

There are several potential pathways of extrapelvic spread of pelvic disease. Lateral extension into the gluteal region occurs through the sciatic foramina. It is important to identify extrapelvic spread, as combined trans-abdominal and trans-gluteal surgery may be required. Knowledge of gluteal anatomy is also essential for trans-gluteal biopsy and drainages.

The greater and lesser sciatic notches are noted in the posterior border of the innominate bone separated by the ischial spine.

The greater sciatic foramen (GSF) is bounded antero-superiorly by the greater sciatic notch, postero-superiorly by the sacrum, and inferiorly by the sacrospinous ligament. The piriformis muscle arises from the ventral aspect of the sacrum and passes through the GSF to insert into the greater trochanter. It divides the GSF into two compartments. The suprapiriformis foramen transmits the superior gluteal vessels and nerves. The infrapiriformis foramen transmits the inferior gluteal vessels and nerves, pudendal and sciatic nerves.

The lesser sciatic foramen (LSF) is bounded anteriorly by the lesser sciatic notch, superiorly by the sacrospinous ligament, and postero-inferiorly by the sacrotuberous ligament. The obturator internus tendon, the pudendal nerve, and the internal pudendal vessels pass through the LSF.

Tan CH, Vikram R, Boonsirikamchai P, Faria SC, Charnsangavej C, and Bhosale PR. Pathways of extrapelvic spread of pelvic disease: Imaging findings. *RadioGraphics* 2011; 31: 117–133.

54. C. The umbilical cord inserting at the apex of the hernia.

Omphalocele is the total failure of the midgut to return to the peritoneal cavity during the tenth week of gestation. The contents may vary from a single loop of small bowel to the entire GI tract, including the liver. An omphalocele can be differentiated from a gastroschisis (rupture of the abdominal wall) because in an omphalocele, the herniated structures are covered by peritoneum and amnion, and the umbilical cord inserts at its apex. In gastroschisis, there is a normally positioned umbilicus and the hernia is through a paraumbilcal defect. Because this (probably ischaemic) rupture of the abdominal wall occurs after the bowel has returned to the peritoneal cavity, the protruding viscera are not covered in peritoneum. The contents of the hernia in gastroschisis include stomach, midgut, and occasionally portions of the urinary tract. In omphalocele, there may be associated congenital cardiac anomalies and there is also an association with Beckwith Wiedeman syndrome. There is a low incidence of additional anomalies in gastroschisis.

Blickman H. *Pediatric Radiology: The Requisites*, 2nd edn, Mosby, 1998, Ch 4.

55. C. Pulmonary valve hypoplasia with a VSD and overriding aorta.

These are the features of tetralogy of Fallot. Even in the absence of radiology this represents the most common form of congenital cyanotic heart disease. To help characterize congenital heart disease there are a number of features to note on the radiograph as well as clinically. The presence of cyanosis excludes coarctation, which does not cause cyanosis. Truncus arteriosus (and total anomalous pulmonary venous return (TAPVR)) are associated with increased pulmonary flow, not reduced, as present in this case. Pulmonary valve atresia with an intact ventricular septum does have reduced pulmonary flow, but would present earlier than four days and the heart is typically grossly enlarged, as in this anomaly there is no forward flow of blood out of the right ventricle. D-transposition of the great arteries is classically described as giving an egg-on-a-string appearance due to the narrowed superior mediastinum caused by the abnormal rotation of the great vessels. This appearance is seldom seen as D-transposition presents early with cyanosis and is surgically corrected. The most common CXR appearance in an infant is a normal CXR. The pulmonary vascularity on the radiograph is either normal or increased, not decreased.

Donnelly L. *Fundamentals of Pediatric Radiology*, Saunders, 2001, pp. 74–92.

56. B. Calcification.

This is the most specific feature of retinoblastoma and is apparent in 95% of cases. Other features of retinoblastoma include hyperattenuating mass extending into the vitreous and secondary retinal detachment. Contrast enhancement is seen in <30% of cases. The globe is normal sized. The non-neoplastic causes of leucocoria, the so-called pseudoretinoblastomas, include persistent hyperplastic primary vitreous (PHPV), Coat's disease, and toxocara endophthalmitis. CT findings in PHPV include micro-opthalmia and an enhancing retrolental mass. Coat's disease is a vascular malformation of the retina and presents with a hyperattenuating globe and an enhancing subretinal exudate on CT. CT features of toxocara are non-specific and similar to Coat's disease. Secondary retinal detachment may be seen. None of the pseudoretinoblastomas exhibit calcification.

Chung EM, Specht CS, and Schoeder JW. Pediatric orbit tumors and tumorlike lesions: neuroepithelial lesions of the ocular globe and optic nerve. *RadioGraphics* 2007, 27, 1159–1186.

57. C. Posterior dislocation and medial epicondyle fracture.

The elbow is the most commonly dislocated joint in children (in adults the shoulder and interphalangeal joints are more common). A supracondylar fracture of the elbow is more common in children (65% of elbow fractures) than in adults, who generally suffer a radial head injury (50%). However, in both groups of patients, if dislocation occurs it tends to be posterior dislocation of the radial head and ulna with respect to the distal humerus (85–90%). The most common fracture seen in association with elbow dislocation in children is a fracture of the medial epicondyle or separation of the medial epicondyle. The second most common fracture involves the radial head and neck. In terms of total paediatric elbow fractures, those involving the lateral epicondyle (15%) are next most common after the supracondylar fracture; medial epicondyle fractures comprise approximately 10%.

Rogers LF. *Radiology of Skeletal Trauma*, 3rd edn, Churchill Livingstone, 2001, pp. 683–778.
Manaster BJ, May DA, and Disler DG. *Musculoskeletal Imaging: The Requisites*, 3rd edn, Mosby, 2007, pp. 117–125.

58. A. Congenital megacalyces

This is a rare developmental abnormality of the renal medulla. Imaging demonstrates dilated, multifaceted, or polygonal calyces as opposed to spherical calyces of obstructive hydronephrosis. In addition, the infundibula, renal pelvis, and ureter are normal in calibre in congenital hydronephrosis. The affected kidneys may demonstrate cortical thinning but the renal function is preserved.

Bekele W and Sanchez TR. Congenital megacalyces presenting as neonatal hydronephrosis. *Pediatric Radiology* 2010; 40: 1579.

59. C. Pancreatic duct dilatation.

In cases of acute pancreatitis in children, the echogenicity of the pancreas on ultrasound is not a helpful diagnostic feature and pancreatic enlargement is absent in 50% of the patients. The most useful diagnostic feature is dilatation of the pancreatic duct (>1.5 mm at 1–6 years of age, >1.9 mm at 7–12 years, and >2.2 mm at 13–18 years).

Pancreatic ductal dilatation may also be seen in chronic pancreatitis. Pancreatic atrophy and parenchymal calcifications are more typically associated with chronic disease.

Nievelstein RAJ, Robben SGF, and Blickman JG. Hepatobiliary and pancreatic imaging in children – techniques and overview of non-neoplastic disease entities. *Pediatric Radiology* 2011; 41: 55–75.

60. B. Type B.

Tracheoesophageal fistulae are classed depending on the communications present between the trachea and the oesophagus. In types A–D the mid-portion of the oesophagus is absent. Type A are not truly fistulae, but consist of an absence of the mid-portion of the oesophagus. In type B the proximal oesophageal bud communicates with the trachea and in type C it is the distal bud that has a tracheal fistula. Type C is the most common subtype. Both proximal and distal buds have fistulous connections with the trachea in type D. Type E (or H type) tracheoesophageal fistulae have complete trachea and oesophagus with a fistulous connection between them resembling the letter H.

Dahnert W. *Radiology Review Manual*, 6th edn, Lippincott Williams & Wilkins, 2007, 806–808.

61. C. Langerhans cell histiocytosis (LCH).

The radiographic description is typical for skull involvement in LCH. The bevelled edge results from uneven destruction of the inner and outer skull tables. They are more likely to present with pain than any other lesion. Marginal sclerosis may be seen with healing lesions. Epidermoids are oval-shaped lytic lesions, but tend to have sclerotic margins. Neuroblastoma metastases are also lytic lesions, but with a sunburst periosteal reaction. Sutural diastasis may be seen due to dural involvement. Haemangiomas exhibit a coarse trabecular pattern radiating from an oval defect. Osteomas appear as a dense homogenous focus.

Willatt JMG and Quaghebeur G. Calvarial masses of infants and children. a radiological approach. *Clinical Radiology* 2004; 59: 474–486.

62. E. None of the above.

The correct answer is to do nothing. This is the classical description of a non-ossifying fibroma (NOF). These and fibrous cortical defects are common in children and adolescents, and are usually a painless, incidental finding. They are eccentric, well-defined, cortically-based lesions with marginal sclerosis. They can be expansile. They are most common in the femur and tibia. Fibrous cortical defects measure less than 2 cm whereas NOFs are larger. They routinely heal by sclerosis and disappear. An IBS can show uptake during healing and a CT scan can show apparent cortical breakthrough. Thus the correct management is to do nothing. If there are atypical features, such as pain or periostitis, then additional investigation is indicated.

Helms C. *Fundamentals of Skeletal Radiology*, 3rd edn, Elsevier, 2005, 16–17.

63. B. CF.

Bilateral seminal vesicle agenesis is frequently associated with bilateral agenesis of the vas deferens and mutations in the CF transmembrane conductance regulator gene (64–73%). It is thought to be related to luminal obstruction by thick secretions. Bilateral agenesis of the vas deferens is seen in 99% of CF in males. The affected patients usually have normal kidneys.

Unilateral seminal vesicle agenesis and seminal vesicle cyst are commonly associated with ipsilateral renal agenesis. Bilateral calcified vas deferens is commonly seen in diabetics.

Kim B, Kawashima A, Ryu J, Takahashi J Hartman RP, and King BF Jr. Imaging of the seminal vesicle and vas deferens. *RadioGraphics* 2009; 29: 1105–1121.

64. C. Water-soluble contrast enema.

This is rarely, if ever, indicated in the acute phase of necrotizing enterocolitis (NEC). It may be used for the evaluation of the presence of strictures, usually approximately 6–12 months after the acute phase of NEC.

Supine AXR is the primary method used to evaluate NEC. A 'jumbled' pattern may be seen secondary to bowel wall oedema, which either compresses the lumen in some areas or causes an ileus appearance in other areas. Pneumatosis may be seen, which is either 'bubbly' or linear. This can lead to air in the portal venous system, which does not appear to alter the morbidity or mortality.

Perforation may occur and this may be demonstrated on the supine AXR by Rigler's sign (air on both sides of the bowel wall) or the 'football sign' (air outlining the falciform ligament). The left lateral decubitus and supine cross-table AXRs may both be used to detect small quantities of free air.

Abdominal ultrasound may be helpful in the acute setting of NEC, as it can depict intra-abdominal fluid, bowel wall thickening, assess bowel wall perfusion, and may also detect small quantities of free air and portal venous gas.

Epelman M, Daneman A, Navarro OM, Morag I, Moore AM, Kim JH, Faingold R, Taylor G, and Gerstle JT. Necrotizing enterocolitis: review of state of the art imaging findings with pathologic correlation. *RadioGraphics* 2007; 27: 285–305.

65. B. Partial anomalous pulmonary venous return (PAPVR).

This most commonly involves the right superior pulmonary vein, but in this case involves the inferior vein. This condition may remain asymptomatic for a number of years, depending on the amount of blood that returns anomalously. PAPVR can drain into the superior vena cava (SVC), right atrium, or IVC on the right and into the brachocephalic vein or coronary sinus on the left.

Scimitar syndrome is a subtype of PAPVR that is associated with ipsilateral lung hypoplasia (hence alternative name hypogenetic lung syndrome) and occasionally dextrocardia. As noted in the history, the lungs were normal. Extralobar sequestrations have aberrant pulmonary arterial supply, not present in this case. Total anomalous pulmonary venous return presents in the neonatal period, commonly with cyanosis and plethora on CXR. Patient survival depends on the presence of an ASD or PDA. No atrial abnormalities were noted to indicate cor triatriatum, although this is another disorder in the spectrum of pulmonary venous developmental anomalies.

Dillman J, Yarram S, and Hernandez R. Imaging of pulmonary venous developmental anomalies. *American Journal of Roentgenology* 2009; 192(5): 1272–1285.

66. D. Pleomorphic adenoma.

This is the most common benign salivary gland tumour in children and usually appears in later childhood or adolescence. The tumour originates in the parotid gland in up to 90% of cases. Haemangiomas are the next most common benign lesion. They are usually seen in the first 6 months of life and have a female predilection. They are hypoechoic and display a variable degree of abnormal vasculature. Parotitis is usually due to mumps and results in a tender gland, which is diffusely enlarged with a heterogenous echotexture on ultrasound. Warthin tumour is a well-circumscribed cystic solid lesion, usually towards the tail of the parotid gland. It is the most common lesion to manifest as multifocal or bilateral masses. Primary lymphoma of the salivary glands is rare, but most often involves the parotid. Ultrasound will show an enlarged, diffusely infiltrated gland.

Garcia CJ, Flores PA, Arce JD, Chuaqui B, and Schwartz DS. Ultrasonography in the study of salivary gland lesions in children. *Pediatric Radiology* 1998; 28: 418–425.
Lowe LH, Stokes LS, Johnson JE, Heller RM, Royal SA, Wushensky C et al. Swelling at the angle of the mandible: imaging of the pediatric parotid gland and periparotid region. *RadioGraphics* 2001; 21: 1211–1227.

67. D. Diaphyseal aclasia.

The description is classic for multiple hereditary osteochondromas/exostoses, also known as diaphyseal aclasia.

Osteochondromas are the result of displaced growth plate cartilage, which causes lateral bone growth from the metaphysis. They typically point away from the epiphysis. There is continuity of the normal marrow, cortex, and periosteum between the exostosis and the host bone. The cartilage cap, which is the source of growth, may have some chondoid matrix, but the appearance is otherwise of a deformed but normal bone. They are normally found in the extremities, with 36% around the knee. Their growth normally ceases at skeletal maturity.

Symptoms are related to pressure effects on adjacent neural or vascular structures. Less than 1% of solitary osteochondromas undergo malignant transformation to chondrosarcoma. Findings that should alert to this are destruction of exostosis bone, destruction of matrix in the cartilage cap, irregular or thick (>2 cm in adults, >3 cm in children) cap, or growth of the cap after skeletal maturity.

Multiple hereditary osteochondromatosis is an uncommon autosomal dominant condition. Patients present with multiple osteochondromas, which cause short stature. The elbow and wrist joints are often deformed. There is a higher risk of malignant transformation than in solitary osteochondromas, probably 2–5%.

Ollier disease is the presence of multiple enchondromas and Mafucci syndrome requires, in addition, multiple soft-tissue haemangiomas. Morquio and Hunter syndromes are mucopolysaccharidoses, with their own musculoskeletal abnormalities, which often make an appearance in exams.

Manaster BJ, May DA, and Disler DG. *Musculoskeletal Imaging: The Requisites*, 3rd edn, Mosby, 2007, pp. 445–450.
Wootton-Gorges SL. MR imaging of primary bone tumours and tumour-like conditions in children. *Radiologic Clinics of North America* 2009; 47: 957–975.

68. C. Intercornual distance of more than 4 cm.

Incomplete fusion of the Mullerian ducts results in bicornuate uterus. MRI demonstrates divergent uterine horns with an external fundal cleft that is more than 1 cm deep and an intercornual distance of more than 4 cm. In bicornuate bicollis uterus, two separate cervical canals are seen. This is distinguished from uterus didelphys by a greater degree of fusion between the horns in the lower uterine segment.

Septate uterus results from incomplete septal resorption following Mullerian duct fusion. It is the most common uterine anomaly (55%). At MRI, the external fundal countour may be convex, flat, or minimally concave (less than 1 cm deep). MRI is also useful in characterizing the type (fibrous/muscular) and extent of the septum. Differentiation between bicornuate and septate uterus is important, as septate uterus is amenable to surgical management.

Steinkeler JA, Woodfiled CA, Lazarus E, and Hillstrom MM. Female infertility: a systematic approach to radiologic imaging and diagnosis. *RadioGraphics* 2009; 29: 1353–1370.

69. B. Gastric mucosa.

The most sensitive and specific evaluation for a Meckel's diverticulum is a ^{99m}Tc pertectnetate scan. This is positive only if gastric mucosa is present (in approximately 20% of patients). However, ectopic gastric mucosa is present in nearly all cases of Meckel's diverticulum that bleed, as it is the ulcerated ectopic gastric mucosa that is the source of the haemorrhage. Ectopic pancreatic and colonic mucosa can occur in a Meckel's divericulum, but are not typically associated with haemorrhage. Ectopic thyroid tissue is not usually found in a Meckel's diverticulum.

Other complications of a Meckel's diverticulum include obstruction (either volvulus or intussusception) and diverticulitis.

Blickman H. *Pediatric Radiology: The Requisites*, 2nd edn, Mosby, 1998, Ch 4.

70. D. Thymic/nodal malignant infiltration.

The first step in this question is to localize the lesion. The posterior displacement of the trachea indicates an anterior mediastinal position. It is then necessary to consider the common causes of anterior mediastinal masses in children, which are: normal thymus and thymic/nodal infiltration (leukaemia, lymphoma), with other causes (lymphangioma and teratoma) being much less common. A normal thymus would not be expected to cause significant posterior displacement of the trachea. On plain film it would not be possible to differentiate thymic infiltration from anterior mediastinal nodal infiltration. TB in children would be uncommon in the anterior mediastinum, especially when no abnormality is noted in the hila.

Adam A and Dixon A. *Grainger and Allison's Diagnostic Radiology. A textbook of medical imaging, Vol 2*, 5th edn, Churchill Livingstone, 2008, Ch 64.

71. E. Delayed sulcation.

Signs of ACC include absence of the cavum septum pellucidum, colpocephaly, high-riding third ventricle, and widening of the inter-hemispheric fissure. ACC is reported to be isolated in <10% on foetal MR imaging. Sulcation delay is present in most foetuses with ACC (particularly those imaged at <30 weeks gestation), including those with good neurodevelopmental outcome, implying a global white matter dysgenesis. Periventricular nodular heterotopia and parenchymal T2WI signal hypointensity are usually seen in association with abnormal sulcal morphology. Associated posterior fossa abnormalities are also common, with cerebellar hemispheric abnormalities seen more than abnormalities of the vermis. Brainstem abnormalities typically occur in association with a cerebellar abnormality.

Tang PH, Bartha AI, Norton ME, Barkovich AJ, Sherr EH, and Glenn OA. Agenesis of the corpus callosum: an MR imaging analysis of associated abnormalities in the fetus. *American Journal of Neuroradiology* 2009; 30: 257–263.

72. B. Achondroplasia.

This question tests knowledge of the severe skeletal dysplasias. Achondroplasia is the most common cause of dwarfism and is hereditary. The humeri and femora are more profoundly affected than the other long bones, although the entire skeleton is abnormal. Narrowing of the interpedicular distance as one progresses caudally down the spine is unique to this condition. Other features include a large skull with a small skull base, square iliac wings with a 'champagne-glass' pelvic cavity, and widened metaphyses.

Thanatophoric dysplasia results in early death. Features include severe platyspondyly and 'telephone receiver' femora. Chondrodysplasia punctata results in stippled epiphysis and rhizomelic dwarfism. Jeune syndrome (asphyxiating thoracic dystrophy) results in respiratory distress, very short ribs, metaphyseal irregularity/beaking, and trident acetabulum. Cleidocranial dysplasia is characterized by lack of development of the pubic bones bilaterally. There is also absence or hypoplasia of the clavicles and the presence of wormian bones in the skull.

Markowitz RL and Zackai E. A pragmatic approach to the diagnosis of pediatric syndromes and skeletal dysplasias. *Radiologic Clinics of North America* 2001; 39: 791–802.
Donnelly LF. *Fundamentals of Pediatric Radiology*, Saunders, 2001, pp. 197–199.

73. A. Enlarged ovary.

Ovarian torsion can occur in all age groups, with the highest prevalence in the reproductive age group. Large heavy cysts and cystic neoplasms commonly predispose to ovarian torsion. Torsion of normal ovaries is unusual but more common in adolescents. Clinical symptoms are often non-specific and therefore imaging is routinely requested.

On ultrasound, an enlarged ovary is the most constant finding. The enlarged ovary may be heterogenous due to haemorrhage and oedema. Other findings include multiple small cysts aligned in the periphery of the enlarged ovary (string of pearls sign), coexistent mass, pelvic free fluid, and twisted ovarian pedicle. Benign cystic teratoma is the most common tumour predisposed to ovarian torsion.

Absent arterial flow is described as the classic colour Doppler finding. However, the most frequent Doppler finding is decreased or absent venous flow with or without reduced arterial flow. A twisted ovarian pedicle with a 'whirlpool' sign is a useful finding on colour Doppler.

Chang HC, Bhatt S, and Dogra VS. Pearls and pitfalls in diagnosis of ovarian torsion. *RadioGraphics* 2008; 28: 1355–1368.

74. E. Peutz–Jehger's syndrome.

This is an autosomal dominant disease with incomplete penetrance characterized by intestinal polyposis and mucocutaneous pigmentation. It is the most frequent of the polyposis syndromes to involve the small intestine. When symptomatic, the most common presentation is abdominal pain (due to small bowel intussusception in up to 50%). There may also be GI haemorrhage. There is an increased risk of malignancy of the GI tract, pancreas, and breast, even though the polyps are hamartomas.

Cronkhite–Canada syndrome is non-neoplastic, non-hereditary inflammatory polyposis associated with ectodermal abnormalities. It usually occurs in the middle-aged to elderly and the polyps are more common in the stomach and colon than in the small bowel. Intussusception is not a typical presentation.

Gardner syndrome is an autosomal dominant disease characterized by a triad of colonic polyposis, osteomas, and soft-tissue tumours (including desmoid tumours). Age at presentation is 15–30 years. The location of the polyps is colon (100%), duodenum (90%), stomach (5–58%), and the remainder of the small bowel (<5%). Small bowel intussusception is therefore a very rare presentation. There is a very high risk of malignant transformation of the colonic polyps if left untreated. Treatment is prophylactic total colectomy.

Familial adenomatous polyposis syndrome is an autosomal dominant disease. The polyps start to appear around puberty and have a similar distribution/location to those in Gardner syndrome. Again there is a high risk of malignant transformation of these adenomatous polyps.

Cowden disease is multiple hamartoma syndrome. It causes hamartomatous neoplasms of the skin and mucosa, GI tract, bones, CNS, eyes, and genitourinary tract. There may be associated malignant tumours of the breast and thyroid.

Dahnert W. *Radiology Review Manual*, 3rd edn, Williams and Wilkins, 1996, Ch Gastrointestinal Tract.

75. A. Posterior rib fracture.

Metaphyseal corner fractures (or bucket handle fractures) and posterior rib fractures are the most specific for NAI. The other injuries given in the stem are also worrisome for NAI, particularly when observed in infants. Posterior rib fractures are sometimes relatively occult on plain film and scintigraphy is more sensitive. They occur when the chest is squeezed tightly, e.g. when a child is shaken. Shaking can also result in a thoraco-lumbar compression fracture. Spiral fractures of long bones are suspicious in infants, but in ambulatory children the 'toddler's' spiral fracture of the tibia is common and often has no memorable preceding trauma.

Duodenal haematoma and jejunal perforation are both recognized sequelae of NAI: the small bowel is the most injured organ in child abuse.

Lonergan GJ, Baker AM, Morey MK, and Boos SC. Child abuse: radiologic-pathologic correlation. *RadioGraphics* 2003; 23: 811–845.

chapter 6

CENTRAL NERVOUS AND HEAD AND NECK

QUESTIONS

1. **A 9-year-old male presents to the paediatric A&E department with a history of increasing drowsiness over the last 24 hours. Neurological assessment reveals that there is absence of upward gaze. A CT brain is requested which reveals hydrocephalus, with marked dilatation of the lateral and third ventricles. The fourth ventricle is unremarkable and there is obliteration of the ambient cistern due to mass effect from a hyperdense mass noted posterior to the third ventricle. This mass has some central areas of calcification. There is no evidence of haemorrhage. An MRI is carried out following insertion of a shunt to decompress the ventricles. On sagittal sequences a lesion is located between the splenium of the corpus callosum and the tectal plate, which exerts mass effect. This lesion is of intermediate signal intensity on both T1WI and T2WI, and displays avid contrast enhancement. Enhancing meningeal lesions are also noted in the spinal cord, indicating seeding. What is the most likely diagnosis?**

   A. Pituitary teratoma.
   B. Meningioma.
   C. Pineoblastoma.
   D. Germinoma.
   E. Pineal cyst.

2. **A patient presents with recent onset neurological symptoms suspicious of an acute presentation of multiple sclerosis (MS). Which of the following anatomical sites of plaque involvement is least consistent with this?**

   A. Corpus callosum.
   B. Spine involvement in the absence of brain involvement.
   C. Cerebral cortex.
   D. Symmetrical involvement of cerebral white matter.
   E. Floor of the fourth ventricle.

3. A 45-year-old female patient is referred to you with a history of mild confusion and new onset seizures. This patient has a history of breast cancer and is currently undergoing chemotherapy following a wide local excision with axillary radiotherapy. The patient has a low-grade pyrexia and a low neutrophil count. An MRI reveals a solitary lesion in the right frontal lobe, which is low/intermediate signal on T1WI and high signal on T2WI. The lesion demonstrates ring enhancement. Diffusion-weighted imaging (DWI) reveals slightly increased signal on B1000 imaging, with increased signal on B0 imaging, and this area is bright on the apparent diffusion coefficient (ADC) map. What is the most likely diagnosis?

A. Abscess.
B. Metastasis.
C. Glioblastoma multiforme.
D. Infarct.
E. Radiotherapy change.

4. A 69-year-old lady was admitted 10 days ago following an acute intracerebral haematoma diagnosed on CT. What are the most likely radiological findings on the follow-up MRI scan of brain?

A. Haematoma hypointense to grey matter on T1WI, hyperintense on T2WI.
B. Haematoma hyperintense to grey matter on both T1WI and T2WI.
C. Haematoma hyperintense to grey matter on T1WI, hypointense on T2WI.
D. Haematoma hypointense to grey matter on both T1WI and T2WI.
E. Haematoma isointense to grey matter on both T1WI and T2WI.

5. A 40-year-old man is being investigated by the neurologists for new onset epilepsy. An electroencephalogram (EEG) indicates an epileptogenic focus in the left temporal lobe. An MRI is carried out. The hippocampal structures are unremarkable. A 2-cm lesion is noted in the subcortical region of the left temporal lobe. This lesion demonstrates mild enhancement. Areas of low signal on T1WI and T2WI are felt to represent foci of calcification. There is also an area of high signal on T1WI and T2WI seen inferiorly within the lesion, which probably represents an area of haemorrhage. There is a rim of surrounding oedema noted on T2WI and fluid-attenuated inversion recovery (FLAIR). What is the most likely diagnosis?

A. Haemangioblastoma.
B. Desmoplastic infantile ganglioglioma (DIG).
C. Dysembryoplastic neuroepithelial tumour (DNET).
D. Pleomorphic xanthoastrocytoma (PXA).
E. Oligodendroglioma.

6. A 52-year-old man is investigated by MRI of brain for a possible transient ischaemic attack (TIA). Focal lesions of CSF signal intensity are identified adjacent to the anterior commissures. The referring neurologist suspects that these lesions are chronic lacunar infarcts. What MRI finding suggests that these are in fact prominent perivascular spaces?

A. No restricted diffusion on DWI.
B. Hypointense on T1WI.
C. Hyperintense on T2WI.
D. Suppress on FLAIR.
E. Normal surrounding brain parenchyma.

7. A patient with a known diagnosis of a neurocutaneous syndrome is having a routine follow-up MRI scan. This patient is noted to have a history of right retinal calcifications. On MRI a retinal lesion is noted in the right eye, which is increased signal on T1WI. The scan shows a 2-cm lesion in the left lateral cerebellar hemisphere. This is predominantly low on T1WI and high on T2WI, but has a peripheral nodular area, which has a central signal void and demonstrates enhancement on T1WI. A further small enhancing lesion is noted in the cervical spinal cord, with an associated syrinx. The appearances are unchanged from previous imaging. Based on these findings, which neurocutaneous syndrome does this patient have?

A. Neurofibromatosis type 1 (NF-1).
B. Neurofibromatosis type 2 (NF-2).
C. Tuberous sclerosis.
D. Sturge Weber syndrome.
E. Von Hippel–Lindau syndrome.

8. A 32-year-old man presents with recent onset of migraine and TIAs. He also reports some cognitive decline. Cerebral angiogram is normal. An MRI of brain reveals discrete hyperintensities in the anterior temporal poles and external capsules. What is the most likely diagnosis?

A. Cerebral autosomal dominant arteriopathy with subcortical infarcts and leukoencephalopathy (CADASIL).
B. Mitochondrial myopathy, encephalopathy, lactic acidosis, and stroke (MELAS).
C. Myoclonic epilepsy with ragged red fibres (MERRF).
D. Sporadic subcortical arteriosclerotic encephalopathy (sSAE).
E. Protein S deficiency.

9. **A 36-year-old patient with known AIDS is admitted to your hospital with a right-sided hemiparesis. His wife gives a history of cognitive decline, headache, and lethargy for the past few weeks, but with an acute deterioration in the last 36 hours. His CD4 counts are between 200 and 500 (category B). An MRI is carried out which shows multiple ring-enhancing lesions in the brain. These lesions are high signal on T2WI/FLAIR, but demonstrate a low intensity peripheral ring. Lesions are noted in the basal ganglia bilaterally. The cortical region and subcortical U-fibres are spared. A thallium SPECT is also carried out that shows abnormal uptake in the brain, which correlates with the areas identified on MRI. What is your primary diagnosis?**

   A. Nocardia abscesses.
   B. Toxoplasmosis.
   C. Progressive multifocal leukoencephalopathy.
   D. Primary CNS lymphoma.
   E. Cerebral cryptococcus infection.

10. **A 50-year-old male patient is referred from A&E for a CT brain. He has a history of headache for 2 months and increasing clumsiness. The CT shows a lesion abutting the sphenoid in the anterior cranial fossa. It measures 4 cm in size and demonstrates heterogeneous enhancement. There is no evidence of calcification. The lesion is displacing and effacing the third ventricle, causing mild hydrocephalus in the lateral ventricles. An MRI is performed. The lesion is isointense on T1WI and T2WI, and demonstrates an enhancing dural tail and broad dural base. Again the enhancement pattern is heterogeneous. A number of flow voids are noted in the lesion. There is little peritumoural oedema noted. An MR angiogram is performed, which indicates dual supply to the lesion from the internal and external carotid artery. What lesion typically demonstrates these imaging findings?**

    A. WHO 1 meningioma.
    B. WHO 3 meningioma.
    C. Haemangiopericytoma.
    D. Melanocytoma.
    E. Schwannoma.

11. **A patient is referred to your neurointerventional team for embolization of a meningioma prior to surgical resection. The lesion is based on the tentorium. What is the likely feeding vessel (parent vessel is named in brackets)?**

    A. Anterior meningeal artery (vertebral).
    B. Middle meningeal artery (external carotid artery (ECA)).
    C. Posterior meningeal artery (variable).
    D. Bernasconi–Casanari artery (Internal carotid artery (ICA)).
    E. Dorsal meningeal artery (ICA).

12. A 7-year-old girl is brought into A&E with a history of headache of 4 hours' duration, associated with neck stiffness. The parents noted a petechial rash and are concerned about the possibility of meningitis. There is no photophobia and no other neurological signs are present. A&E have requested a CT scan to rule out raised intracranial pressure and to diagnose meningitis, whilst also commencing antibiotic therapy for presumed meningitis. The CT scan is normal. As it is a normal working day, A&E have also requested an MRI scan to diagnose meningitis. This was not carried out as the child was agitated. The following day the child develops a pyrexia and a right unilateral aspect to the headache, with decreased GCS. An MRI is carried out and demonstrates features of developing right temporal lobe empyema. Which of the following is an appropriate indication for imaging in the investigation of meningitis?

A. CT to rule out raised intracranial pressure.
B. CT to diagnose meningitis.
C. MRI to diagnose meningitis.
D. MRI due to deterioration in clinical course.
E. All of these.

13. A 13-year-old boy is brought to your paediatric hospital with a recent history of headache and high fever. The child is becoming progressively drowsy and demonstrates rigidity and tremor on neurological examination. An MRI is requested. Relevant past medical history on the request form is of recent travel to Asia, history of measles as a 6-year-old and recent viral infection. The MRI scan shows increased signal on T2WI and FLAIR sequences in the hippocampal regions of the temporal lobes. There is also increased FLAIR signal in the thalami and putamina bilaterally. Small foci of increased T1WI signal within these regions are felt to represent haemorrhage. What diagnosis would you place at the top of your differential list?

A. Herpes simplex type 1 encephalitis.
B. Herpes simplex type 2 encephalitis.
C. Japanese encephalitis.
D. Varicella Zoster encephalitis.
E. Subacute sclerosing panencephalitis (SSPE).

14. An 8-year-old female patient presents to your paediatric neurology service with a history of increasing ataxia, repeated headaches, and vomiting, increasing in severity over the last 5 months. Clinical examination reveals marked cerebellar signs of past pointing and dysdiadochokinesis. An MRI is requested, which shows a solid mass in the posterior fossa measuring 2 cm in size. This mass arises in the left cerebellar hemisphere and displaces the fourth ventricle. It is of low intensity on T1WI and high signal on T2WI. There is only a small rim of surrounding oedema. The lesion demonstrates relatively homogeneous moderate enhancement. There is no evidence of subarachnoid seeding. What is the most likely diagnosis?

A. Pilocytic astrocytoma.
B. Ependymoma.
C. Medulloblastoma.
D. Metastasis.
E. Lhermitte–Duclos syndrome.

15. A 30-year-old male patient is referred from ENT for an MRI with a history of tinnitus and slight hearing loss on the left side. A lesion is noted in the left cerebellopontine angle. This extends along the nerve and expands the internal auditory canal. A separate nerve is noted to enter the anterior superior portion of the internal auditory canal. The lesion is isointense to the pons on all pulse sequences. The lesion makes an acute angle with the petrous bone. There is no evidence of a dural tail following enhancement. What is the most likely cause?

A. Meningioma.
B. Facial nerve schwannoma.
C. Vestibular nerve schwannoma.
D. Epidermoid.
E. Arachnoid cyst.

16. An MRI is carried out for your neurology service on a 30-year-old male patient. The most pertinent abnormality is of thick smooth meningeal enhancement following the dural-arachnoid around the convexity, falx, and tentorium without extension into the basal ganglia or ventricles. The referring clinician arrives to discuss the findings, but has mislaid the request form and clinical information. While he is looking for it, what do you think the most likely clinical presentation is?

A. Neck stiffness, photophobia, raised WCC, petechial rash.
B. Neck stiffness, drowsiness, with history of breast cancer.
C. Acute limb weakness on right side 3 days previously, not resolving.
D. Recent back surgery complicated by ongoing CSF leak.
E. Possible fungal meningitis in immunocompromised patient.

17. A patient is having an MRI scan carried out to investigate a possible right frontal astrocytoma, incidentally detected on CT following a head injury. The MRI features are typical of an astrocytoma, with no evidence of necrosis or callosal involvement to indicate glioblastoma multiforme (GBM). MRS has been carried out to help assess the grade of this tumour. What MRS features would indicate a high grade lesion?

A. Elevated choline, reduced N-acetyl aspartate (NAA), choline/creatine (Cho/Cr) ratio of 1.
B. Elevated choline, reduced NAA, Cho/Cr ratio of 2.
C. Normal choline, elevated NAA.
D. Reduced choline, reduced NAA. Cho/Cr ratio of 1.2.
E. All normal, these are unaffected by tumour grade.

18. Which one of the following orbital pathologies typically arises from the intraconal compartment?

A. Cavernous haemangioma.
B. Adenocystic carcinoma.
C. Rhabdomyosarcoma.
D. Dermoid.
E. Orbital pseudotumour.

19. A 35-year-old man presents with tinnitus and hearing loss in the right ear. Investigations include an MRI of the internal auditory meati. This demonstrates an expansile lesion in the right petrous apex, without bone destruction. The lesion is of increased signal on T1WI, increased signal on T2WI, and non-enhancing. What is the most likely diagnosis?

A. Cholesteatoma.
B. Petrous apex cephalocele.
C. Mucocele.
D. Petrous apicitis.
E. Cholesterol granuloma.

20. A 54-year-old lady with a history of exophthalmos undergoes a CT scan of orbits for assessment. There is spindle-shaped enlargement of extra-orbital musculature that does not involve the tendinous insertions. Which pair of muscles is most likely to be involved?

A. Superior and inferior.
B. Superior and medial.
C. Superior and lateral.
D. Inferior and medial.
E. Inferior and lateral.
F. Medial and lateral.

21. A 7-year-old boy presents with rapid onset right proptosis. CT shows an extraconal mass in the right orbit with irregular margins. There is evidence of intraconal and intracranial extension. On MRI, the lesion is of decreased signal on T1WI, increased signal on T2WI, and shows relatively uniform enhancement. What is the most likely diagnosis?

A. Retinoblastoma.
B. Non-Hodgkin lymphoma.
C. Capillary haemangioma.
D. Ruptured dermoid cyst.
E. Rhabdomyosarcoma.

22. A 10-year-old girl presents with gradual onset proptosis in the left eye and is noted to have restricted left eye movements. An MRI scan is performed and this demonstrates a poorly circumscribed lobulated lesion that involves both the intraconal and extraconal compartments. The lesion has mixed signal intensity on T1WI, with areas of increased and decreased signal. It is mostly of increased signal on T2WI and there are areas containing a fluid–fluid level. Post contrast, there is heterogenous enhancement. What is the most likely diagnosis?

A. Venous-lymphatic malformation.
B. Orbital varix.
C. Cavernous haemangioma.
D. Capillary haemangioma.
E. Haemangiopericytoma.

23. A 20-year-old female with a history of neurofibromatosis presents with reduced visual acuity in the right eye. She subsequently has CT and MR imaging of the orbits to assess for a tumour relating to the right optic nerve. Which of the following findings on imaging would be more suggestive of the presence of an optic nerve glioma, rather than a meningioma arising from the optic nerve sheath?

A. Presence of the 'tram-track' sign.
B. Presence of optic canal widening.
C. Presence of marked intense tumour enhancement.
D. Presence of calcification.
E. Presence of bony hyperostosis.

24. A 45-year-old man has a severe head injury and is noted to have a left facial nerve palsy. Following stabilization, a subsequent HRCT scan of the temporal bone is performed. This demonstrates a fracture of the left temporal bone, involving the course of the left facial nerve. Which orientation of fracture and which segment of the facial nerve are most likely to be involved?

A. Transverse/internal auditory canal.
B. Longitudinal/internal auditory canal.
C. Transverse/labyrinthine.
D. Longitudinal/labyrinthine.
E. Transverse/mastoid.
F. Longitudinal/mastoid.

25. A 42-year-old woman has a CT scan of brain performed for the investigation of headache. A lesion with density similar to cerebrospinal fluid is noted at the right cerebellopontine angle. A subsequent MRI scan is performed and this shows that the lesion is well defined, of decreased signal on T1WI and increased signal on T2WI. You think the lesion is most likely an epidermoid cyst, but wish to exclude an arachnoid cyst. Which of the following further MRI sequences will be most helpful in achieving this aim?

A. Proton density.
B. STIR.
C. T1 with fat suppression.
D. FLAIR.
E. T1 post gadolinium.

26. A 45-year-old man presents with a 4-month history of worsening lower back pain radiating into the right lower extremity with weakness. An MRI scan of lumbar spine shows a 3-cm well-defined ovoid lesion eccentrically placed at the conus medullaris, the location of which is felt to be intradural and extramedullary. It is hypointense on T1WI and hyperintense on T2WI. There are flow voids and haemorrrhage within the lesion. It enhances avidly post injection of contrast. Which of the following lesions fits best with the imaging findings?

A. Meningioma.
B. Schwannoma.
C. Neurofibroma.
D. Paraganglioma.
E. Metastasis.

27. A 45-year-old woman presents with a several month history of neck pain and gradually progressive weakness and paraesthesia in the upper limbs. An MRI scan of the cervical spine is performed and this shows a well-defined central intramedullary mass in the mid-cervical spinal cord. The mass is generally slightly hyperintense on T2WI, but also has a few low signal peripheral areas. It enhances homogeneously with gadolinium. What is the most likely diagnosis?

A. Astrocytoma.
B. Metastasis.
C. Haemangioblastoma.
D. Ganglioglioma.
E. Ependymoma.

28. A 30-year-old male patient attends A&E 30 minutes after a head injury. He has consumed alcohol. You are contacted by the A&E doctor, who requests a CT brain. At this time, which of the following is a correct indication for immediate scanning?

A. Two episodes of vomiting.
B. GCS 13.
C. Loss of consciousness.
D. Amnesia for 20 minutes before accident.
E. Visual hallucinations.

29. A 27-year-old female patient undergoes urgent neuroimaging following loss of consciousness as a result of an RTA. CT is unremarkable. MRI reveals multiple small areas of increased signal on T2WI in the white matter near the grey–white matter junction within the frontal and temporal lobes. In the same locations, DWI reveals areas of increased signal on the B1000 image and reduced signal on the ADC map. What is the most likely diagnosis?

A. Subarachnoid haemorrhage.
B. Extradural haematoma.
C. Subdural haematoma.
D. Hypoxic brain injury.
E. Diffuse axonal injury.

30. A 34-year-old man undergoes MRI of brain after admission for head trauma. Which of the following sequences is most sensitive for subarachnoid haemorrhage?

A. T1WI.
B. T1WI with fat saturation.
C. T2WI.
D. FLAIR.
E. Proton density.

31. A 58-year-old patient is found at home with a reduced GCS. CT brain reveals atrophy only. MRI brain reveals hyperintensity in the tegmentum (except for the red nucleus) and hypointensity of the superior colliculus on T2WI, as well as hyperintensity in the basal ganglia. What is the most likely cause?

A. Cocaine abuse.
B. Methanol poisoning.
C. Primary basal ganglia haemorrhage.
D. Wilson's disease.
E. Carbon monoxide poisoning.

32. A 27-year-old man suffers a head injury. A CT brain is performed. Which of the following features favours a subdural haematoma (SDH) over an extradural haematoma (EDH)?

A. The haematoma measures 50 HU.
B. The presence of a temporal skull fracture.
C. The haematoma crosses the midline over the falx.
D. The collection has a biconvex configuration.
E. The haematoma crosses sutures.

33. A 65-year-old woman with a history of previous subarachnoid haemorrhage presents with slowly progressive cognitive decline and worsening gait. A CT brain reveals ventricular dilatation with rounded frontal horns and periventricular hypodensity. What is the most likely diagnosis?

A. Heavy metal toxicity secondary to aneurysm clip.
B. Parkinson's disease.
C. Alzheimer's disease.
D. Normal pressure hydrocephalus.
E. Binswanger's disease.

34. A 34-year-old liver transplant recipient presents to hospital with confusion and seizures. A CT brain reveals low attenuation in the deep and subcortical white matter of the occipital and parietal lobes bilaterally. There is no abnormal enhancement post IV contrast administration. As the reporting radiologist, you advise that the clinical team first:

A. measure blood glucose
B. measure serum alpha-feta protein
C. measure blood pressure
D. send coagulation screen
E. measure d-dimer.

35. A 34-year-old female presents with neurological symptoms suggestive of MS and is referred for an MRI of brain by the neurology team. Which of the following sequences is most useful for determining if there are plaques of differing ages (i.e. dissemination in time)?

A. FLAIR.
B. T2WI.
C. Pre- and post-contrast T1WI.
D. Proton density.
E. STIR.

36. A 34-year-old woman presents with a seizure. She has a history of migraine and low mood over the preceding year, and reported occasional episodes of confusion. On examination there is slight left-sided motor weakness. An MRI of brain reveals small multifocal frontal and parietal subcortical white matter T2WI hyperintensities, and a few areas of restricted diffusion in the right cerebral hemisphere on DWI. What is the most likely diagnosis?

A. Multiple sclerosis (MS).
B. SLE.
C. Small vessel ischaemia.
D. Susac syndrome.
E. Lyme disease.

37. A 73-year-old has been referred for assessment of cognitive decline. A CT brain reveals cerebral atrophy and a dementia specialist refers her for PET-CT brain. Which of the following findings is most consistent with early Alzheimer's disease?

A. Diffuse reduced activity.
B. Reduced activity in the precuneus and posterior cingulate gyrus.
C. Reduced activity in the frontotemporal regions.
D. Reduced activity in the caudate and lentiform nuclei.
E. Reduced activity bilaterally in the occipital cortex.

38. A 15-year-old male presents with a history of recurrent epistaxis and nasal obstruction. MRI demonstrates a lesion centred at the sphenopalatine foramen, which is hypointense on T1WI and heterogeneously intermediate signal on T2WI. Intense lesional enhancement and multiple flow voids are noted on post-gadolinium T1WI. What is the diagnosis?

A. Ludwig angina.
B. Nasopharyngeal carcinoma.
C. Inverted papilloma.
D. Juvenile angiofibroma.
E. Glomus jugulare.

39. A 50-year-old male presents with a history of intermittent epistaxis, nasal obstruction, and frontal headache. He undergoes a CT of the sinuses that demonstrates an isodense soft-tissue mass filling the right maxillary antrum with extension through the infundibulum into the nasal cavity. There is associated bony remodelling of the infundibulum. On MRI, the mass is isointense to muscle on T1WI and T2WI, and demonstrates a convoluted cerebriform pattern on enhanced T1WI. The remainder of the sinuses are unremarkable. What is the diagnosis?

A. Juvenile angiofibroma.
B. Inverted papilloma.
C. Antrochoanal polyp.
D. Invasive fungal sinusitis.
E. Nasal carcinoma.

40. A 45-year-old female patient presents with recurrent frontal sinusitis following functional endoscopic sinus surgery (FESS). Which of the following CT findings is not commonly associated with postoperative frontal recess stenosis?

A. Inadequate removal of the agger nasi and frontal recess cells.
B. Retained superior portion of the uncinate process.
C. Medialization of middle turbinate.
D. Osteoneogenesis due to chronic inflammation or mucosal stripping.
E. Scarring or inflammatory mucosal thickening.

41. A 12-year-old male with a history of gelastic seizures is referred for MRI of the brain. Which of the following statements regarding hamartomas of the tuber cinereum is true?

A. No change in size, shape, or signal intensity on follow-up MRI.
B. Demonstrate homogenous contrast enhancement.
C. Calcification is a common finding.
D. Hyperintense on T1WI and T2WI, and hypointense on fat suppressed sequences.
E. Located in the sella turcica.

42. You are reporting a CT scan of neck in a patient with a head and neck cancer. You see an enlarged necrotic jugulo-digastric lymph node on the right side and wish to describe the appropriate level of this lymph node in your report. What is the correct level?

A. I.
B. II.
C. III.
D. IV.
E. V.
F. VI.
G. VII.

43. A 4-week-old infant with a history of breech delivery is brought to the A&E department with a history of swelling in the left side of the neck and torticollis. An ultrasound of the neck demonstrates a non-tender, focal fusiform enlargement of the lower half of the left sternocleidomastoid muscle. No other abnormality is identified. What is the diagnosis?

A. Fibromatosis colli.
B. Lymphoma.
C. Rhabdomyosarcoma.
D. Cystic hygroma.
E. Branchial cleft cyst.

44. A 60-year-old female presents with a history of facial pain and diplopia. Clinical examination reveals palsies of the III, IV, and VI cranial nerves, Horner's syndrome, and facial sensory loss in the distribution of the ophthalmic and maxillary divisions of the trigeminal (V) cranial nerve. Where is the causative abnormality located?

A. Dorello's canal.
B. Cavernous sinus.
C. Superior orbital fissure.
D. Inferior orbital fissure.
E. Meckel's cave.

45. A 50-year-old male undergoes an MR carotid angiogram on which an incidental soft-tissue mass is noted in right parapharyngeal soft tissue. The mass displaces the right parapharyngeal space anteromedially. What is the location of the soft-tissue mass?

A. Masticator space.
B. Carotid space.
C. Retropharyngeal space.
D. Mucosal space.
E. Parotid space.

46. A 55-year-old man undergoes ^{99m}Tc scintigraphy on which incidental note is made of multiple foci of increased tracer uptake in the parotid regions. Ultrasound of the parotid glands demonstrates bilateral multiple hypoechoic lesions with anechoic areas. On MRI, the lesions are of intermediate signal intensity on T1WI and intermediate signal intensity with focal areas of hyperintensity on T2WI. There is no enhancement following contrast administration. What is the likely diagnosis?

A. Pleomorphic adenomas.
B. Warthin tumours.
C. Lipomas.
D. Haemangiomas.
E. Mucoepidermoid carcinomas.

47. A 60-year-old woman presents with a painless, slowly growing mass in the lateral aspect of the neck. The patient is referred for imaging with a clinical diagnosis of carotid body paraganglioma. Which of the following is a distinctive feature of carotid body paraganglioma on imaging?

A. Soft-tissue mass in the carotid space.
B. Intense enhancement after IV contrast administration.
C. High signal on T2WI.
D. Splaying of the internal and external carotid arteries.
E. Low signal on T2WI.

48. A 22-year-old woman presents with upper and lower limb neurological symptoms and signs. She is subsequently discovered on MRI to have a mass in the cervical spinal cord. Which of the following features on MRI is going to point more towards a diagnosis of spinal cord astrocytoma, rather than ependymoma?

A. Predominant T2WI high signal.
B. Homogeneous enhancement post gadolinium.
C. Short segment of cord involvement.
D. Eccentrically placed lesion in the cord.
E. Sharply marginated lesion.

49. A 52-year-old woman presents with gradually increasing gait disturbance and lower limb sensory symptoms. An MRI of her spine is performed and this shows an anteriorly placed intradural, but extramedullary spinal mass. It is fairly markedly low signal on T1WI and T2WI, and shows only miminal patchy enhancement post administration of intravenous gadolinium. What is the most likely diagnosis?

A. Neurofibroma.
B. Schwannoma.
C. Lymphoma.
D. Metastasis.
E. Meningioma.

50. You are asked to protocol an MRI scan that is specifically being performed to look for vertebral metastatic disease. The radiographer complains that you have asked for too many sequences. Which of the following sagittal sequences is likely to be least helpful for the purposes of your examination?

A. STIR.
B. T2 fast SE with fat saturation.
C. T2 fast SE.
D. T1 fast SE.
E. T1 GE out of phase.

51. A 44-year-old woman presents with severe facial injuries following an RTA. CT of the facial bones demonstrates multiple maxillofacial fractures in keeping with a Le Fort configuration. Which of the following statements regarding Le Fort fractures is false?

A. Any combination of Le Fort I, II, and III fractures can occur.
B. Disruption of pterygoid plates from the posterior maxilla is an essential finding in Le Fort fractures.
C. Le Fort fractures by definition refer to fractures involving the maxilla bilaterally.
D. Craniofacial separation is noted in Le Fort III pattern.
E. Le Fort fracture associated with a palate fracture will result in widening of the maxillary arch.

52. A 25-year-old woman is brought to the A&E department following an RTA. CT of brain and facial bones are requested for assessment of head and facial injuries. On the CT studies, incidental note is made of dense calcification of the falx cerebri, midface hypoplasia, and prognathism. Multiple cystic lesions are also noted in the mandible, which are associated with cortical expansion. Some of the lesions break through the cortex. Following contrast administration there is minimal peripheral enhancement. What is the underlying mandibular abnormality?

A. Radicular cyst.
B. Keratocystic odontogenic tumour.
C. Dentigerous cyst.
D. Stafne cyst.
E. Ameloblastoma.

53. A 45-year-old female undergoes an MRI of the pituitary that demonstrates a kidney-shaped lesion located centrally in the pituitary fossa in the axial plane. It is hyperintense on T1WI and hypointense on T2WI. There is no enhancement following gadolinium administration and no fluid–fluid level. What is the diagnosis?

A. Rathke cleft cyst.
B. Craniopharyngioma.
C. Cholesterol granuloma.
D. Haemorrhagic adenoma.
E. Lipoma.

54. A 30-year-old male presents with a fluctuant swelling in the right side of the neck. On ultrasound examination, an anechoic lesion with posterior acoustic enhancement is noted along the anteromedial margin of the sternocleiodomastoid muscle, posterior to the submandibular gland and superficial to the carotid artery and internal jugular vein. There is no increased surrounding vascularity on power Doppler. What is the likely diagnosis?

A. Dermoid cyst.
B. Lymphangioma.
C. First branchial cleft cyst.
D. Abscess.
E. Second branchial cyst.

55. A 5-year-old girl with a clinical suspicion of retropharyngeal abscess is referred for MRI of the neck. Which of the following features on MRI is useful in differentiating retropharyngeal abscess from retropharyngeal suppurative lymph node?

A. Enhancing wall.
B. Rounded or ovoid configuration.
C. Mass effect.
D. Filling of retropharyngeal space from side to side.
E. Primary infection source such as otitis media or tonsillitis.

56. A 42-year-old male patient of African-Caribbean ethnicity presents to the neurologists with a history of facial paraesthesia and slight weakness, headache, lethargy, and neck stiffness. He also has a history of mild dyspnoea. An MRI is requested, which shows left frontal leptomeningeal thickening, with an apparent dural mass noted along the falx. There is increased T2WI/FLAIR signal in the cortex adjacent to this area of meningeal disease. There is also thickening and enhancement noted of the right trigeminal and facial nerves on post-contrast T1WI. Further enhancement is also noted along the parasellar region on the left. Multiple non-enhancing high T2WI/FLAIR periventricular white matter lesions are noted. Abnormality is noted in the skull vault, where there is an expanded diploic space over the right occipital region, with associated apparent thinning of the outer table, although this is hard to define on MRI. Due to concern with regard to multifocal meningioma the patient is started on steroids to reduce the mass effect from the frontal lesion and referred to neurosurgery. A CT is non-contributory. An MRI is repeated, which shows only mild meningeal thickening. What is the most likely diagnosis?

A. NF-2.
B. Neurosarcoid.
C. Neurotoxoplasmosis.
D. Tuberous sclerosis.
E. Multiple sclerosis.

57. A 62-year-old man presents with tremor and incontinence. Examination reveals bradykinesia and gait ataxia. He is also noted to have a reduced mini mental state examination (MMSE) and postural hypotension. He has an MRI scan of brain as part of the diagnostic workup. On the axial T2WI a cruciform hyperintensity in the pons is noted. Which of the following is the most likely diagnosis?

A. Parkinson's disease.
B. Multisystem atrophy (MSA).
C. Progressive supranuclear palsy (PSP).
D. Cryptobasal degeneration.
E. Lewy body dementia.

58. A 56-year-old man with chronic alcohol dependence presents with progressive cognitive impairment, gait disturbance, and signs of interhemispheric disconnection. An MRI scan of brain demonstrates increased T2WI signal lesions without mass effect within the corpus callosum and dorsal part of the external capsule. Which of the following is the most likely diagnosis?

A. Wernicke's encephalopathy.
B. Osmotic myelinolysis.
C. Marchifava–Bignami disease.
D. Alcohol withdrawal syndrome.
E. Chronic hepatic encephalopathy.

59. A 74-year-old woman is admitted with acute left-sided hemiplegia of 2 hours onset. On assessment by the stroke team she is deemed suitable for thrombolysis and referred for CT. As part of your institution's work-up, CT perfusion (CTP) is performed following the unenhanced study. Which of the following CTP findings with regards to cerebral blood flow (CBF), cerebral blood volume (CBV) and mean transit time (MTT) are consistent with infarction?

A. Decreased CBF/decreased CBV/increased MTT.
B. Decreased CBF/increased CBV/increased MTT.
C. Decreased CBF/decreased CBV/decreased MTT.
D. Increased CBF/increased CBV/decreased MTT.
E. Increased CBF/decreased CBV/decreased MTT.

60. An immunocompetent 24-year-old patient presents with an acute history of right-sided limb weakness which has rapidly progressed. The patient now also has mixed sensory symptoms and poorly controlled seizures. Basic observations and initial blood results are normal. An MRI is carried out which shows a large mass-like lesion in the right posterior frontal lobe. There is mild mass effect associated with this lesion on the adjacent parenchyma, with mild compression of the right lateral ventricle. The lesion is also noted to involve the corpus callosum and cross the midline into the left cerebral hemisphere. This lesion is bright on FLAIR imaging. On post-contrast T1WI the lesion has peripheral rim enhancement. Vascular structures are noted to pass through the lesion. There is no evidence of necrosis or haemorrhage. On DWI, the b1000 sequence reveals increased signal in the lesion. Other high T2WI lesions are noted in the cerebellum, with a further lesion in the spinal cord. What is the most likely diagnosis based on this information?

A. MS.
B. Glioblastoma multiforme.
C. High-grade astrocytoma.
D. Lymphoma.
E. Abscess.

61. A 32-year-old woman of 38 weeks gestation presents with seizure following a headache. She is referred for CT querying venous thrombosis. Unenhanced CT brain demonstrates bilateral low attenuation change within the thalami. Given this location, where is the most likely site of thrombosis?

A. Superior sagittal sinus.
B. Transverse sinus.
C. Sigmoid sinus.
D. Straight sinus.
E. Cavernous sinus.

62. A 36-year-old man is admitted following a seizure. Unenhanced CT demonstrates a right frontal mixed attenuation lesion, which avidly enhances post contrast. Multiple flow voids are seen on MRI of brain. What finding on catheter angiography differentiates arteriovenous malformation (AVM) from other vascular lesions of the brain?

A. Early venous drainage.
B. Arterial stenoses of feeder vessels.
C. External carotid transdural supply.
D. Dilated medullary veins (caput medusa).
E. Dilated cortical veins.

63. You are contacted by the A&E department requesting a CT brain for a 28-year-old female presenting with headache which reached peak intensity 15 minutes after onset. The headache came on during sexual activity and is associated with vomiting. Which feature in the clinical history is most predictive of subarachnoid haemorrhage?

A. Female sex.
B. Age <40 years.
C. 15 minute onset to peak intensity.
D. Onset during sexual activity.
E. Association with vomiting.

64. A 54-year-old female is admitted following a seizure. CT of the brain demonstrates a rounded, 2-cm hyperdense lesion within the right temporal lobe, which exhibits calcification. No enhancement is seen post contrast. On follow-up MRI of brain, the lesion is of mixed intensity on T1WI. The lesion has a hypointense rim on T2WI. Prominent susceptibility effect is noted on T2* GE imaging. DWI is normal and no enhancement is demonstrated on T1WI post gadolinium. Based on the imaging findings, what is the most likely diagnosis?

A. AVM.
B. Haemorrhagic neoplasm.
C. Cavernous malformation (cavernoma).
D. Amyloid angiopathy.
E. Capillary telangiectasia.

65. A 42-year-old man is admitted with sudden onset headache suspicious of subarachnoid haemorrhage. There is no loss of consciousness. Unenhanced CT demonstrates blood in the cisterns around the midbrain and into the anterior part of the interhemispheric fissure. Subsequent CT angiogram (CTA) is negative. What is advised next for this patient?

A. Lumbar puncture.
B. MRA.
C. Catheter angiography.
D. Repeat CTA in 1 week.
E. No further investigation necessary (perimesencephalic haemorrhage).

66. A 74-year-old man with a history of diabetes presents with a history of slurred speech and right-sided weakness, which spontaneously resolved over 1–2 hours. Initial unenhanced CT is normal. Further investigation by MRI is requested. What sequence is most sensitive for diagnosing acute ischaemia?

A. T2WI.
B. FLAIR.
C. DWI.
D. GE imaging.
E. T1WI post gadolinium.

67. A 16-year-old female is referred for MRI after presenting with an increasing number of cutaneous neurofibromata. As a child she had been noted to have a cafe-au-lait spot on her back. What MRI finding would confirm the diagnosis of NF-1?

A. Multiple hyperintense white matter foci on T2WI.
B. Bilateral vestibular schwannomas.
C. Meningioma.
D. Optic nerve glioma.
E. Multiple ependymomas.

68. A 16-year-old male with a history of epilepsy is investigated via MRI. Axial T2WI demonstrates a cystic space within the left frontal lobe isointense to CSF. This is causing local mass effect and there is adjacent enlargement of the left lateral ventricle.
What is the most likely diagnosis?

A. Porencephalic cyst.
B. Arachnoid cyst.
C. Schizencephaly.
D. Hydranencephaly.
E. Ependymal cyst.

69. A 32-year-old man presents with schizophrenic-like psychosis and parkinsonian-type movement disorder. There is a family history of neuropsychiatric disturbance. An initial CT is requested which demonstrates heavy bilateral, symmetric calcifications within the globus pallidus, thalami, putamen, and cerebellum. There is no enhancement post contrast. Which of the following suggests a diagnosis of Fahr disease over pseudohypoparathyroidism?

A. Involvement of the globus pallidus.
B. Involvement of the thalami.
C. Involvement of the putamen.
D. Involvement of the cerebellum.
E. Normal calcium-phosphorus metabolism.

70. A 29-year-old female complains of increasing headache, followed by generalized seizure activity 24 hours after giving birth. She is noted to be hypertensive. MRI demonstrates bilateral parieto-occipital T2WI hyperintense cortical and subcortical lesions. ADC is elevated. Similar lesions are noted in the anterior watershed zones. What is the most likely diagnosis?

A. Hypotensive cerebral infarction.
B. Postpartum cerebral angiopathy.
C. Posterior reversible encephalopathy syndrome (PRES).
D. Progressive multifocal leucoencephalopathy (PML).
E. Gliomatosis cerebri.

71. A 62-year-old man is referred for MRI of brain after presenting with cognitive decline, gait apraxia, and urinary incontinence. There is a preceding history of chronic headache. Ventriculomegaly is noted on initial CT. Which of the following conventional MRI findings distinguishes aqueductal stenosis from normal pressure hydrocephalus?

A. Periventricular T2WI hyperintensity.
B. Normal sulci.
C. Aqueductal flow void.
D. Funnel-shaped aqueduct.
E. Relatively normal calibre fourth ventricle.

72. A 24-year-old male boxer is admitted with concussion following a head injury. His admission CT does not demonstrate any evidence of intracranial injury, but the A&E physician asks you about a midline CSF space. You explain that this is a cavum velum interpositum. What distinguishes this CSF space from cavum septum pellucidum and cavum vergae?

A. Position between the frontal horns of the lateral ventricles.
B. Posterior extension between the fornices.
C. Does not extend anterior to foramen of Monro.
D. Mildly hyperdensity to CSF in lateral ventricles.
E. Absent septum pellucidum.

73. A 42-year-old male is admitted with first presentation of a seizure. There is no significant past medical history. CT demonstrates a mass lesion within the right frontal lobe. He is further investigated via MRI, which includes MR perfusion and spectroscopy. The neurosurgical team are keen to biopsy this lesion if there is radiological suspicion of a high-grade lesion. Which of the following radiological findings is most consistent with a high grade lesion?

A. Relative cerebral blood volume (rCBV) 1.5 on MR perfusion.
B. Lactate peak on MRS.
C. Elevated ADC on DWI.
D. Peritumoral hyperintensity on T2WI.
E. Nodular enhancement on T1WI post gadolinium.

74. A 54-year-old man presents with hearing loss in the left ear, which is of the sensori-neural type. He undergoes an MRI scan of the internal auditory meati and subsequently a full MRI scan of brain. A large extra-axial mass lesion is identified at the left cerebellopontine angle. Which of the following features on MR imaging will be most helpful in indicating that this is probably a large vestibular schwannoma, rather than a meningioma?

A. Enhancing dura adjacent to the mass.
B. Erosion of the adjacent porus acousticus.
C. Tumour within the adjacent internal auditory meatus.
D. Intense enhancement within the mass.
E. Hyperostosis in the adjacent petrous temporal ridge.

75. A 32-year-old female is referred to neurology complaining of visual disturbance and headache. She is 4 months postpartum. On examination a bitemporal hemianopia is noted. Hormonal testing reveals hypoadrenalism and hypothyroidism. A dedicated MRI of her pituitary gland is requested. Which of the following features is suggestive of autoimmune hypophysitis over pituitary adenoma?

A. Asymmetric pituitary enlargement.

B. Heterogenous gadolinium enhancement.

C. Loss of the posterior pituitary bright spot.

D. Sphenoid sinus mucosal thickening.

E. Age >30.

chapter 6 CENTRAL NERVOUS AND HEAD AND NECK

ANSWERS

1. D. Germinoma.

The lesion is described in the pineal region, so the differential of pineal tumours should be considered. These are differentiated between germ cell tumours and pineal cell tumours. Germinomas account for 40% of all pineal region masses and are much more frequent in males than females. They are also the most common germ cell tumour, with teratomas and choriocarcinoma having different imaging characteristics. The main differential in this case is between pineoblastoma and germinoma, as both occur in patients of this age group and both are hyperdense on CT. Imaging features described to help differentiate are the avid enhancement, which is more characteristic of germinomas, but can occur in either. Central calcification is seen commonly in germinomas, but is uncommon in pineoblastomas, and when it occurs is often peripheral, giving the impression of an 'exploded' pineal gland. Subarachnoid seeding is seen in both tumours and if present CSF sampling can yield a tissue diagnosis. Pineocytomas occur in an older age group and infrequently cause subarachnoid seeding.

Smirniotopoulos J, Rushing E, and Mena H. Pineal region masses: differential diagnosis. *RadioGraphics* 1992; 12(3): 577–596

Grossman R and Yousem D. *Neuroradiology: The Requisites*, 2nd edn, Mosby, 2003, pp. 156–162.

2. D. Symmetrical involvement of cerebral white matter.

Symmetrical involvement of the cerebral hemispheres or cerebellar peduncles is unusual in MS and is occasionally seen in acute disseminated encephalomyelitis (ADEM). ADEM can mimic an acute presentation of MS both clinically and in terms of imaging findings. The monophasic nature of ADEM can be deduced both from the uniformity of lesional oedema and contrast enhancement in the acute phase. Lesions in ADEM resolve on follow-up, and although enhancing and non-enhancing lesions can coexist for a period, new lesions should not appear.

MS plaques are classically seen in the periventricular and juxtacortical white matter. The other options in the question are all common plaque locations. Involvement of the corpus callosum is characteristic. Other common supratentorial sites include the white matter abutting the temporal horns and trigones of the lateral ventricles. Cortical lesions are less conspicuous on MRI than white matter lesions, but their detection is improved by the inclusion of a FLAIR sequence. Juxtacortical white matter lesions are highly suggestive of MS, as lesions are not commonly seen in this region in normal ageing. Twelve per cent of patients have lesions on MRI limited to the spine without brain involvement.

Pretorius PM and Quaghebeur G. The role of MRI in the diagnosis of MS. *Clinical Radiology* 2003; 58: 434–448.

3. B. Metastasis.

The answer options give some of the classical radiological differentials for a ring-enhancing lesion in the brain: MAGIC DR (metastasis, abscess, glioblastoma multiforme, infarct, contusion, demyelinating conditions and post-radiotherapy change). The clinical history should steer the reader toward the first two. DWI is reasonably useful at differentiating between these two (exceptions being in some fungal infections and toxoplasmosis), with necrotic metastasis having unrestricted diffusion and abscess having restricted diffusion. The appearances in this case are slightly confused by the DWI b1000 imaging showing increased signal. However, the presence of increased signal on the ADC map correctly identifies this as being T2 shine through, showing the importance of checking both sequences.

Chapman N and Nakielny R. *Aids to Radiological Differential Diagnosis*, 4th edn, Saunders, 2003, p. 433.
Grossman R and Yousem D. *Neuroradiology: The Requisites*, 2nd edn, Mosby, 2003, p. 143.

4. B. Haematoma hyperintense to grey matter on both T1WI and T2WI.

The MRI appearances of intracranial haemorrhage are determined primarily by the state of the haemoglobin (Hb), which evolves with age. This can be staged as hyperacute (first few hours), acute (1–3 days), early subacute (3–7 days), late subacute (4–7 days to 1 month), or chronic (1 month to years). Table 6.1 illustrates the sequential signal intensity changes of the evolving intracerebral haematoma.

Table 6.1 The sequential signal intensity changes of the evolving intracerebral haematoma

	Hyperacute	**Acute**	**Early subacute**	**Late subacute**	**Chronic**
State of Hb	Intracellular oxy-Hb	Intracellular deoxy-Hb	Intracellular met-Hb	Extracellular met-Hb	Haemosiderin
Magnetic properties	Diamagnetic	Paramagnetic	Paramagnetic	Paramagnetic	Superpara-magnetic
T1 Signal intensity	↔/↓	↔/↓	↑↑	↑↑	↔/↓
T2 Signal intensity	↑	↓	↓↓	↑↑	↓↓

Data from Parizel PM, Makkat S, Van Miert E, Van Goethem JW, van den Hauwe L, and De Schepper AM. Intracranial hemorrhage: principles of CT and MRI interpretation. *European Radiology* 2001; 11: 1770–1783.

5. E. Oligodendroglioma.

Prior to evaluating the imaging characteristics, the patient's demographics should be considered in this case, as in all cases of intracranial masses, as it will help limit the differential diagnosis significantly. The patient is an adult, thus making DIG and DNET unlikely. Secondly, consider the temporal lobe location. Haemangioblastomas are usually infratentorial in location, especially in the absence of a history of von Hippel–Lindau syndrome. All the other lesions are classical temporal lobe tumours. Finally, considering the imaging characteristics, both PXA and oligodendrogliomas may be entirely solid, but cysts are commonly seen in PXAs. Calcification is seen in 60–80% of oligodendrogliomas, but is rarely seen in PXAs. Similarly haemorrhage, while not typical of oligodendrogliomas, is rare in PXAs.

Grossman R and Yousem D. *Neuroradiology: The Requisites*, 2nd edn, Mosby, 2003, pp. 137–141.

6. E. Normal surrounding brain parenchyma.

Perivascular spaces (Virchow–Robin spaces) are pial lined interstitial fluid structures that accompany penetrating arteries, but do not communicate directly with the subarachnoid space. They can occur anywhere, but typically cluster around the anterior commissure. They follow CSF signal intensity, suppress on FLAIR, and do not exhibit restricted diffusion. They can occasionally be giant when located within the midbrain. Lacunar infarcts will also be hypointense on T1WI and hyperintense on T2WI. Restricted diffusion will be seen when acute/subacute. They are typically of increased signal on FLAIR, although will suppress if there is central encephalomalacia. A halo of surrounding high signal on T2WI and FLAIR is typical of lacunar infarction, although up to 25% of prominent perivascular spaces can also demonstrate a slight halo of increased signal. Lacunar infarcts are also more typically seen in the setting of more extensive white matter disease.

Osbom AG, Blaser SI, Salzman KL, Katzman GL, Provenzale J, Castillo M et al. *Diagnostic Imaging: Brain*, Amirsys, 2004, I-7: 22–25.

7. E. Von Hippel–Lindau syndrome.

This syndrome is characterized by retinal lesions variously described as being retinal angiomas, retinal haemangiomas, or retinal hamartomas. These lesions (Lindau tumours) cause retinal calcification, although this is also seen in NF-1 and tuberous sclerosis (TS) from other causes. The findings describe the classical appearance of a cerebellar haemangioblastoma. These lesions can also be entirely cystic or solid in a minority of cases. A signal void and lack of dural enhancement help differentiate this from other infratentorial masses in adults. Twenty per cent of haemangioblastomas are associated with Von Hippel–Lindau syndrome and 80% of Von Hippel–Lindau syndrome patients have this tumour. The spinal finding also indicates a further haemangioblastoma in the cord. Unlike in the posterior fossa, these seldom have flow voids, but are associated with the development of a syrinx.

Leung R, Biswas S, Duncan M, and Rankin S. Imaging features of von Hippel-Lindau Disease. *RadioGraphics* 2008; 28(1): 65–79.
Grossman R and Yousem D. *Neuroradiology: The Requisites*, 2nd edn, Mosby, 2003, pp. 456–457.
Chapman S and Nakielny R. *Aids to Radiological Differential Diagnosis*, 4th edn, Saunders, 2003, pp. 450–451.

8. A. Cerebral autosomal dominant arteriopathy with subcortical infarcts and leukoencephalopathy (CADASIL).

This is a hereditary small vessel disease, which causes stroke in young adults. The genetic mutation is found on chromosome 19. Presentation can include migraine, cognitive decline, psychiatric disturbance, TIAs, and stroke, the latter usually with substantial/complete recovery after individual strokes, particularly early in the disease process.

Imaging reveals subcortical lacunar infarcts and leukoencephalopathy in young adults. The frontal lobe has the highest lesion load, followed by the temporal lobe and insula. Anterior temporal pole and external capsule lesions have higher sensitivity and specificity for CADASIL. The cerebral cortex is usually spared. MRI is the investigation of choice: CT will reveal only areas of hypodensity and angiography is normal.

sSAE is associated with hypertension and results in multiple lacunar infarcts in the lenticular nuclei, pons, internal capsule, and caudate nuclei. MELAS and MERRF are mitochondrial disorders. MELAS results in bilateral multiple cortical and subcortical hyperintense lesions on FLAIR images; MERRF has a propensity for the basal ganglia and caudate nuclei, and watershed ischaemia/infarcts are common. Hypercoagulable states such as protein S deficiency result in cortical and lacunar infarcts of various sizes, but the cerebral angiogram is abnormal.

Osbom AG, Blaser SI, Salzman KL, Katzman GL, Provenzale J, Hedlund GL et al. *Diagnostic Imaging: Brain*, Amirsys, 2004, I-4: 62–65.

9. B. Toxoplasmosis.

This is the most common intracranial opportunistic infection in AIDS patients and the most common cause of intracranial mass lesions in this population, with lymphoma second and cryptococcus third. Differentiating toxoplasmosis from lymphoma has been the subject of much debate in the literature and ultimately there is no definitive means of differentiating them on imaging alone. As described toxoplasmosis causes multiple ring-enhancing lesions and often affects the basal ganglia. Lymphoma tends to involve the subependymal regions and can cause leptomeningeal enhancement. Lymphoma can cause encasement of the ventricle, which is not seen with toxoplasmosis. Toxoplasmosis tends to be higher intensity on T2WI/FLAIR than lymphoma.

PET and thallium SPECT have also been reported to show abnormal uptake in lymphoma, but not toxoplasmosis, although exceptions exist. Response to anti-toxoplasma treatment is often used as a clinical differentiator.

Cryptococcus classically causes dilatation of Virchow–Robin spaces. PML is a demyelinating condition secondary to JC virus of oligodendrocytes and is differentiated from other HIV-related demyelinating conditions by affecting the subcortical U fibres.

Offiah C and Turnbull I. The imaging appearances of intracranial CNS infections in adult HIV and AIDS patients. *Clinical Radiology* 2006; 61: 393–401.
Buerger J. Mass lesions of the brain in AIDS: the dilemmas of distinguishing toxoplasmosis from primary CNS lymphoma. *American Journal of Neuroradiology* 2003; 24(4): 554–555.
Grossman R and Yousem D. *Neuroradiology: The Requisites*, 2nd edn, Mosby, 2003, p. 297.

10. C. Haemangiopericytoma.

The imaging findings clearly describe an extra-axial tumour. These are classed as either lesions of meningeal origin or tumours of neurogenic origin. The broad dural base and dural tail indicates that this is a tumour of meningeal origin. Meningioma is the most common of these tumours, but the imaging characteristics are not typical. World Health Organization (WHO) 1 and 2 meningiomas demonstrate uniform enhancement, although haemorrhage into meningiomas is recognized. WHO 3 meningiomas (malignant meningiomas) are indicated on imaging when there is invasion of the adjacent parenchyma, which is not described. Otherwise the diagnosis of malignant meningioma is made by an aggressive pattern of growth on serial imaging and biopsy. The dual arterial supply is also atypical. While meningiomas can have dual supply, they more typically derive their arterial supply from the external carotid (via the meningeal artery). Melanocytomas are suggested on imaging by increased signal on T1WI and are more commonly infratentorial. Without this the diagnosis is again reached most commonly following biopsy. All the features described are typical of haemangiopericytoma.

Sibtain N, Butt S, and Connor S. Imaging features of central nervous system haemangiopericytomas. *European Radiology* 2007; 17: 1685–1693.
Grossman R and Yousem D. *Neuroradiology: The Requisites*, 2nd edn, Mosby, 2003, 99–105.

11. D. Bernasconi–Casanari artery (ICA).

The majority of meningiomas occur in the parafalcine region, along the convexity or around the sphenoid. These all derive their supply from the ECA, although parafalcine meningiomas can also receive supply from a branch of the ophthalmic artery. Tentorial or cerebellopontine angle (CPA) tumours are classically fed by the Bernasconi–Casanari artery, a branch of the meningohypophyseal trunk of the ICA. Lesions around the foramen magnum, clivus, and posterior fossa are fed by branches of the vertebral artery (anterior and posterior meningeal) and meningohypophyseal trunk of the ICA.

Grossman R and Yousem D. *Neuroradiology: The Requisites*, 2nd edn, Mosby, 2003, p. 104.

12. D. MRI due to deterioration in clinical course.

In the absence of clinical features of raised intracranial pressure a CT is not necessarily indicated prior to lumbar puncture to exclude raised intracranial pressure. CT is also insensitive at diagnosing meningitis, being normal in most uncomplicated cases. MRI is also negative in 50% of cases of uncomplicated meningitis. The value of imaging is in the detection of complications of meningitis, including hydrocephalus, abcess, cerebritis, venous thrombosis, and infarction.

Hughes D, Raghavan A, Mordekar S, Griffiths P, and Connolly D. Role of imaging in the diagnosis of acute bacterial meningitis and its complications. *Postgraduate Medical Journal* 2010; 86(1018): 478–485.

13. C. Japanese encephalitis.

Japanese encephalitis and herpes simplex virus (HSV) encephalitis both present with similar acute and rapidly progressive neurological symptoms. The key differentiator is involvement of the basal ganglia, which is typical in Japanese encephalitis but rare in HSV. Both commonly involve the hippocampi, this being the classical appearance of HSV encephalitis. HSV type 1 is the subtype that affects adult and older children. HSV type 2 causes neonatal and *in utero* infection. Herpes varicella zoster virus (VZV) infection can be seen in immunocompromised children, but in the immunocompetent population is more typically seen in elderly patients, often, but not exclusively, in the presence of cutaneous shingles. It causes a vasculitis, which can be seen angiographically and causes bilateral increased T2WI/FLAIR foci and gyriform enhancement in the distribution of the vasculitis. SSPE presents with a more protracted history of neurological decline.

Andreula C. Cranial viral infections in the adult. *European Radiology* 2004; 14: E132–E144.
Grossman R and Yousem D. *Neuroradiology: The Requisites*, 2nd edn, Mosby, 2003, 288–304.

14. A. Pilocytic astrocytoma.

This question deals with the classical neurological differential diagnosis of a posterior fossa mass in a child. While there are many causes, pilocytic astrocytoma and medulloblastoma account for over 60% of all childhood posterior fossa masses. Pilocytic astrocytomas have a classical appearance of being cystic lesions with an avidly enhancing mural nodule. However, 30% of pilocytic astrocytomas are solid tumours. In differentiating them from medulloblastomas, pilocytic astrocytomas often arise more peripherally and displace the fourth ventricle, whereas medulloblastomas usually arise centrally from the vermis. Subarachnoid seeding is seen in up to 50% of cases of medulloblastoma. Ependymomas are also included in the differential. As these arise from the ependyma lining the ventricle, they tend to be centred on the fourth ventricle in children. Metastases are the most common cause of a posterior fossa mass in adults, but are less common in children.

Brant W and Helms C. *Fundamentals of Diagnostic Radiology*, Lippincott Williams & Wilkins, 2006, pp. 135–142.

15. C. Vestibular nerve schwannoma.

Even in the absence of the imaging findings this would be a reasonable bet as it accounts for 75% of CPA tumours. However, assessment of the imaging characteristics increases the likelihood of this diagnosis. The second most common cause of CPA tumour is meningioma (10%). Differentiating features are lack of a dural tail, acute angle with the petrous bone (seen in schwannomas, less commonly with meningiomas, which make an obtuse angle), and, most importantly, expansion of the internal auditory canal (IAC). Facial nerve schwannomas can appear in the same site and appear identical, but they only constitute 4% of lesions in this site and as such would not be the most likely cause. The facial nerve lies in the antero-superior portion of the IAC, although it cannot usually be separated from the mass in the IAC on imaging.

Grossman R and Yousem D. *Neuroradiology: The Requisites*, 2nd edn, Mosby, 2003, pp. 105–108.

16. D. Recent back surgery complicated by ongoing CSF leak.

The key feature is the pattern of meningeal enhancement. It is important to recognize that the imaging findings describe pachymeningeal, not leptomeningeal, enhancement and as such the causes of leptomeningeal enhancement (bacterial or fungal meningitis) can be discounted. Similarly a recent stroke can cause gyriform enhancement, not pachymeningeal enhancement. Breast cancer is the most common malignancy to cause pachymeningeal enhancement, but this would usually be more nodular than smooth. CSF leak or any cause of intracranial hypotension will be associated with smooth pachymeningeal thickening, primarily over the convexities and falx. This enhances, not because of any inflammatory process, but because this part of the meninges has no blood–brain barrier, unlike the leptomeninges.

Smirniotopoulos J, Murphy F, Rushing E, Rees J, and Shroeder J. Patterns of contrast enhancement in the brain and meninges. *RadioGraphics* 2007; 27: 525–551.

17. B. Elevated choline, reduced NAA, Cho/Cr ratio of 2.

NAA is thought to be a marker of neuronal integrity, choline indicates cell turnover, and creatine indicates cell metabolism. Lactate is not detectable in normal brain spectra but is elevated in inflammation, infarction, and some neoplasms. Most brain conditions, whether neoplastic, vascular, or demyelinating, are associated with a reduction in NAA. A notable exception is Canavan's disease, which causes a rise in NAA. Choline is elevated in many disorders, but is markedly increased in high-grade neoplasms. It has been reported that the ratio of choline to creatine can be used to help grade tumours, with a ratio over 1.5 indicating high grade in the majority of cases. A reduced choline and NAA in an area of tumour can indicate necrosis.

Soares D and Law M. Magnetic resonance spectroscopy of the brain: review of metabolites and clinical applications. *Clinical Radiology* 2009; 64(1): 12–21.
Fayed N, Davila J, Medrano J, and Olmos S. Malignancy assessment of brain tumours with magnetic resonance spectroscopy and dynamic susceptibility contrast MRI. *European Journal of Radiology* 2008; 67(3): 427–433.

18. A. Cavernous haemangioma.

The orbital compartments are split up into extraconal, conal, intraconal, and globe. The extraconal compartment consists of fat, lacrimal gland, and bony orbit. Pathology in this region includes infection, neurofibroma, adenocarcinoma, mucoepidermoid and adenoid cystic carcinoma, neoplasia of bone, and lymphoma.

Conal pathology (muscle) includes rhabdomyosarcoma, thyroid eye disease, and idiopathic orbital inflammation (pseudotumour).

The intraconal compartment consists of fat, lymph nodes, vessels, nerves, and the optic nerve sheath complex. Pathology in this region includes venolymphatic malformation, haemangioma, arteriovenous malformation, optic nerve meningioma/glioma, and lymphoma.

Pathology in the globe includes retinoblastoma, metastasis, and melanoma.

Aviv RI and Miszkiel K. Orbital imaging Part2. Intraorbital pathology. *Clinical Radiology* 2005; 60: 288–307.

19. E. Cholesterol granuloma.

The findings described are typical of cholesterol granuloma. A critical distinction is between this and a petrous carotid artery aneurysm, which may show similar features of increased T1WI signal. However, the presence of flow void, lesion centred on the carotid canal, and additional complex areas of signal due to blood products of varying ages might be expected in an aneurysm.

A petrous apex cephalocele is an area of fluid signal (hypointense T1WI, hyperintense T2WI) adjacent to the petrous apex that is in communication with Meckel's cave.

A mucocele of the petrous apex may cause benign bony expansion and is typically of decreased signal on T1WI and increased signal on T2WI, and is non-enhancing. A cholesteatoma may have similar T1WI and T2WI signal characteristics, but these entities may be differentiated by DWI. On DWI, cholesteatoma is typically of increased signal, whereas a mucocele is of decreased signal.

Petrous apicitis is an aggressive process that typically enhances with gadolinium and is secondary to infection. There may be an accompanying history of infection, middle ear disease, diabetes, or immunocompromise.

Connor SEJ, Leung R, and Natas S. Imaging of the petrous apex: a pictorial review. *British Journal of Radiology* 2008; 81: 427–435.

20. D. Inferior and medial.

The question refers to Graves ophthalmopathy, where enlargement of the extraocular muscles is observed, with sparing of the tendinous insertions. This is in distinction to idiopathic orbital inflammatory syndrome, where the muscle swelling typically involves the tendinous insertions.

In Graves ophthalmopathy, the extra-orbital muscles are involved with decreasing frequency as follows: inferior, medial, superior, and lateral recti.

LeBedis CA and Sakai O. Nontraumatic orbital conditions: diagnosis with CT and MR imaging in the emergent setting. *RadioGraphics* 2008; 28: 1741–1753.

21. E. Rhabdomyosarcoma.

The clinical and radiological features described are typical of rhabdomyosarcoma. It usually presents in the first decade of life with a rapidly growing mass causing proptosis. The globe is often distorted and displaced, but rarely invaded. The lesion is aggressive and there may be extension into the sinuses or intracranial compartment, and bony destruction can occur.

NHL is usually found in older adults, but it can occur in older children or adolescents. Unlike rhabdomyosarcoma, NHL commonly causes lacrimal gland involvement, may be hypointense on T2WI, and encases rather than distorts the globe.

Capillary haemangioma typically presents in the first few months of life. They have a proliferative phase for approximately 12 months following diagnosis and then are stable, before gradually involuting over a period of years. These lesions show rapid and persistent enhancement on CT and MRI. On unenhanced MRI, it is typically iso- to hyperintense relative to muscle on T1WI and moderately hyperintense on T2WI, with flow voids at the periphery of or within the tumour.

A ruptured dermoid cyst can mimic a rhabdomyosarcoma both clinically and radiologically, but one might expect to see calcification or fatty or cystic components in the native lesion. Retinoblastoma is an intraorbital lesion.

Chung EM, Smirniotopoulos JG, Specht CS, Schroeder JW, and Cube R. Pediatric orbit tumors and tumorlike lesions: nonosseous lesions of the extraocular orbit. *RadioGraphics* 2007; 27: 1777–1799.

22. A. Venous-lymphatic malformation.

Venous-lymphatic malformation (previously known as a lymphangioma) typically has a presentation in childhood. MRI is the modality of choice for diagnosis, as fluid–fluid levels are almost pathognomic of this condition and these represent areas of haemorrhage of varying ages. The MRI findings are as those described and there are typically no large feeding vessels or flow voids. The lesion is predominantly extraconal, but can insinuate into the intraconal compartment.

Capillary haemangioma also presents in childhood, but may be apparent clinically and on MRI there are not typically fluid–fluid levels, but there may be flow voids within the lesion from prominent vessels. Also, enhancement is usually more rapid and persistent in capillary haemangioma than in venous-lymphatic malformation.

Orbital varices usually present in young adults and on imaging have the appearance of dilated, tortuous vessels.

Cavernous haemangioma typically presents in adulthood. They are usually well-circumscribed and most often occur in the lateral aspect of the retrobulbar intraconal space. On CT, they are slightly hyperattenuating prior to contrast and may contain phleboliths. On MRI, they are iso-intense to muscle on T1WI and hyperintense on T2WI. They show progressive enhancement on multiphase dynamic imaging.

Haemangiopericytomas are rare vascular tumours that are more often seen in adults than children. Large lesions may show bony erosion and they do not typically have fluid–fluid levels on CT or MRI.

Smoker WRK, Gentry LR, Yee NK, Reede DL, and Nerad JA. Vascular lesions of the orbit: more than meets the eye. *RadioGraphics* 2008; 28: 185–204.

23. B. Presence of optic canal widening.

The presence of a widened optic nerve canal occurs in up to 90% of cases of optic nerve glioma. While it can also occur in meningioma, it is more common in glioma and some cases of meningioma may even have a narrowed canal secondary to bony hyperostosis.

The 'tram-track' sign is typically associated with meningioma and refers to the more avidly enhancing meningioma surrounding the non-enhancing optic nerve on axial CT and MR imaging of the orbit. Although both meningioma and glioma enhance following intravenous contrast, it is meningioma that is more typically associated with marked intense enhancement.

Calcification and bony hyperostosis are features associated with meningioma. Calcification is rare in gliomas, unless they have previously undergone radiotherapy.

Goh PS, Gi MT, Charlton A, Tan C, Gangadhara Sundar JK, and Amrith S. Review of orbital imaging. *European Journal of Radiology* 2008; 66: 387–395.
Aviv RI and Miszkiel K. Orbital imaging Part2. Intraorbital pathology. *Clinical Radiology* 2005; 60: 288–307.

24. C. Transverse/labyrinthine.

Transverse temporal bone fractures are more commonly associated with facial nerve paralysis (approximately up to 50%) than longitudinal temporal bone fractures (approximately up to 20%). The labyrinthine segment is the most likely segment of the facial nerve to be associated with facial paralysis.

Jager L and Reiser M. CT and MR imaging of the normal and pathologic conditions of the facial nerve. *European Journal of Radiology* 2001; 40: 133–146.

25. D. FLAIR.

On a FLAIR sequence, epidermoid cysts can be differentiated from arachnoid cysts because the former show mixed iso- to hyperintense signal, but with poor demarcation, while the signal of the latter is suppressed, like the signal of CSF.

DWI offers a finding specific for extra-axial epidermoid cysts by showing very high signal. Restricted ADC compared to CSF, almost comparable to that of the brain and T2 shine-through effect, both play an important role in the high signal intensity of epidermoid cyst at DWI. This can therefore be useful in helping to distinguish them from arachnoid cyst.

Bonneville F, Savatovsky J, and Chiras J. Imaging of cerebellopontine angle lesions: an update. Part 2: intra-axial lesions, skull base lesions that may invade the CPA region, and non-enhancing extra-axial lesions. *European Radiology* 2007; 17: 2908–2920.

26. D. Paraganglioma.

Paragangliomas are rare intradural extramedullary tumours that are usually benign and have imaging characteristics as those described. Schwannomas, neurofibromas, and meningiomas are much more common, but do not typically contain vascular flow voids or areas of haemorrhage. Meningiomas may have a dural tail or foci of calcification. Schwannomas and neurofibromas can be difficult to distinguish on imaging. They are typically isointense on T1WI and markedly hyperintense on T2WI. Enhancement may be intense and homogenous or peripheral. Neurofibromas tend to encase, rather than displace, nerve roots.

Leptomeningeal metastases present with three different imaging patterns:
1) Diffuse, thin enhancing coating of the surface of the spinal cord and nerve roots.
2) Multiple small enhancing nodules on the surface of the cord and nerve roots.
3) A single mass in the lowest part of the thecal sac.

Abul-Kasim K, Thurnher MM, McKeever P, and Sundgren PC. Intradural spinal tumors: current classification and MRI features. *Neuroradiology* 2008; 50: 301–314.

27. E. Ependymoma.

Ependymoma is the most common intramedullary neoplasm in adults. It tends to be centrally located within the cord, unlike astrocytoma, which can be eccentric. Astrocytoma can have a longer segment of cord involvement than ependymoma and may have a more infiltrative margin. The peripheral low signal areas seen on T2WI in ependymoma are related to haemosiderin deposition from prior haemorrhage.

Haemangioblastoma is more often seen in the dorsal cord than the cervical cord and is typically a small well-defined lesion. It may have an associated cord cyst or syrinx. Flow voids may be seen within the lesion, from dilated vascular channels.

Ganglioglioma is a very rare, slow-growing tumour of low malignant potential. The imaging appearance is non-specific, but there are some findings that may suggest the diagnosis. Compared with other spinal cord tumors, gangliogliomas are more likely to involve long segments of the cord (greater than four levels, up to the whole cord), to be associated with bone erosion or scalloping, to have tumoral cysts, and to have areas of mixed high signal on precontrast T1WI.

Intramedullary metastasis represents less than 5% of intramedullary lesions. They usually occur in the setting of advanced malignant disease, typically from a lung or breast primary. The spinal cord oedema can seem out of keeping with the small size of the metastatic lesion.

Smith JK, Lury K, and Castillo M. Imaging of spinal and spinal cord tumors. *Seminars in Roentogenology* 2006; 41: 274–293.

28. A. Two episodes of vomiting.

Almost anything will buy you a CT brain these days, but surprisingly, the GCS must be less than 13 in the A&E department within 2 hours of the injury under NICE guidelines to warrant one. After 2 hours have passed, a GCS of anything less than normal is an indication for scanning. Other factors which require a CT within 1 hour are suspected open or depressed skull fracture, sign of fracture at skull base, post-traumatic seizure, focal neurological deficit and amnesia, or loss of consciousness **and** coagulopathy. Additional factors which necessitate a CT brain within 8 hours are amnesia of events for greater than 30 minutes before impact, and if there is any amnesia or loss of consciousness **and** the patient is older than 65/dangerous mechanism of injury. Note that, perversely, even if the scan can be delayed but be performed within 8 hours, the guidelines state it should be requested immediately. Prepare to be awoken from your sleep!

NICE Guideline on Head Injury: triage, assessment, investigation and early management of head injury in infants, children and adults. September 2007. Quick reference guide. Available online at: http://www.nice.org.uk/nicemedia/live/11836/36257/36257.pdf.

29. E. Diffuse axonal injury (DAI).

CT is initially often normal (up to 80% of cases) in DAI. If positive, it may reveal small low attenuation foci (oedema) or high attenuation foci of petechial haemorrhage. The gray/white matter interface of the frontotemporal lobes, corpus callosum (especially the splenium), and brainstem are the most commonly involved sites in DAI. MRI is much more sensitive and is the investigation of choice.

The signal on MRI depends on the age of the lesion and whether haemorrhage is present, but classically hyperintense foci on T2WI sequences are seen acutely. In the more chronic phase, the lesions may only be detected as hypointense foci at characteristic locations on GE sequences: this appearance may remain for years. DWI reveals hyperintense foci of restricted diffusion on B1000 images, with corresponding low signal on the ADC map. The findings on DWI are easily distinguishable from extradural haematoma/subarachnoid haemorrhage/subdural haematoma/ generalized oedema, which are discussed in other questions in this chapter.

Osborn AG, Blaser SI, Salzman KL, Katzman GL, Provenzale J, Hedlund GL et al. *Diagnostic Imaging: Brain*, Amirsys, 2004, I-2: 30–33.

30. D. FLAIR.

Although CT is generally used for investigating acute subarachnoid haemorrhage (SAH), FLAIR sequence on MRI has been suggested as being as sensitive as or more sensitive than CT. It is particularly useful in regions where CT may be limited due to beam hardening artefacts or if there is a very small amount of blood. Acute SAH appears as high intensity on FLAIR within the cisterns and sulci. Subacute SAH may be better appreciated on MRI because of its high signal intensity when the blood is isointense to CSF on CT. SAH differs from intra-parenchymal haemorrhage in that the mix of blood with high-oxygen tension CSF delays generation of paramagnetic deoxyhaemoglobin, and oxyhaemoglobin remains present longer than in intra-parenchymal haemorrhage. This contributes to continued T2 prolongation. Beware that there are other pathological (meningitis, leptomeningeal metastases, acute stroke, fat-containing tumour/dermoid rupture) and benign (artefact, supplemental oxygenation) causes of FLAIR hyperintensity in the subarachnoid space.

Chronic haemorrhage from SAH is best detected on GE sequences, resulting in marked subarachnoid low signal (the blooming of superficial siderosis).

Stuckey SL, Goh TD, Heffernan T, and Rowan D. Hyperintensity in the subarachnoid space on FLAIR MRI. *American Journal of Roentgenology* 2007; 189: 913–921.

31. D. Wilson's disease.

Hyperintensity in the tegmentum (except for the red nucleus) and hypointensity of the superior colliculus are described as the 'face of the giant panda sign' and are seen in axial T2WI sections of the midbrain in Wilson's disease. A 'double panda sign' has also been described, with a second 'panda cub face' in the pons. Abnormal signal can also be seen in the basal ganglia and thalamus in Wilson's disease (putamen most commonly). The signal abnormalities are due to copper deposition. Signal is generally reduced on T1WI sequences, although it may be increased due to the paramagnetic effects of copper and also due to the hepatic component of Wilson's disease (a portocaval shunt can produce this latter finding). Signal is generally increased on T2WI sequences, but it can be of mixed or reduced intensity. Similarly carbon monoxide poisoning and methanol poisoning can cause increased or reduced signal on T1WI. Methanol poisoning typically causes abnormal signal in the putamen, with haemorrhagic necrosis being more typical, whereas carbon monoxide poisoning typically affects the globus pallidus. The latter would be expected to cause low attenuation in the basal ganglia on CT.

The findings on CT exclude basal ganglia haemorrhage. Amphetamine and cocaine abuse can cause high T2WI signal in the basal ganglia due to small areas of infarction, but are not associated with the midbrain changes.

Jacobs DA, Markowitz CE, Liebeskind DS, and Galetta SL. The 'double panda sign' in Wilson's disease. *Neurology* 2003; 61: 969.

32. E. The haematoma crosses sutures.

An SDH will cross suture lines and may extend over the whole cerebral hemisphere; an EDH will not. Only an EDH can cross the midline, and this usually occurs at the vertex in the setting of a venous EDH. EDHs are more usually arterial bleeds and associated with temporal skull fractures, which disrupt the adjacent middle meningeal artery. The latter are typically biconvex; SDHs are typically lentiform in shape. Both measure 50–60 HU if acute. Chronic SDHs may be iso- or hypodense to brain, although anaemia or clotting disorders can produce a similar appearance. EDH is a neurosurgical emergency more so than SDH because of the potential lucent period followed by sudden deterioration as arterial bleeding continues after having stripped the dura from the inner table of the skull.

Barr RM, Gean AD, and Tuong HL. Craniofacial trauma. In: Brant WE and Helms CA (eds), *Fundamentals of Diagnostic Radiology*, 3rd edn, Lippincott, Williams & Wilkins, 2007, pp. 57–59.

33. D. Normal pressure hydrocephalus.

Fifty per cent of cases of normal pressure hydrocephalus (NPH) are idiopathic, while 50% have a cause, e.g. meningitis, neurosurgery, head trauma, or, as in the current vignette, previous subarachnoid haemorrhage. The imaging reveals dilated ventricles with rounded frontal horns, which are enlarged out of proportion to the degree of sulcal enlargement (as one would see in cerebral atrophy). On CT there may be periventricular low attenuation in the frontal and occipital regions, representing transependymal CSF flow. The MRI equivalent is periventricular high signal and there are other MRI findings, including upward bowing of the corpus callosum and the aqueductal flow void sign (reflecting increased CSF velocity through the cerebral aqueduct).

The bradykinesia and gait apraxia of NPH may mimic Parkinson's disease, although there is typically no associated tremor. Binswanger's disease (also known as subcortical arteriosclerotic encephalopathy) is a continuous, irreversible ischaemic degeneration of periventricular and deep white matter. MRI reveals extensive periventricular and deep white matter hyperintensities, which reflect microinfarctions and demyelination, and enlarged ventricles.

Hathout GM. *Clinical Neuroradiology: A case based approach*, Cambridge University Press, 2009, p. 106.
Osborn AG, Blaser SI, Salzman KL, Katzman GL, Provenzale J, Hedlund GL et al. *Diagnostic Imaging: Brain*, Amirsys, 2004, II-1: 24–27.

34. C. Measure blood pressure

The CT findings are consistent with PRES. This is a usually reversible neurological syndrome with a variety of presenting symptoms ranging from altered mental status to seizures, headache, and loss of vision. Common causes include hypertension, eclampsia and preeclampsia, immunosuppressive medications such as cyclosporine, various antineoplastic agents (including interferon), SLE, and various causes of renal failure. Hypertension is common in PRES, but may be mild and is not universally present, especially in the setting of immunosuppression. However, in the vignette given, hypertension is a possible cause and should be sought. Cyclosporin or tacrolimus might be causes; the former is thought to result in PRES both via a direct neurotoxic effect and by causing hypertension.

The condition is not always reversible and may result in haemorrhagic infarcts. The classic MRI finding is of hyperintensity on FLAIR in the parieto-occipital and posterior frontal cortical and subcortical white matter. Less commonly the brainstem, basal ganglia, and cerebellum are involved. Atypical imaging appearances include contrast enhancement, haemorrhage, and restricted diffusion on MRI. Abnormalities can often be seen on CT, as described in the vignette.

McKinney AM, Short J, Truwit CL, McKinney ZJ, Kozak OS, SantaCruz KS et al. Posterior reversible encephalopathy syndrome: incidence of atypical regions of involvement and imaging findings. *American Journal of Roentgenology* 2007; 189: 904–912.

35. C. Pre- and post-contrast T1WI.

MS plaques are generally most conspicuous on FLAIR sequences. However, if there are enhancing and non-enhancing plaques on T1WI post-contrast, this indicates plaques of differing ages, i.e. dissemination in time. While this is not diagnostic of MS (imaging alone never is), it is very suggestive.

Proton density sequences are useful, but not quite as useful as FLAIR sequences, in showing periventricular lesions. T2WI sequences are superior to FLAIR sequences when it comes to detection of lesions in the posterior fossa and spinal cord. T2W STIR is probably superior to standard T2WI sequences in detecting spinal cord lesions, but is not routinely used. STIR sequences or fat suppression are useful when imaging the optic nerves, as contrast between lesions and the surrounding orbital fat is increased.

Pretorius PM and Quaghebeur G. The role of MRI in the diagnosis of MS. *Clinical Radiology* 2003; 58: 434–448.

36. B. SLE.

The combination of white matter hyperintensities and focal infarcts (indicated by the areas of restricted diffusion) in combination with established neurology and neuropsychiatric symptoms, in a woman of child-bearing age, strongly suggests the diagnosis of cerebral lupus. SLE is an autoimmune disorder that affects many organ systems, including the CNS. Clinical presentation can include migraine, seizures, stroke, chorea, psychosis, mood disorder, acute confusional state, cognitive dysfunction, transverse myelopathy, cranial neuropathies, and aseptic meningitis. The CNS pathology includes vasculitis, dural venous sinus thrombosis, cerebritis, intracranial haemorrhage, infarction, and infection. Infarction can occur as a result of direct thrombosis as well as embolism from Libman–Sacks endocarditis. Diffuse neuropsychiatric symptoms are attributed to direct neuronal damage mediated by antibodies.

The most common imaging finding is small multifocal T2WI or FLAIR hyperintense white matter lesions. Focal infarcts and grey matter lesions may also be seen, as well as diffuse steroid responsive subcortical lesions. Acute lesions may enhance. MR angiography and venography may show thrombotic lesions of vessels and dural venous sinus thrombosis, respectively. When a patient with SLE presents with an acute neurological deterioration, it is crucial to image them promptly: initially with unenhanced CT to exclude haemorrhage and then with MRI (including post-contrast sequences) to evaluate for stroke or abscess. Note that a negative brain MRI cannot exclude cerebral lupus. Treatment consists of immunosuppression, with anticoagulation for thrombotic events.

Stroke is atypical for MS. Small vessel ischaemia should not occur in such a young age without an underlying cause and is not a satisfactory diagnosis. Susac syndrome is a triad of encephalopathy, branch retinal artery occlusions, and hearing loss. It is a microangiopathy of unknown aetiology and results in multiple T2WI hyperintense deep white matter and corpus callosum lesions. Lyme disease results in T2WI hyperintense periventricular white matter lesions, which may enhance, and it may resemble ADEM or MS.

Lalani TA, Kanne JP, Hatfield GA, and Chen P. Imaging findings in systemic lupus erythematosus. *RadioGraphics* 2004; 24: 1069–1086.
Osborn AG, Blaser SI, Salzman KL, Katzman GL, Provenzale J, Hedlund GL et al. *Diagnostic Imaging: Brain*, Amirsys, 2004, I-4: 54–57.

37. B. Reduced activity in the precuneus and posterior cingulate gyrus.

FDG-PET-CT has been shown to have a sensitivity and specificity of 93% for mild to moderate Alzheimer's disease. The technique has been shown to provide important prognostic information so that a negative PET-CT scan is indicative of unlikely progression of cognitive impairment for a mean follow-up of 3 years in those patients who initially present with cognitive symptoms of dementia. The more specific findings on PET-CT in Alzheimer's disease are early reduced activity in the precuneus/posterior cingulate gyrus and the superior, middle, and inferior temporal lobe gyrus, with relative sparing of the primary sensorimotor and visual cortex, and sparing of the striatum, thalamus, and cerebellum.

Diffuse reduced activity of the cortical/subcortical regions and cerebellum is more typical of multiinfarct dementia. Reduced activity in the fronto-temporal regions is more consistent with fronto-temporal dementia. Reduced activity in the occipital cortex reflects the visual problems encountered in lewy body dementia. Reduced activity in the caudate and lentiform nuclei is more typical of Huntingdon's chorea.

Silverman DHS and Thompson PM. Structural and functional neuroimaging: focussing on mild cognitive impairment. *Applied Neurology* 2006; Feb: 10–24.

38. D. Juvenile angiofibroma.

Juvenile angiofibromas are benign but locally aggressive tumours with high vascularity. They typically occur in adolescent boys and present with recurrent epistaxis and nasal obstruction. They are centred within the sphenopalatine foramen and involve the pterygopalatine fossa, producing a bowed appearance of the posterior wall of maxillary sinus and widening of pterygopalatine fossa, inferior orbital, and pteryogomaxillary fissures. Osseous erosion is commonly seen.

The specific differentiating feature on MRI is the presence of multiple flow voids on T2WI and enhanced T1WI.

Momeni A, Roberts C, and Chew F. Imaging of chronic and exotic sinonasal disease: self-assessment module. *American Journal of Roentgenology* 2007; 189: S46–S48.
Ludwig B, Foster B, Saito N, Nadgir RN, Castro-Aragon I, and Sakai O. Diagnostic imaging in nontraumatic pediatric head and neck emergencies. *RadioGraphics* 2010; 30: 781–799.

39. B. Inverted papilloma.

Inverted papillomas are uncommon benign epithelial neoplasms with significant malignant potential. They arise from the lateral nasal wall or maxillary sinus. They are most commonly seen in 40–70-year-olds with a male to female ratio of 2–4:1. CT demonstrates a soft-tissue mass centred in the middle meatus associated with bone remodelling. Stippled calcification is seen in 20% of cases. On MRI, it is isointense on T1WI and iso/hypointense on T2WI. Heterogenous enhancement is seen in 50% of cases. A convoluted cerebriform pattern on T2WI or enhanced T1WI is typical of inverted papillomas.

Juvenile angiofibromas are seen in younger patients and are located in the posterior nasal cavity. They demonstrate intense enhancement and flow voids on MRI. Antrochoanal polyps are homogenously hyperintense on T2WI. Invasive fungal sinusitis is primarily seen in immunosuppressed patients. They are frequently bilateral. CT findings include complete opacification of sinuses by hyperdense mass, erosion or remodelling of sinuses, and intrasinus calcification. They are hypointense on T2WI. Nasal carcinomas cause bone erosion/destruction rather than remodelling.

Momeni A, Roberts C, and Chew F. Imaging of chronic and exotic sinonasal disease: self-assessment module. *American Journal of Roentgenology* 2007; 189: S46–S48.

40. C. Medialization of middle turbinate.

FESS is the treatment of choice for patients with medically refractory sinusitis. Obstruction of the frontal recess is the main cause for medically refractory frontal sinusitis. The frontal recess is considered a difficult area to treat with FESS and it is also prone to re-stenosis.

All of the above options are commonly associated with postoperative frontal recess stenosis except medialization of middle turbinate. Medialization ('Bolgerization') is performed to treat a lateralized middle turbinate, which is a well-recognized cause of frontal recess stenosis.

Huang B, Lloyd K, DelGaudio JM, Jablonsowski E, and Hudgins PA. Failed endoscopic sinus surgery: spectrum of CT findings in the frontal recess. *RadioGraphics* 2009: 29: 177–195.

41. A. No change in size, shape, or signal intensity on follow-up MRI.

Hypothalamic hamartomas are developmental malformations located in the tuber cinereum of the hypothalamus. The typical patient is male, in the first or second decade of life, presenting with precocious puberty or gelastic seizures.

On MRI, they appear as well-defined pedunculated or sessile lesions that are iso/mildly hypointense on T1WI and iso/hyperintense on T2WI, with no contrast enhancement or calcification. Lack of interval change strongly supports the diagnosis.

Saleem S, Ahmed-Hesham MS, and Lee DH. Lesions of the hypothalamus: MR imaging diagnostic features. *RadioGraphics* 2007; 27: 1807–1108.

42. B. II.

Lymph nodes in the neck have been divided into seven levels, generally for the purpose of squamous cell carcinoma staging. This is, however, not all inclusive, as the parotid nodes and retropharyngeal space nodes are not included in this system.

Level I: Below mylohyoid to hyoid bone anteriorly
- Level Ia: Submental
- Level Ib: Submandibular

Level II: Jugulodigastric (base of skull to hyoid)
Level III: Deep cervical (hyoid to cricoid)
Level IV: Virchow (cricoid to clavicle)
Level V: Posterior triangle groups
- Level Va: Accessory spinal (posterior triangle), superior half
- Level Vb: Accessory spinal (posterior triangle), inferior half

Level VI: Prelaryngeal/pretracheal/Delphian node
Level VII: Superior mediastinal (between common carotid arteries (CCAs), below top of manubrium)

Lymph node levels of the neck. Radiopaedia.org.

43. A. Fibromatosis colli.

Fibromatosis colli or pseudotumour of the sternocleidomastoid muscle is a benign self-limiting condition that occurs in the first 2–4 weeks of life. It is often associated with breech or forceps delivery. It is thought to result from pressure necrosis and subsequent fibrocollagenous infiltration of the sternocleidomastoid muscle.

Typical presentation is with a firm and non-tender mass in the lower two-thirds of the sternocleidomastoid muscle. It may be associated with torticollis in approximately 20% of cases. It usually resolves spontaneously in the first year of life.

Typical findings on ultrasound include focal or diffuse enlargement of the sternocleidomastoid with variable echogenicity. The clinical history and ultrasound appearances are so typical that no further investigation is usually necessary.

Ludwig B, Foster B, Saito N, Nadgir RN, Castro-Aragon I, and Sahai O. Diagnostic imaging in nontraumatic pediatric head and neck emergencies. *RadioGraphics* 2010; 30: 781–799.

44. B. Cavernous sinus.

Cranial nerves III, IV, and VI, and ophthalmic (V1) and maxillary (V2) divisions of the V cranial nerve course through the cavernous sinus along with the internal carotid artery. The V2 division of the trigeminal nerve passes through the inferior portion of the cavernous sinus and exits via the foramen rotundum. The remainder of the cranial nerves mentioned above enter the orbit via the superior orbital fissure.

The cavernous sinus location accounts for these features. Palsies of cranial nerves III, IV, and VI result in ophthalmoplegia. Involvement of V1 and V2 divisions of the trigeminal nerve produces facial pain and sensory loss; involvement of sympathetic nerves around the internal carotid artery results in Horner's syndrome. This cluster of findings is found in Tolosa Hunt syndrome, an idiopathic inflammatory process involving the cavernous sinus.

Hoang J, Eastwood J, and Glastonbury C. What's in a name? Eponyms in head and neck imaging. *Clinical Radiology* 2010; 65: 237–245.

45. E. Parotid space.

Loss of symmetry and displacement of the parapharyngeal space are useful for lesion identification and localization in the parapharyngeal soft tissues. A thorough knowledge of the anatomical relationship between the spaces is essential.

The parapharyngeal space is shaped like an inverted pyramid with the apex pointing inferiorly toward the greater cornu of the hyoid bone and the skull base demarcates the base superiorly. A lesion arising from the parotid space displaces the fat in the parapharyngeal space anteromedially. A lesion in the masticator space displaces the parapharyngeal fat posteromedially. Carotid space lesions displace it anteriorly, mucosal space lesions displace it posterolaterally, and retropharyngeal space lesions displace it anterolaterally.

Posterior displacement of the carotid space or parapharyngeal fat completely surrounding a lesion localizes it to the parapharyngeal space.

Bahrami S and Yim C. Blind spots at brain imaging. *RadioGraphics* 2009; 29: 1877–1896.

46. B. Warthin tumours.

Warthin tumour or adenolymphoma is the second most common benign tumour of the parotid gland. It is usually solitary. Multiple or bilateral parotid masses and increased uptake on ^{99m}Tc are strongly suggestive of Warthin tumour. Warthin tumours do not enhance following gadolinium administration.

Pleomorphic adenomas are usually solitary and unilateral. They appear as hypoechoic, lobulated, well-defined lesions with posterior acoustic enhancement on ultrasound scan (USS).

On MRI, they are of intermediate signal on T1WI and hyperintense on T2WI. They demonstrate homogenous enhancement following gadolinium administration.

Mucoepidermoid carcinomas vary in appearances. Low-grade tumours are similar to pleomorphic adenomas. High-grade tumours are heterogenous with low to intermediate signal intensity on T1WI and T2WI. They demonstrate infiltrating margins and heterogenous enhancement following gadolinium administration.

Soler R, Bargiela A, Requejo I, Rodriguez E, Rey JL, and Sancristan F. Pictorial review: MR imaging of parotid tumours. *Clinical Radiology* 1997; 52: 269–275.
Bialek EJ, Jakubowski W, Zajkowski P, Szopinski KT, and Osmolski A. US of the major salivary glands: anatomy and spatial relationships, pathologic conditions, and pitfalls. *RadioGraphics* 2006; 26: 745–763.

47. D. Splaying of the internal and external carotid arteries.

Carotid body tumour or paraganglioma is the most common paraganglioma of the head and neck. It arises from the paraganglionic cells located on the medial aspect of the carotid bifurcation. On MRI, they are of low to intermediate signal intensity on T1WI and hyperintense on T2WI. They are hypervascular and demonstrate intense enhancement after contrast administration. Splaying of the internal and external carotid arteries and multiple flow voids producing a 'salt and pepper' appearance are distinctive features on imaging.

Lee KY, Oh Y-W, Noh HJ, Lee YJ, Yong HS, and Kang EY. Extraadrenal paragangliomas of the body: imaging features. *American Journal of Roentgenology* 2006; 187: 492–504.

48. D. Eccentrically placed lesion in the cord. Table 6.2 illustrates the diagnostic features of astrocytoma and ependymoma.

Table 6.2 Diagnostic features of astrocytoma and ependymoma

	Astrocytoma	**Ependymoma**
Age	Children	Adults
Region	C > T > L	C > T = L
Location in cord	Eccentric	Central
Margins	Infiltrating	Sharp
Other findings	Long segment involved	Peripheral low T2WI signal
Associated syndrome	Neurofibromatosis-1	Neurofibromatosis-2

Smith JK, Lury K, and Castillo M. Imaging of spinal and spinal cord tumors. *Seminars in Roentogenology* 2006; 41: 274–293.

49. E. Meningioma.

Spinal meningiomas are typically iso- to hypointense on T1WI and slightly hyperintense on T2WI. There is usually strong and homogeneous enhancement with gadolinium. However, some meningiomas may contain calcification and are typically the only intradural extramedullary tumours to do so. Some meningiomas can be heavily calcified and such a meningioma is being described in the question. These will remain dark on all MRI sequences and demonstrate only little contrast uptake (in the non-calcified areas).

Schwannomas, neurofibromas, and metastases would not typically be hypointense on T2WI. Meningeal lymphomas are very rare and usually manifest as diffuse thickening of nerve roots and/or multiple enhancing nodules.

Abul-Kasim K, Thurner MM, McKeever P, and Sundgren PC. Intradural spinal tumours: current classification and MRI features. *Neuroradiology* 2008; 50: 301–314.

50. C. T2 fast SE.

T2 fast SE is probably the least useful sequence when specifically looking for vertebral marrow deposits because the metastases are less conspicuous, typically being high signal on a background of high-signal fatty marrow. On STIR and T2 fast SE with fat saturation, the metastases typically stand out as being of increased signal on a background of dark marrow because of the fat saturation techniques. On T1 fast SE sequences, the metastases typically stand out as being low signal on a background of high-signal fatty marrow.

Finally, T1 GE out–of-phase imaging is also good for looking for vertebral metastatic disease. This is a sequence with a specific echo time corresponding to the time it takes for water and fat protons to move exactly 180° out of phase. In the normal adult human, the medullary bone of the vertebral bodies contains approximately equal amounts of water and fat protons. In out-of-phase conditions, the signal of both will cancel out, leaving the vertebrae completely black. In the case of vertebral pathology, however, the signal will increase and, as such, vertebral metastases (or other lesions) will clearly stand out.

Van Goethem JWM, Van den Hauwe L, Ozsarlak O, De Schepper AMA, and Parizel PM. Spinal tumours. *European Journal of Radiology* 2004; 50: 159–176.

51. C. Le Fort fractures by definition refer to fractures involving the maxilla bilaterally.

Separation of all or a portion of the maxilla from the skull base is described as a Le Fort fracture. This can be unilateral when it is associated with sagittal or parasagittal fractures of the palate.

Le Fort fractures by definition involve the posterior maxillary buttress at the junction of the posterior maxillary sinus and the pterygoid plates of the sphenoid. This may be either through the pterygoid plates or through the posterior walls of the maxillary sinus.

Once a pterygomaxillary disruption has been identified, the remaining facial buttresses are inspected to identify the type of Le Fort fracture. In Le Fort I fracture, the maxillary arch will move in relation to the rest of the face and skull. In Le Fort II fracture, the entire maxilla will move in relation to the skull base. In Le Fort III, there is complete craniofacial separation.

Any combination of Le Fort I, II, and III can occur. Posterior extension of Le Fort fracture into the hard palate results in widening of the maxillary arch and dental malocclusion.

Hopper RA, Salemy S, and Sze RW. Diagnosis of midface fractures with CT: what the surgeon needs to know. *RadioGraphics* 2006; 26: 783–793.

52. B. Keratocystic odontogenic tumour.

These are benign but locally aggressive developmental tumours affecting adults in the second to fourth decades. They are most commonly located in the mandibular ramus and body, and are associated with an impacted tooth. They may be unilocular or multilocular and often contain daughter cysts extending into the surrounding bone. They can be associated with cortical expansion and erosion. They demonstrate minimal peripheral enhancement with contrast.

The presence of multiple keratocystic odontogenic tumours raises the possibility of Gorlin basal cell nevus syndrome, which is an autosomal dominant disorder. Associated features include multiple basal cell carcinomas of the skin, mental retardation, midface hypoplasia, frontal bossing and prognathism, calcification of the falx and dura, and bifid ribs.

Devenney-Cakir B, Subramaniam RM, Reddy SM, Imsande H, Gohel A, and Sakai O. Cystic and cystic-appearing lesion of the mandible: Review. *American Journal of Roentgenology* 2001; 196: WS66–WS77.

53. A. Rathke cleft cyst.

These are benign cystic lesions of the pituitary fossa derived from the Rathke pouch. They are usually asymptomatic. Rathke cleft cysts are located in the midline between the anterior and posterior pituitary lobes and have a characteristic kidney shape on axial images. They are homogenously hyperintense on T1WI, due to high protein concentration, and hypointense on T2WI, due to low intracystic water content. They do not enhance following contrast administration.

Absence of a fluid–fluid level is helpful in differentiating Rathke cleft cyst from hemorrhagic adenoma. Acute haemorrhage has heterogenous signal on T2WI and may demonstrate thin peripheral enhancement on T1WI. Craniopharyngiomas have variable solid, cystic, and calcified components. They demonstrate heterogenous enhancement following contrast. They may be intrasellar or suprasellar. A pseudo-fluid–fluid level may occasionally be seen in craniopharyngioma. Lipoma and cholesterol granuloma are hyperintense on both T1WI and T2WI.

Bonneville F, Cattin F, Marsot-Dupuch K, Dormont D, Bonneville J-F, and Chiras J. T1 signal hyperintensity in the sellar region: spectrum of findings. *RadioGraphics* 2006; 26: 93–113.

54. E. Second branchial cleft cyst.

The majority of branchial cleft anomalies arise from the second branchial cleft. The described findings are typical of a second branchial cleft cyst. Similar ultrasound appearances may be seen in a first branchial cleft cyst or a dermoid cyst. The anatomical location is the key to the diagnosis. Dermoid cysts are typically midline in location in the neck and first branchial cleft cysts are located in the region of parotid gland, external auditory canal, and angle of mandible.

Lymphangiomas are typically located in the posterior triangle. On ultrasound, they appear multiloculated with intervening thin septa. Abscesses appear as ill-defined, irregular collections with thick walls and internal debris. Surrounding soft-tissue oedema, hyperaemia, and enlarged adjacent lymph nodes are also noted.

Wong KT, Lee YYP, King AD, and Ahuja AT. Imaging of cystic and cyst-like neck masses. *Clinical Radiology* 2008; 63: 613–622.

55. D. Filling of retropharyngeal space from side to side.

Understanding the retropharyngeal space anatomy is crucial in differentiating retropharyngeal space abscess and retropharyngeal suppurative lymph node. The retropharyngeal space is bounded by visceral fascia covering the pharynx and oesophagus anteriorly, the prevertebral fascia covering the prevertebral muscles posteriorly, and the carotid sheaths laterally.

A retropharyngeal suppurative lymph node is unilateral, whereas a retropharyngeal abscess fills the entire retropharyngeal space from side to side. The differentiation is important because many cases of suppurative lymph nodes do not have purulent material at surgery. The treatment for suppurative lymph nodes is a trial of antibiotics if the patient is stable. Surgical drainage is considered if there is progression or if the suppurative lymph node is large at presentation. The volume of central low density is a better predictor of purulence than the mere presence of rim enhancement and low-density centre.

Hoang JK, Branstetter IV BF, Eastwood JD, and Glastonbury CM. Multiplanar CT and MRI of collections in the retropharyngeal space: Is it an abscess? *American Journal of Roentgenology* 2011; 196: W426–W432.

56. B. Neurosarcoid.

Whilst primary neurosarcoid is rare, it is not uncommon for the systemic disease to present via its neurological manifestations. The findings of neurosarcoid are non-specific, with the common manifestations mirroring those described in this patient. Leptomeningeal thickening and enhancement are classical. Involvement of the perivascular spaces adjacent to this can cause increased signal in the adjacent cortex. This appearance can mimic meningioma.

Multifocal meningiomas and nerve sheath schwannomas are features of NF-2, but this would not be expected to resolve with steroid therapy. The features described are not typical of TS.

The meningeal disease would make MS unlikely, even given the periventricular high-signal lesions, which are the most common intraparenchymal finding in neurosarcoid.

Sarcoid involving the skull table is not directly related to the neurosarcoid and is more commonly seen with other manifestations of musculoskeletal sarcoid.

Toxoplasmosis, in the absence of immunocompromise, is unlikely.

Overall the response to steroid, along with the wide variation of CNS disease described, are the strongest indicators for sarcoid. Whilst neurosarcoid does typically respond well to steroid therapy, it has a high recurrence rate.

Lury K, Smith K, Matheus M, and Castillo M. Neurosarcoidosis – review of imaging findings. *Seminars in Roentgenology* 2004; 39(4): 495–504.

57. B. Multisystem atrophy (MSA).

T2WI cruciform hyperintensity or the 'hot cross bun' sign within the pons, is suggestive of MSA, although it is not specific, as it also occurs in spinocerebellar ataxia. Other MRI features include hyperintensity within the putamen. Patients with MSA typically have parkinsonian features poorly responsive to levodopa therapy and autonomic disturbance. MRI features of Parkinson's disease are generally non-specific, but narrowing of the pars compacta of the substantia nigra may be seen on T2WI. Substantia nigra atrophy is also a feature of Lewy body dementia. T2WI hypointensity of the putamen due to iron deposition is a feature of progressive supranuclear palsy.

Gilman S, Wenning GK, Low PA, Brooks DJ, Mathias CJ, and Trojanowski JQ. Second consensus statement on the diagnosis of multiple system atrophy. *Neurology* 2008; 71(9): 670–676 .

58. C. Marchifava–Bignami disease.

This is a rare complication of chronic alcohol consumption characterized by demyelination and necrosis of the corpus callosum, although other white matter tracts (such as the external capsule) may be involved. Bilateral and symmetrical T2WI hyperintensities within the thalami, periaqueductal grey, and mammillary bodies are seen in Wernicke's encephalopathy. Osmotic myelinolyis is usually secondary to rapid changes in serum sodium and results in increased T2WI signal within the central pons. Extrapontine myelinolysis is rare. In alcohol withdrawal syndrome, patients present with seizures and delirium tremens. MRI may show volume loss in the temporal cortex and anterior hippocampus. Hepatic encephalopathy secondary to hepatocellular failure may produce T1WI hyperintensity within the caudate nucleus, globus pallidus, putamen, and anterior midbrain due to increased concentration of manganese.

Geibprasert S, Gallucci M, and Krings T. Alcohol induced changes in the brain as assessed by MRI and CT. *European Radiology* 2010; 20: 1492–1501.

59. A. Decreased CBF/decreased CBV/increased MTT.

In identifying the ischaemic penumbra, CT perfusion offers promise in improved patient selection for thrombolysis beyond a rigid time window. In the infarct core (tissue which is not salvageable) both CBF and CBV are decreased with a corresponding increase in MTT. Penumbral tissue (which is potentially recoverable by thrombolysis) exhibits a CBF/CBV mismatch with an increased CBV, but decreased CBF (and increased MTT). An increase in CBF and CBV with decreased MTT is a feature noticed in tumours secondary to angiogenesis and microvascular permeability.

Hoeffner EG, Case I, Jain R, Gujar SK, Shah GV, Deveikis JP et al. Cerebral perfusion CT: technique and clinical applications. *Radiology* 2004; 231: 632–644.

60. A. MS.

The key feature in this clinical vignette is the identification of the mass lesion crossing the midline. Only a few lesions demonstrate this ability and they are GBM, lymphoma, metastases, MS and other white matter disorders, lipoma, stroke, and shearing injuries. Abscess is thus excluded and would be unlikely given the clinical features. GBM is unlikely given the absence of necrosis and would be rare in a patient of this age group. High-grade astrocytomas do not involve the corpus callosum and cross the midline. Lymphoma exhibiting these features would be uncommon in immunocompetent patients, being more typically associated with HIV-related lymphoma. Tumefactive MS typically presents with an acute clinical history and frequently displays the imaging features described. The presence of vascular structures crossing the lesion also indicates this diagnosis, as these would be displaced by neoplastic lesions.

Grossman R and Yousem D. *Neuroradiology: The Requisites*, 2nd edn, Mosby, 2003, pp. 139–145, 153–155.

61. D. Straight sinus.

Pregnancy is a risk factor for both venous sinus thrombosis and hypertensive haemorrhage secondary to eclampsia. Hyperattenuating thrombus within the occluded sinus is classical on the unenhanced CT, but is seen in only 25% of cases. On the contrast-enhanced study, a central filling defect surrounded by enhancing dura (empty delta sign) is present in over 30%. Most of the superior cerebrum is drained by the superior sagittal sinus. The transverse sinuses receive blood from the temporal, parietal, and occipital lobes. The transverse sinuses drain into the sigmoid sinuses and on into the internal jugular veins. The straight sinus forms from the confluence of the inferior sagittal sinus and vein of Galen. The vein of Galen is part of the deep venous system, which drains the corpus callosum, basal ganglia, thalami, and upper brainstem. Cavernous sinus thrombosis presents with proptosis and cranial nerve palsies (usually cranial nerve VI first). The cavernous sinus receives the petrosal sinuses and middle cerebral veins.

Leach JL, Fortuna RB, Jones BV, and Gaskill-Shipley MF. Imaging of cerebral venous thrombosis: current techniques, spectrum of findings and diagnostic pitfalls. *RadioGraphics* 2006; 26: S19–S41.

62. A. Early venous drainage.

Brain AVMs are abnormal connections between arteries that would normally supply the brain tissue and veins that normally drain the brain, resulting in shunting with an intervening network of vessels within the brain parenchyma. The finding of early venous drainage is important in differentiating brain AVMs from other vascular lesions. Cortical venous drainage may be seen in superficial lesions. Recruitment of transdural supply is observed in large lesions, although this is a more typical feature of proliferative angiopathy, which is a diffuse type of AVM. Classically, in this condition, normal brain parenchyma is interspersed between the abnormal vessels. Stenoses of feeder vessels are also often identified in proliferative angiopathy. The caput medusa of dilated medullary veins is a feature of DVAs, a normal variant. Dilated cortical veins are seen in dural arteriovenous fistulas (DAVFs), which are abnormal connections between arteries that normally supply the meninges (but not the brain) and small venules within the dura.

Geibprasert S, Pongpech S, Jiarakongmun P, Shroff MM, Armstrong DC, and Krings T. Radiologic assessment of brain arteriovenous malformations: what clinicians need to know. *RadioGraphics* 2010; 30: 483–501.

63. E. Association with vomiting.

Headache accounts for approximately 2% of all A&E department visits, yet subarachnoid haemorrhage accounts for less than 3% of these headaches. Up to half of all patients with subarachnoid haemorrhage, however, will be alert and neurologically intact. A recent study prospectively assessed neurologically intact patients presenting with headache peaking within 1 hour to determine which variables are predictive of subarachnoid haemorrhage. High-risk variables include age >40, neck pain, witnessed loss of consciousness, onset with exertion (but not sexual activity), arrival by ambulance, vomiting, and blood pressure >160/100 mmHg. The presence of one or more of these findings in a patient with an acute non-traumatic headache reaching maximum intensity within 1 hour should prompt further investigation.

Perry JJ, Stiell IG, Sivilotti MLA, Bullard MJ, Lee JS, Eisenhauer M et al. High risk clinical characteristics for subarachnoid haemorrhage in patients with acute headache: prospective cohort study. *British Medical Journal* 2010; 341: c5204.

64. C. Cavernous malformation (cavernoma).

This is a benign vascular hamartoma, which can occur anywhere throughout the CNS, although spinal cord involvement is rare. It is typically a discrete, lobulated mass <4 cm containing blood products at different stages of evolution. On MRI they are described as having a 'popcorn' appearance of mixed signal intensity with a hypointense haemosiderin rim. They display little to no enhancement. Prominent susceptibility effect on T2* GE is typical. AVMs will demonstrate multiple flow voids. Haemorrhagic neoplasms will exhibit strong enhancement and an incomplete haemosiderin rim. Multiple 'black dots' are a feature of amyloid angiopathy. Capillary telangiectasias are poorly demarcated lesions, usually <1 cm, demonstrating 'brush-like' enhancement on T1WI post contrast. They are not usually identified on CT.

Osborn AG, Blaser SI, Salzman KL, Katzman GL, Provenzale J, Castillo M et al. *Diagnostic Imaging: Brain*, Amirsys, 2004, I-5: 24–27.

65. C. Catheter angiography.

Perimesencephalic haemorrhage is confined to the cisterns around the midbrain. In some cases the only blood is found anterior to the pons. Some sedimentation into the lateral ventricles may occur, but frank haemorrhage into the ventricles and/or extension into the sylvian fissure or anterior interhemispheric fissure (as in this case) indicates arterial haemorrhage. Catheter angiography following a negative CTA in the setting of a perimesencephalic bleed arguably does not have any extra diagnostic yield. However, catheter angiography remains the gold standard for detecting aneurysms, and in this case an anterior communicating artery aneurysm requires exclusion.

Van Gijn J and Rinkel CJE. Subarachnoid haemorrhage: diagnosis, causes and management. *Brain* 2001; 124: 249–278.

66. C. DWI.

The sensitivity and specificity of DWI in detecting acute ischaemia are 88–100% and 86–100%, respectively, and DWI is established as better than other conventional MRI techniques. In addition, acute from chronic ischaemia can be differentiated. DWI is a measure of the Brownian motion of water molecules within a tissue. Two sets of images are acquired; the DWI and the quantitative ADC map. Chronic lesions may appear bright on the DWI (T2 shine through), but only acute lesions with restricted diffusion will be dark on the ADC map. It should be noted, however, that high signal intensity on DWI with low ADC has been reported in a variety of conditions such as abscess, lymphoma, and gliomas. GE is useful for identifying microbleeds that may influence antithrombotic treatment.

Wallis A and Saunders T. Imaging transient ischaemic attack with diffusion weighted magnetic resonance imaging. *British Medical Journal* 2010; 340: c2215.

67. D. Optic nerve glioma.

NF-1 is an autosomal dominant neurocutaneous disorder. The gene locus is located on 17q11.2. Diagnosis of NF-1 requires two or more of the following: six or more cafe-au-lait spots, two or more neurofibromas (or one plexiform neurofibroma), axillary/inguinal freckling, optic nerve glioma, sphenoid wing dysplasia or a first-degree relative with NF-1. The classic imaging appearance is multiple focal areas of white matter and deep gray matter signal abnormality. Other potential findings include intracranial stenoses and moyamoya type proliferation. NF-2 characteristically presents with multiple intracranial schwannomas, meningiomas and ependymomas (MISME). Bilateral vestibular schwannomas is diagnostic of NF-2.

Osborn AG, Blaser SI, Salzman KL, Katzman GL, Provenzale J, Castillo M et al. *Diagnostic Imaging: Brain*, Amirsys, 2004, I-1: 78–85.

68. A. Porencephalic cyst.

Porencephaly is a congenital/acquired cystic cavity within the brain parenchyma with adjacent enlargement of the lateral ventricle. They develop *in utero* or early infancy. Arachnoid cysts are also CSF isointense, but are extra-axial, displacing the brain away from the adjacent skull. Ependymal cysts are intraventricular and the surrounding brain is usually normal. Schizencephaly is characterized by an intraparenchymal cleft extending from the ventricular surface to the brain surface lined by gray matter. Hydranencephaly results from an early destructive process of the developing brain. The cranial vault is CSF filled with absence of the cortical mantle and ventricles (water-bag brain). Death in infancy is typical.

Osborn AG, Blaser SI, Salzman KL, Katzman GL, Provenzale J, Castillo M et al. *Diagnostic Imaging: Brain*, Amirsys, 2004, I-7: 36–39.

69. E. Normal calcium-phosphorus metabolism.

Fahr disease is a rare degenerative neurological disorder characterized by extensive bilateral basal ganglia calcifications that can lead to progressive dystonia, parkinsonism, and neuropsychiatric manifestations. CT has higher diagnostic specificity for basal ganglia calcification over MRI. The distribution of calcifications is similar in endocrinological disorders such as hyperparathyroidism, hypoparathyroidism, and pseudohypoparathyroidism. The calcium–phosphorus metabolism is usually normal in Fahr disease. In pseudohypoparathyroidism the serum calcium is low with an appropriately high parathyroid hormone (PTH), due to PTH resistance.

Osborn AG, Blaser SI, Salzman KL, Katzman GL, Provenzale J, Castillo M et al. *Diagnostic Imaging: Brain*, Amirsys, 2004, I-10: 16–19.

70. C. Posterior reversible encephalopathy syndrome (PRES).

This is a disorder of cerebrovascular autoregulation and is associated with eclampsia, which is defined clinically as seizure or coma with pregnancy-induced hypertension. There is a predilection for the posterior circulation and watershed zones, possibly due to its sparse vasomotor sympathetic innervation. T2WI hyperintense lesions within the posterior cortex and subcortical white matter, without diffusion restriction, are typical. Diffusion restriction/low ADC will be found in infarction. The diagnosis of postpartum cerebral angiopathy should be considered in normotensive postpartum women presenting with intracerebral haemorrhage. Reversible high T2WI signal abnormalities may also be seen in the cortex and subcortical white matter. Multifocal stenoses and beading of the intracranial vasculature are also a feature. PML presents with asymmetrical T2WI hyperintensity in the periventricular and subcortical white matter, with cortical sparing. It is seen in the immunocompromised. Gliomatosis cerebri is a diffusely infiltrating tumour involving two or more lobes and is frequently bilateral. Enlargement of the involved structures is seen. It can mimic brainstem PRES.

Zak IT, Dulai HS, and Kish KK. Imaging of neurologic disorders associated with pregnancy and the postpartum period. *RadioGraphics* 2007; 27: 95–108.
Osbom AG, Blaser SI, Salzman KL, Katzman GL, Provenzale J, Castillo M et al. *Diagnostic Imaging: Brain*, Amirsys, 2004, I-10: 28–31.

71. D. Funnel-shaped aqueduct.

Aqueductal stenosis is a focal reduction in aqueduct size, which can be congenital or acquired. Stenosis occurs at the level of the superior colliculi or at the intercollicular sulcus. The best diagnostic clue is a funnel-shaped aqueduct. There is resultant ballooning of the lateral and third ventricles. The fourth ventricle is normal distal to the obstruction. The most specific finding is lack of CSF flow through the aqueduct on phase contrast MRI. Other findings include thinning of the corpus callosum and downward displacement of the internal cerebral veins and third ventricular floor. In older patients it can present similarly to NPH. Imaging findings in NPH include ventriculomegaly (with relative sparing of the fourth ventricle) out of proportion to sulcal enlargement, with normal hippocampi. The aqueductal 'flow-void' sign reflects increased CSF velocity through the aqueduct, although this can be observed in normal individuals.

Osbom AG, Blaser SI, Salzman KL, Katzman GL, Provenzale J, Castillo M et al. *Diagnostic Imaging: Brain*, Amirsys, 2004, II-1: 20–27.

72. C. Does not extend anterior to the foramen of Monro.

Cavum septum pellucidum (CSP), cavum vergae (CV), and cavum vellum interpositum (CVI) are all considered normal variants, although CSP is possibly more prevalent in boxers due to repeated head trauma, most famously referred to in *Rocky V*. CSP is universal in foetuses, but decreases with age. CSP is an elongated finger-shaped CSF collection between the frontal horns of the lateral ventricles. Posterior extension between the fornices is referred to as CV. CV almost never occurs in the absence of CSP. CVI, however, is a triangular-shaped CSF space between the lateral ventricles that does not extend anterior to the foramen of Monro. Absent septum pellucidum can look like CSP/CV on sagittal imaging. It is commonly associated with other congenital anomalies.

Osbom AG, Blaser SI, Salzman KL, Katzman GL, Provenzale J, Castillo M et al. *Diagnostic Imaging: Brain*, Amirsys, 2004, II-1: 8–11.

73. B. Lactate peak on MR spectroscopy.

Neuroepithelial tumours are either low grade (WHO I and II) or high grade (WHO III and IV). The classification relies on pathology, but as this requires brain biopsy it is not without significant risk. Advanced MRI techniques play an increasing role in helping to differentiate these lesions, as low-grade lesions may be managed via a 'watch and wait' approach. Conventional MRI is poorly sensitive for glioma grading, as low-grade gliomas can enhance (in up to 20%) and up to 30% of non-enhancing gliomas are malignant. MR perfusion can help differentaiate, as rCBV tends to increase with tumour grade. A threshold of 1.75 is commonly utilized to separate low- from high-grade gliomas, but low-grade oligodendrogliomas can give misleadingly elevated rCBV values. The classic MR spectroscopy features of high-grade lesions are elevated choline and reduced NAA.

In addition an elevated lactate signal is typical of high-grade lesions secondary to the anaerobic environment. ADC is usually lower in high-grade lesions, but there is considerable overlap and so ADC maps are insufficient on their own for predicting tumour grade.

Al-Okaili RN, Krejza J, Wang S, Woo JH, and Melhem ER. Advanced MR imaging techniques in the diagnosis of intraaxial brain tumors in adults. *RadioGraphics* 2006; 26: S173–S189.
Law M, Yang S, Wang H, Babb JS, Johnson G, Cha S et al. Glioma grading: sensitivity, specificity and predictive values of perfusion MR imaging and proton MR spectroscopic imaging compared with conventional MR imaging. *American Journal of Neuroradiology* 2003, 24: 1989–1998.

74. B. Erosion of the adjacent porus acousticus.

A large meningioma at the cerebellopontine angle can easily grow into the adjacent internal auditory meatus (IAM), but typically does so without causing any enlargement or erosion of this structure. Most vestibular schwannomas arise from the inferior vestibular nerve within the IAM and as they grow they smoothly erode the posterior edge of the porus acousticus.

Although dural enhancement has been described adjacent to vestibular schwannomas, an enhancing 'dural tail' would be a finding more commonly associated with a lesion arising from the dura, typically a meningioma.

Bony hyperostosis is a finding that is associated with meningioma. Both meningiomas and vestibular schwannomas typically show avid enhancement with intravenous gadolinium.

Bonneville F, Savatovsky J, and Chiras J. Imaging of cerebellopontine angle lesions: an update. Part 1: enhancing extra-axial lesions. *European Radiology* 2007; 17: 2472–2482.

75. C. Loss of the posterior pituitary bright spot.

Autoimmune hypophysitis (AH) and non-secreting pituitary adenomas can only be differentiated with certainty on histology. As a result, approximately 40% of patients with AH are misdiagnosed as having pituitary macroadenoma and undergo unnecessary surgery. Hormone production is compromised in both conditions, although a history of infertility is common with adenomas, whereas patients with AH typically achieve spontaneous pregnancy. In an attempt to develop a scoring system to differentiate the two conditions, a recent study found that features significantly associated with AH over adenoma were age <30, relation to pregnancy, homogenous gadolinium enhancement, loss of the posterior pituitary bright spot, and enlarged stalk. Features consistent with adenoma were asymmetrically enlarged pituitary, size >6 cm^3, and associated sinus mucosal thickening. The normal posterior pituitary gland is bright on T1WI due to the rich content of vasopressin neurosecretory granules. This is frequently lost in AH due to direct autoimmune involvement of the neurohypophysis, whereas it is conserved in the majority of adenomas, even when displaced by large tumour size.

Gutenberg A, Larsen J, Lupi I, Rohde V, and Caturegli P. A radiologic score to distinguish autoimmune hypophysitis from nonsecreting pituitary adenoma preoperatively. *American Journal of Neuroradiology* 2009; 30: 1751–1753.

INDEX

Note: page numbers in **bold** refer to answers. References to questions may not explicitly refer to the index heading.

Printed and bound by CPI Group (UK) Ltd, Croydon, CR0 4YY